HEALTHCARE TECHNOLOGIES SERIES 23

Advances in Telemedicine for Health Monitoring

Other volumes in this series:

IET Book Series on e-Health Technologies – Call for Authors

Book Series Editor: Professor Joel P. C. Rodrigues, the National Institute of Telecommunications (Inatel), Brazil and Instituto de Telecomunicações, Portugal

While the demographic shifts in populations display significant socio-economic challenges, they trigger opportunities for innovations in e-Health, m-Health, precision and personalised medicine, robotics, sensing, the Internet of Things, cloud computing, Big Data, Software Defined Networks, and network function virtualization. Their integration is however associated with many technological, ethical, legal, social and security issues. This new Book Series aims to disseminate recent advances for e-Health Technologies to improve healthcare and people's wellbeing.

Topics considered include Intelligent e-Health systems, electronic health records, ICT-enabled personal health systems, mobile and cloud computing for eHealth, health monitoring, precision and personalized health, robotics for e-Health, security and privacy in e-Health, ambient assisted living, telemedicine, Big Data and IoT for e-Health, and more.

Proposals for coherently integrated International multi-authored edited or co-authored handbooks and research monographs will be considered for this Book Series. Each proposal will be reviewed by the Book Series Editor with additional external reviews from independent reviewers. Please email your book proposal for the IET Book Series on e-Health Technologies to: Professor Joel Rodrigues at joeljr@ieee.org or joeljr@inatel.br

Advances in Telemedicine for Health Monitoring

Technologies, Design and Applications

Edited by
Tarik A. Rashid, Chinmay Chakraborty and Kym Fraser

The Institution of Engineering and Technology

Published by The Institution of Engineering and Technology, London, United Kingdom

The Institution of Engineering and Technology is registered as a Charity in England & Wales (no. 211014) and Scotland (no. SC038698).

First published 2020

The Institution of Engineering and Technology
Michael Faraday House
Six Hills Way, Stevenage
Herts, SG1 2AY, United Kingdom

www.theiet.org

British Library Cataloguing in Publication Data
A catalogue record for this product is available from the British Library

ISBN 978-1-78561-986-1 (hardback)
ISBN 978-1-78561-987-8 (PDF)

Typeset in India by MPS Limited

Contents

Foreword

I am delighted to write the foreword for this edited book on "Advances in Telemedicine for Health Monitoring: Technologies, Design, and Applications". This book highlights various new biomedical tools and technologies which can be applied to assist doctors and health professionals to diagnose medical conditions remotely.

Telemedicine is used to improve human health outcomes via the prevention, diagnosis, monitoring, treatment of disease, illness, injury, including physical and mental impairment. To accomplish successful outcomes many biomedical data must be known about a patient. Patient-centric clinical data such as image, text, sound, electrical signals, etc. are transferred via telemedicine platforms. To access and apply information about a patient from such heterogeneous data is a large and complicated task, requiring many tools and techniques.

The range of topics covered in this book is quite extensive. For example, contributors address the development, management, and research-related aspects of telemedicine. The book discusses different forms of data analysis regarding EEG signals, image, ultrasound, data mining, data security, Internet of Medical Things, manual observations, etc. Critical factors, challenges, applications, telemedicine mapping with the Internet of Things and future directions have also been covered. The book describes and explains various telemedicine approaches over various medical data types. It also focuses on the different statistical, evolutionary and hybrid techniques for the decision-making process.

This book provides a window to the field of medical and healthcare data analysis in a comprehensive way and enumerates the evolutions of such tools and techniques. In this new age of global interconnectivity and interdependence, it is necessary to provide practitioners, health professionals and students with state-of-the-art knowledge on the frontiers of information processing in the field of telemedicine and remote healthcare.

I recommend this book to a variety of readers, including healthcare practitioners, information and communication technology specialists, academics and medical students. It is my hope and expectation that this book will provide an effective learning experience and reference for health professionals interested in the integration of technology, information, and medicine.

Joel J. P. C. Rodrigues
Federal University of Piauí (UFPI), Teresina – PI, Brazil
Instituto de Telecomunicações, Portugal

About the editors

Tarik A. Rashid is a professor in the Computer Science and Engineering Department, School of Science and Engineering, University of Kurdistan Hewler, Erbil, KRG, Iraq. He received his Ph.D. degree in computer science and informatics from the Computer Science and Informatics Department, College of Engineering, Mathematical, and Physical Sciences, University College Dublin (UCD) in 2006. He was a Postdoctoral Fellow of the Computer Science and Informatics School, University College Dublin (UCD) from 2006 to 2007. His research covers three fields of interest. The first field is the expansion of machine learning and data mining to deal with time series applications. The second field is the development of DNA computing, optimization, swarm intelligence, and nature-inspired algorithms and their applications. The third field is networking, telecommunication and telemedicine applications. He has established collaborative relationships with several international research institutions and published over 100 research articles in internationally refereed books, journals and conferences.

Chinmay Chakraborty is an Assistant Professor (Sr.) in the Department of Electronics and Communication Engineering, BIT Mesra, India. His primary areas of research include wireless body area network, internet of medical things, energy-efficient wireless communications and networking and point-of-care diagnosis. He authored the books "*PSTN-IP Telephony Gateway for Ensuring QoS in Heterogeneous Networks*" (2014), "*Advanced Classification Techniques for Healthcare Analysis*" (2019) and "*Smart Medical Data Sensing and IoT Systems Design in Healthcare*" (2019). He is an Editorial Board Member in the *Journal of Wireless Communication Technology*, *Int. Journal of Telecomm. Engg.*, etc. and also a member of the International Advisory Board for Malaysia Technical Scientist Congress and the Machine Intelligence Research Labs. He received a young research excellence award, Global Peer Review Award, Young Faculty Award and Outstanding Researcher Award.

Kym Fraser is a researcher at the Future Industries Institute, University of South Australia, Adelaide, Australia. He also holds professorships at the University of Brawijaya, Indonesia, University of Kurdistan Hewler, Iraq and Aalborg University, Denmark. Before becoming an academic, he spent 25 years in practice in the areas of operations, service and quality management. Since entering academia his research efforts have tended to fall within the broad field of business and management. He has published in top-tier journals such as *International Journal of Production Research, Journal of Biomedical Science; Computer Methods and Programs in Biomedicine, Sustainability, Studies in Higher Education* to name a few. He has established collaborative relationships with five international research institutions and published over 80 research articles in internationally refereed books, journals and conferences.

Preface

Recent advances in medical sciences, biomedical engineering, information, and communications technologies have enhanced the opportunity for telemedicine applications to impact on improving healthcare outcomes. Telemedicine applications are being developed in areas such as medical monitoring, operations, and providing remote access to patients. These applications are essentially viewed as end-to-end attached sources and sinks (nodes), which can be applied both locally and remotely within healthcare communication systems. These flexible systems can be implemented at economical costs and provide real-time visual awareness and information to patients and physicians. These advances have allowed patient monitoring to be conducted remotely and detect variations in both physiological and non-physiological body parameters as they occur. A significant number of techniques with applications in telemedicine originate from the fields of biomedical sensors, wireless sensor networking, computer-aided diagnosis methods, signal and image processing and analysis, automation, and control, virtual and augmented reality, multivariate analysis, and data acquisition devices. To capture the advances in technologies, design, and applications of health monitoring, this book explores the following:

1. It provides an overview of computational approaches for the control of data collection, big data, and cloud computing, and presents their recent applications in the area of telemedicine.
2. Internet of Medical Things (IoMT), also known as Healthcare IoT, explores medical machine-to-machine communication where captured data can be stored and analysed for further diagnostic processes using intelligent methods.
3. It highlights how bio-inspired algorithms are changing the way medical tests, symptoms, and images are handled and analysed, as these algorithms are derived from biological facts to solve medical issues and are much faster than other traditional methods.
4. Presents advances in both hardware and software used in technological medical facilities to access and treat health conditions and problems in real-time and remotely, therefore reducing the impact of remoteness and distance.

The book presents new methods in the field of telemedicine by advancing data evaluation and diagnosis of medical conditions to improve the quality of life of patients. With the focus on telemedicine advances, the book highlights recent research initiatives by presenting theoretical, methodological, innovative and validated empirical work dealing with different topics. Researchers estimate that the impact of advances in telemedicine will be significant in terms of reducing: per-patient cost, resource load, hospitalisation time, follow up visits, while improving the patient's quality of life.

Keywords: Telemedicine, tele-monitoring, telehealth, medical technologies, biomedical image processing, digital health, tele-social work, biomedical sensors, internet of things in healthcare, artificial intelligence.

Objective

The aim of this book is to highlight the innovation of recent advances in remote healthcare and monitoring using telemedicine applications. In doing so, the book will present robust solutions in the delivery of medical information from patients-to-doctors, with the purpose of enhancing accurate diagnosis without the need for face-to-face contact. It is hoped the book will initiate conversations among technologists, engineers, scientists and clinicians in synergising their efforts into producing low-cost, high-performance, highly efficient, deployable telemedicine applications. The book will additionally investigate the potential for making future advances in a number of scientific disciplines while improving the success of telemedicine and the healthcare sector. The book includes some directions for future research.

Book organisation

The book consists of 13 chapters in the field of telemedicine and healthcare monitoring. A brief summary of each chapter is presented below.

Chapter 1: Critical factors in the development, implementation, and evaluation of telemedicine

The aim of the chapter is to provide an overview of critical factors in the development, implementation, and evaluation of telemedicine. Using a case study approach, which draws on practical examples from the Australian health care sector, this chapter ties together the literature with practical experiences from the frontline of telemedicine. While there is no 'one size fits all' approach, this chapter highlights the critical factors that impact and influence the success and sustainability of telemedicine applications and services. With increasing focus on quality and safety in healthcare, telemedicine is becoming an important tool for healthcare stakeholders in delivering safe, timely, equitable and effective healthcare services. While the positive impacts of telemedicine are well recognised, integrating and operationalising telemedicine within healthcare facilities and systems continues to present many challenges. Identifying the critical factors enhances our understanding of assisting stakeholders to overcome the various challenges in telemedicine.

Chapter 2: Surgical tele-mentoring

In this chapter surgical tele-mentoring is demonstrated and it involves the use of information technology to provide real-time guidance and technical assistance for surgical procedures from an expert surgeon at a different location. The method is a way to overcome the logistical obstacles associated with conventional mentoring while supporting the distribution of advanced surgical techniques. Tele-mentoring has the potential to directly impact patient care by providing immediate access to specialised surgical expertise in locations where qualified surgeons are lacking or not available. With advances in technology, surgical tele-mentoring has made significant improvements in the past two decades and many positive outcomes have been achieved. In spite of this, questions remain regarding ideal videoconferencing methodology, resolution and latency requirements, security and liability issues, and medicolegal issues. This chapter addresses the history and progression, applications, challenges, limitations and future directions of surgical tele-mentoring as a means to distribute advanced surgical expertise around the world.

Chapter 3: Technologies in medical information processing

Advances in health technologies have diversified the sources of information that can be analysed and used for correct diagnostics and decision-making. Researchers and system developers in the field of telemedicine are consciously inventing and improving data generation, collection and processing methods, with the aim to improve the quality of care while reducing the cost and effort needed to provide care. Bringing newly developed technologies, specific to information processing, to the attention of healthcare providers is important to improving the quality of care. In this chapter, the authors explain the importance of a number of health indicators that can be measured for data collection purposes, such as temperature, heart rate, blood pressure, and respiration rate. The chapter also presents the latest technologies that capture data and then process the data to produce meaningful and visual information that can be used for diagnostics and treatment purposes, such as X-ray, computerised tomography scan, magnetic resonance imaging, and ultrasound.

Chapter 4: A comparative note on recent advances of signal/ image processing techniques in healthcare

This chapter deals with the latest advancements in signal and image processing techniques, including network design in healthcare applications. The method involves the integration of cues and modalities of images and visuals, which enhances the performance of processing the visuals and images. This academic and scientific contribution is aimed at fellow researchers who are interested in this emerging area of technology. In addition, the viability/compatibility among electrophysiological signals, such as ECG, EMG, and EEG, along with image processional functionalities have been identified. To enhance the research, real practical case studies in the fields of neuroscience and cardiovascular system have been discussed.

Chapter 5: A real-time ECG processing platform for telemedicine applications

This chapter focuses on the development of an efficient algorithm for automated classification of ECG, which combines feature extraction and classification algorithms, along with the implementation of a microcontroller test platform. The cosine Stockwell transform is used for extracting significant amounts of information from corresponding heartbeats. These features resemble each heartbeat and are further classified using particle swarm optimisation support vector machines into subsequent classes. The proposed method is implemented on a 32-bit advanced RISC machine microcontroller platform. The platform is validated by generating real-time ECG signals using benchmark MIT-BIH data and evaluated under a category-oriented assessment scheme. The platform is interfaced with a Wi-Fi module, which sends the information of classified outputs to a remote microcontroller-based platform. Once an abnormality is detected by the platform, a pop-up message is shown on the display module, interfacing with the platform to acts as an alarm. The test platform has reported accuracy of 95.8% in the category-oriented assessment scheme. Such kind of implementation provides an enriched platform capable of performing real-time diagnosis and can be utilised in hospitals for telemedicine applications.

Chapter 6: Data mining in telemedicine

This chapter discusses the effectiveness of data mining in telemedicine. Due to a wide range of changes occurring in global healthcare systems over the last few decades, medical systems are facing significant challenges. The evolution of data in telemedicine applications requires useful intelligent techniques for diagnosis, health records transmission, and automatic adaptation of biosensors, for extracting meaningful information directly from raw physiological data. In particular, the automated classification of this data has been shown as a promising diagnosis strategy for assisting physicians. The chapter reviews recent advances in data mining techniques, introducing readers to various and new applications, such as feature extraction and selection, artefact removal, artificial intelligence, and machine learning, each assisting in the diagnosis and management of telemedicine applications.

Chapter 7: Social work and tele-mental health services for rural and remote communities

This chapter explores the links between remote and rural social work and information and communication technologies (ICTs), telepsychology and psychiatry. The chapter provides suggestions on how to enhance engagement between social workers and ICT to implement and provide tele-health services tailored to rural and remote community needs. Rural and remote communities often have complex and diverse mental health needs, along with inadequate mental health services and infrastructure. Social work practitioners have additional skills to bring to tele-mental health, and in particular, the socio-cultural dimensions that affect mental health. Therefore, there is a need to recognise and explore these patient's requirements, as well as, the capability to refer patients to resources and services outside of the normal psychology or medical fields. However, despite this potential, a review of international literature reveals that ICTs have not attained widespread uptake in social work practice in rural communities.

Chapter 8: Technology-enhanced social work practice and education

This chapter explores the innovative ways in which tele-social work is being implemented, both in Australian and internationally, to increase the accessibility and flexibility of healthcare services, and thereby improving the health and well-being of users of such services. The potential risks associated with increasing flexibility are also considered. Case studies are provided to demonstrate how tele-social work is being integrated into social work education, drawing on the authors' experience teaching at a higher education institution in Australia.

Chapter 9: Advanced telemedicine system for remote healthcare monitoring

This chapter highlights the advances in telemedicine systems for the monitoring of remotely located patients suffering from a wide range of diseases. Telemedicine systems are used to support various types of biomedical signals, such as electro-encephalography, electrocardiography, and electromyography, along with the integration of modern techniques. The chapter presents standard uses for telemedicine systems, along with special features. A cloud-based workflow model for the monitoring of remote patients has been proposed. For the continuous monitoring and analysis of biomedical signals obtained from remote patients, it is shown that telemedicine system can play a significant role in the technical, social and cultural development of society. The chapter discusses various aspects of monitoring systems and associated issues, including the latest developments and improvements in the field.

Chapter 10: Impact of tone-mapping operators and viewing devices on visual quality of experience of colour and grey-scale HDR images

In this chapter, tone-mapping-operators (TMOs) provide a useful means for converting high dynamic range (HDR) images to low dynamic range images, so they can be viewed on standard displays, but this may affect the visual quality of experience (QoE) of the end-user. There is a need to understand the impact of TMOs to inform the choice of TMO algorithms for different displays, especially for small-screen-devices (SSDs), such as those used in mobile phones. The authors of this chapter evaluate subjectively and objectively, commonly used TMOs in different displays and resolutions for colour and grey-scale HDR images. The results indicate that viewing devices have an influence on the TMO's performance, suggesting the need for a careful choice of TMO to enhance the viewing-quality of experience for end-users. In addition, it was found that Shannon Entropy to be a good objective measure of quality for colour and grey HDR images. This suggests that entropy may find use in automated HDR quality control assessment schemes, while HDR-VDP-2 is a good objective measure for colour HDR image only.

Chapter 11: Modeling the relationships between changes in EEG features and subjective quality of HDR images

This chapter proposes a novel objective QoE model for high dynamic range (HDR) images and is based on the relationship between objective (i.e. delta-beta coupling) and subjective measures (i.e. mean opinion score). The analysis of the results indicates that the proposed QoE model has a strong correlation with mean opinion scores, and therefore can be effectively used in predicting the overall HDR image quality. An advantage of the model is that it is light-weight and it provides a measure of user-perceived quality, but without requiring time-consuming subjective tests. The model has potential applications in several other areas, including QoE control and optimisation. Future mobile providers can benefit from applying the proposed QoE-based model to optimise users' acceptability and satisfaction for different HDR image scenarios.

Chapter 12: IoMT and healthcare delivery in chronic diseases

This chapter discusses the role of the Internet of Medical Things (IoMT) in healthcare for chronic disease monitoring. The IoMT enables machine-to-machine interaction between devices in a patient's body environment and architecture and is predicted to provide higher impact in chronic disease care. Further, the topic broadly reviews the clinical side transformations of technology, explaining how IoT applications would create value for patients in different scenarios, including its relevance in clinical settings. The author proposes technological innovations enabling transformations, such as novel devices and peripheral technologies, and evaluates their impact on existing clinical protocols, value proposition and actual implementation in common chronic disease conditions. The chapter further considers the review of observations on reliability and validation of the technology in diabetes patients, and how IoMT would change the physician's role in healthcare delivery.

Chapter 13: Transform domain robust watermarking method using Riesz wavelet transform for medical data security and privacy

This chapter proposes a new watermarking approach using a transform domain for medical image security. Riesz wavelet transform (RWT) and singular value decomposition (SVD) is employed for embedding the watermarking in the cover medical image from the transmitter side. At the receiver, the embedded information is recovered successfully using the watermarking extraction algorithm. The RWT-SVD algorithm is tested on different types of medical images, like X-ray, CT scan, MRI and retinal images. The watermark is extracted at the receiver without the original image. Imperceptibility evaluation using several metrics shows the improved performance of the proposed approach. In addition, robustness analysis is also carried in terms of the correlation coefficient.

Book target audience

The target audience of this book is broad, ranging from biomedical engineering to technology experts and healthcare researchers, as well as those new or interested in the field. This book could be used as a textbook in both teaching and learning setting or in research-covering areas such as biomedical engineering, technology in healthcare, and advances in telemedicine.

Chapter 1

Critical factors in the development, implementation and evaluation of telemedicine

Saravana Kumar[1] *and Esther Jie Tian*[1]

With increasing focus on the quality and safety of health care, telemedicine has been used as an important tool by health-care stakeholders to support and enhance timely, equitable and effective health service delivery. While the positive impacts of telemedicine are well recognized, operationalizing and integrating telemedicine within health service delivery continues to face numerous challenges. These wide-ranging challenges include issues with technology, integrating with existing, and access to new, infrastructure, legislative and organizational requirements, stakeholder expectations, change management (as telemedicine is often offered as a new model of care) and financial and business considerations. Without explicit recognition of, and targeted strategies for, addressing these challenges, any telemedicine initiative risks not fulfilling its full potential. Similarly, improvements in telemedicine technologies should be complemented by recognition for and understanding of what works at the health service delivery level. The aim of the chapter is to provide a practical resource for stakeholders in telemedicine that outlines the critical factors that are essential in the development, implementation and evaluation of telemedicine. Using a case-study approach, which will draw on a practical example from the South Australian health-care sector, this chapter brings together evidence from the literature as well as experiences from the frontline of telemedicine. While there is no 'one size fits all' approach, this chapter will showcase the critical factors that have been demonstrated to influence the success and sustainability of telemedicine services.

1.1 Introduction

An important challenge that confronts health-care stakeholders and health systems in the twenty-first century is the access to, and availability of, high-quality health care to all consumers [1]. Historically, health-care delivery required the provider and the recipient to be present in the same place and at the same time [2]. However, this creates a barrier to delivering timely, equitable and effective health care to

[1]School of Health Sciences, University of South Australia, Adelaide, Australia

populations who are disadvantaged by location or circumstances, such as rural and remote communities, prisoners and persons in war zones or working at sea [3]. In countries such as Australia, which have been confronted by numerous health-care challenges such as an ageing population, growing burden of chronic diseases, increasing cost of health care, workforce shortage and maldistribution and health-care inequity for disadvantaged population groups, telemedicine has been viewed as a potential solution in tackling some of these challenges. Furthermore, the vast expanse of Australia, from a geographical point of view, creates a tyranny of distance for those seeking health care from rural and remote regions and it is in this context also telemedicine has been seen as an enabling solution. These are not unique to Australia as many western countries experience similar issues with regard to their health systems.

With documented advances in information and communication technology (ICT), there has been a growing interest in using telemedicine as an alternative approach to conventional care as a means of improving access to health-care services. Telemedicine is defined as 'the delivery of health-care services, where distance is a critical factor, by all health-care professionals using information and communication technologies for the exchange of valid information for diagnosis, treatment and prevention of disease and injuries, research and evaluation, and for the continuing education of health-care providers, all in the interests of advancing the health of individuals and their communities' [4]. Such an approach may involve using bi-directional and synchronous real-time (such as videoconferencing) or 'store-and-forward' (such as transmitting medical data through email) communication techniques [5,6].

Despite telemedicine's potential to improve access to, and quality of, health-care services, enable efficiencies and address inequities, operationalizing and integrating telemedicine within health service delivery continue to face numerous challenges [5]. Broadly, these challenges could be grouped into three categories: *technology*, *organizational* and *people*. Despite continued investment in and development of new technology, there continue to be on-going limitations with *technology* (such as availability of reliable and high-speed networks). Even when these networks are available, successfully integrating these with existing *organizational* infrastructure may pose additional challenges. As telemedicine is often underpinned by a different model of care to traditional health-care service delivery, there may be issues with the integration of telemedicine services into existing organizational structures. The structures and processes which underpin telemedicine may be incompatible with existing organizational structures and practices, as well as business models and governing processes between the organizations involved in the delivery of telemedicine. These issues may be in the form of financial and business considerations associated with telemedicine implementation (such as reimbursement and resources), legal concerns especially in relation to medical liability and data security of medical information, just to name a few. As traditional health-care service delivery relies on direct face-to-face contact, health professionals and other providers may view telemedicine as being an inferior service and hence be reluctant to engage with it. Patients and consumers too may express this view although research indicates that while this might be the case in some instances, it can be overcome and not pervasive [5,7–11].

In order for telemedicine to achieve its full potential, it is important challenges such as those highlighted above are identified and addressed through targeted strategies in a timely manner. The aim of the chapter is to provide a practical resource for stakeholders in telemedicine that outlines critical factors that are essential throughout the lifecycle of telemedicine. Our experience of telemedicine is derived from collaboration with colleagues at the Royal Adelaide Hospital (RAH), a tertiary education centre in Adelaide, South Australia, which has used telemedicine as a model of care within its spinal assessment clinic (SAC). The SAC has been in operation since 2007 and its primary role is to identify potential surgical candidates and cases of serious spinal pathology. At the SAC, physiotherapists work in advanced practice roles, where they provide consultations for semi-urgent and non-urgent cases. This was initiated in response to reduced consultant access and increased clinical demands. The videoconferencing at SAC is operated between the RAH site and numerous local sites across rural South Australia. While the processes of, and outcomes from, the telemedicine informed SAC have been positive, we have also learned a number of lessons along the way which have been crucial to the success of this initiative and yet are not often part of the wider narrative on telemedicine. For example, there is a dearth of literature on critical issues that need to be considered before implementing telemedicine initiatives, or how best to implement change management strategies to ensure its success and sustainability. Our experience with the RAH specifically and telemedicine literature more broadly has enabled us to recognize a range of factors that needs to be considered when engaging with telemedicine throughout its lifecycle.

Using a case-study approach, which draws on this practical example from the South Australian health-care sector, this chapter will bring together evidence from the literature as well as experiences from the frontline of telemedicine. While there is no 'one size fits all', by showcasing these critical factors (Figure 1.1), in no particular order, it offers stakeholders in telemedicine (such as health professionals, consumers, managers, administrators, policymakers) a blueprint which can be used during the development, implementation and evaluation of telemedicine services to ensure they are likely to be sustainable and successful in the long term.

1.1.1 Critical factor 1: address a gap in service

Development of telemedicine services should be underpinned by the preliminary work which clearly highlights a gap in service, and not because of its growing popularity, has been mandated or to keep up with other health service organizations. AlDossary *et al.* [12] emphasized this issue by highlighting that the first step for planning for a successful implementation is evaluating needs, especially of health-care professionals and patients and their preference for technology. This view is supported by a systematic review conducted by Obstfelder *et al.* [13], which identified that telemedicine services were developed explicitly to address local challenges such as shortage of specialists, needs of dealing complex medical conditions and reaching isolated populations in remote locations were common characteristics of successfully implemented telemedicine models.

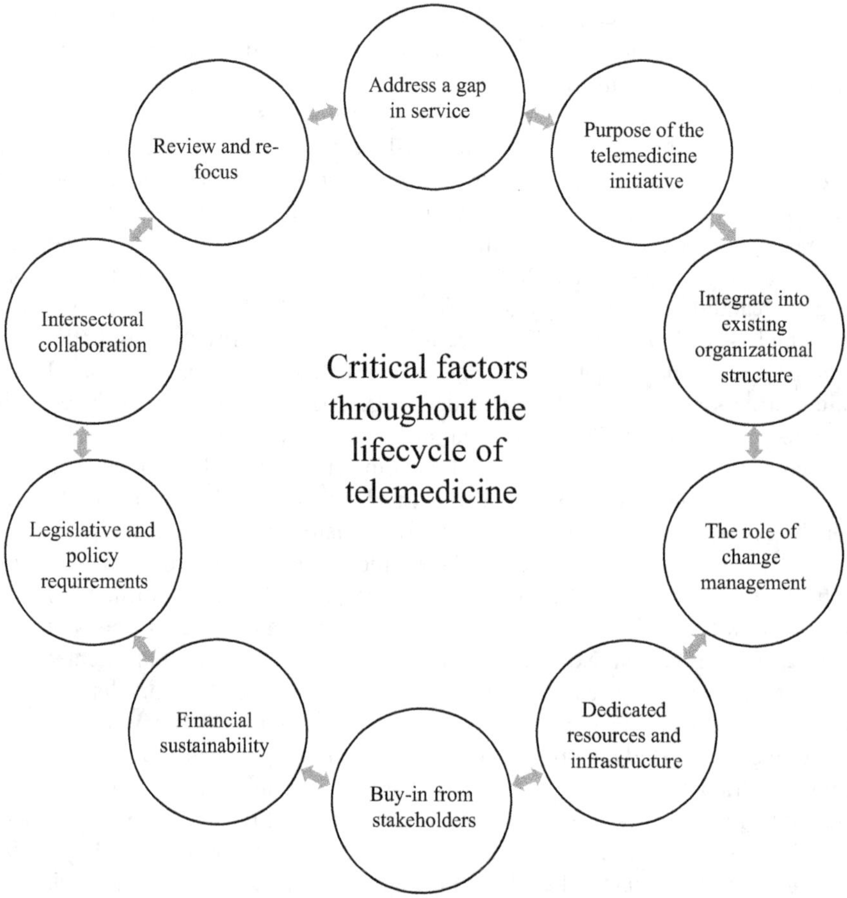

Figure 1.1 An overview of critical factors in the development, implementation and evaluation of telemedicine

Identifying gaps in service and clinical needs can be undertaken through a needs assessment. Needs assessment typically involves consultation with key stakeholders (such as health-care professionals, consumers, managers) from the local community, collection of quantitative (such as utilization rates of health-care services) and qualitative (such as stakeholder's perspectives) data, determining short- and long-term priorities which are supported by and informed through robust evidence, analysis of issues and possible solutions [14]. Conducting needs assessment will enable stakeholders to assess whether telemedicine service is indeed appropriate to meet the local needs and requirements. Furthermore, the mere process of identifying clinical needs appears to facilitate the engagement of key stakeholders, particularly in the early phase of telemedicine development. This early engagement of stakeholders is critical as it ensures stakeholders have buy-in early on, enhances greater acceptance and better adoption of telemedicine, as well as on-going support for the service well into the future [15].

1.1.2 Critical factor 2: clearly defining the purpose of the telemedicine service

Once a gap in service and clinical needs have been identified, it is critically important to explicitly and comprehensively define the specific purpose and objectives of the telemedicine service. The literature supports that establishing a clear vision of what telemedicine is intended to achieve at the planning phase is an essential element of telemedicine service development [15–17]. Given that telemedicine is often underpinned by a different model of care, it is important to consider what impact the introduction of a new model of care may have on the existing structures, processes and the people who operate within it. In order to ameliorate these issues, discussions need to be held with these stakeholders early on and their input sought to explicitly and comprehensively define the specific purpose, objectives of and outcomes from the telemedicine service. The literature on telemedicine is scant in terms of measures of effectiveness but it could range from process measures (such as the use of telemedicine services, improved access, reduced waiting times), clinical outcomes (such as patient health outcomes) and organizational measures (such as cost savings).

Some literature provides suggestions on how this could be operationalized in health-care settings. A pilot project would provide an opportunity to evaluate the viability and capacity of the proposed telemedicine initiative and 'test the waters'. The piloting process can assist in identifying what works, and what does not, for whom and why and what strategies need to be implemented to rectify emergent issues. By identifying these issues during the piloting process, efficient and timely solutions can be implemented. The piloting can, therefore, assist in determining whether the proposed telemedicine model of care can meet its purpose and objectives while trialling and modifying the approach with minimal impact [16].

1.1.3 Critical factor 3: integrate into the organizational structure

Successful models of health service delivery are associated with seamless integration into routine health-care practice. Given the novelty and unfamiliarity of the telemedicine model of care to some organizations, it is vitally important to careful consideration is given on how it will be integrated into the organizational structure and culture. In order for a telemedicine model to operate within an organization, its development needs to align with the organization's strategic plan, vision and mission. Additionally, as telemedicine, especially during the initial stages, will require substantial fanatical and human investment, a convincing business case needs to be established and support the change to current processes [16].

Strong leadership is a commonly recognized component of 'readiness' for integrating telemedicine into existing health systems [18]. For example, an internal champion, such as the chief executive officer (CEO), can ensure that the initiative is properly resourced and supported within the organization [16]. A steering committee, comprising stakeholder representatives, may also be used during this process. The role of the steering committee would be to provide advice and guidance and to ensure appropriate governance and risk-management strategies are in place.

Clinical champions at both the receiving and providing ends of telemedicine are also considered essential [15]. As clinical champions are generally frontline clinicians who are interested in using telemedicine, they are likely to take ownership, act as advocates, drive adoption and support the continued utilization of telemedicine.

A workforce model that is tailored to meet the demands of telemedicine is also recommended in the literature [15,16]. The delivery of telemedicine may require changes to the workforce in terms of who does what, how and when. It may also need to bring in staff from other disciplines (such as technology) which will mean telemedicine workforce will encompass staff with a variety of diverse skills. For example, at the providing end, there will be a need for additional administrative preparation including identifying telemedicine referrals, scheduling clinicians, facilities and equipment, preparing relevant paperwork and providing support on the consultation day. Similarly, the receiving end, additional administrative support may be needed by patients receiving the care (who may be unfamiliar with the telemedicine technology). Therefore, identifying early on the workforce, and the skill sets that will be required, to deliver the telemedicine services is critical.

1.1.4 Critical factor 4: the role of change management

While the pace of change in health care has increased dramatically, health-care organizations face enormous challenges when implementing and sustaining change [19]. As telemedicine is often offered as a new model of care, challenges to its implementation should be expected. While there is no magic bullet or a universally agreed manner by which change can be managed in an organization [20], often resistance to change for telemedicine can arise due to concerns associated with technological difficulties, the need to acquire new skills, uncertainties related to privacy and security, and introduction of new protocols and workplace practice [16]. One way to address these concerns is by engaging with staff throughout the lifecycle of telemedicine. This begins with communicating a clear vision about the change process, outlining the reasons for the change, providing opportunities to capture and respond to concerns, identifying barriers and enacting enabling strategies and monitoring and evaluating the outcomes from the change process. For example, one common concern reported may be a lack of knowledge and skills in the use of telemedicine technology. As part of the change management process, staff could participate in dedicated training sessions to upskill the use of and delivering through telemedicine [15,16]. If this training is underpinned by the competency assessments (not just for knowledge and skills), this expertise could be recognized across jurisdictions.

1.1.5 Critical factor 5: the crucial role of infrastructure

There is consistent literature evidence to indicate that physical and technological infrastructures strongly underpin the successful implementation of a telemedicine service [5,7,15,16,21]. This especially true during the initial stages of setting up, where substantial investment in physical and technological infrastructures is required. These investments may go towards adequate and appropriate consultation rooms that are soundproof, readily equipped with telemedicine technology, easily accessible with booking and having enough space for patients and/or their families to attend the consultation [15]. From a clinician point of view, user-friendly and reliable technological infrastructure (including network and equipment) appears to encourage end-users buy-in. In particular, the technology should be easy, fast and convenient to use, with reliable connections and minimal interruptions to communication. The investment in technology should be about improving efficiency and effectiveness of health-care delivery without placing additional burden on clinicians, particularly in cases of providing time-critical care, such as telestroke care. Yet, due to persistent problems, such as access to high-speed internet in remote Australia, there are on-going concerns about the image quality and break-up during consultations [22].

1.1.6 Critical factor 6: buy-in from stakeholders

A study conducted by Wade *et al.* [23] revealed that *clinician acceptance* is the key factor influencing the success and sustainability of telemedicine services. Interestingly, this research also identified that *clinician acceptance* could overcome barriers associated with low service demands, technological issues, workforce pressure and lack of resources, highlighting the significant enabling effect on driving the adoption of telemedicine services. This highlights the importance of securing buy-in from clinicians early on and keeping them informed and engaged through the lifecycle of telemedicine. Part of this process is understanding that technology should align with, and complement, clinical needs, rather than merely driving the uptake of telemedicine. This ensures that the telemedicine model is appropriate for its intended use and minimizes the risks of overinvestment in technology [15,16]. However, engagement and buy-in should not be limited to clinicians. This is evident in a recent systematic review, which highlighted that *resistance to change* is a commonly reported barrier for staff and programmers to the uptake of telemedicine [10]. Therefore, as a first-step stakeholder mapping may be required to identify anyone who is in a position to facilitate or block tele-medicine services. Once this has occurred, targeted strategies can be implemented, recognizing the needs and requirements of various stakeholders, to ensure their perspectives are captured and buy-in obtained.

1.1.7 Critical factor 7: financial sustainability

The longevity and success of a telemedicine service are often underpinned by financial sustainability as well. A recent systematic review identified that *cost* and *reimbursement* were the two most frequently cited barriers for organizations worldwide in adopting telemedicine services [10]. Therefore, for telemedicine to operate as part of routine health-care delivery, the cost associated with telemedicine delivery needs to be recovered through reimbursement or cost savings produced by the service, as many telemedicine models are funded via seed or grant funding [16]. This is especially important as often there is a large up-front investment in terms of developmental (infrastructure, capital and human) costs.

Reimbursement of telemedicine is generally supported by public, private and third-party organizations, but the level of compensation varies across different countries and jurisdictions [24]. In Australia, health-care professionals such as general practitioners, nurses, midwives, Aboriginal health workers or specialists who deliver video-based consultations are eligible for reimbursement under the medicare benefits schedule (MBS). However, the adoption of telemedicine outside the public hospital system remains low, partly due to the reimbursement is limited to real-time video consultations and is not available for allied health professionals [25]. The current disparity in reimbursement may mean the entire scope of telemedicine may never be fully realized and this should be carefully considered during the developmental stages (as not all clinicians can tap into this resource). A cost-benefit analysis of telemedicine is also recommended in the literature, especially at early stage of establishing telemedicine [16] as a means of evaluating financial sustainability over the short and long term. The process can help to identify the associated costs and the potential cost savings as a result of telemedicine service, which could be used to plan and guide funding allocation and future investments.

1.1.8 Critical factor 8: legislative and policy requirements

While technology has continued to evolve at a rapid pace, its legislative and regulatory frameworks struggle to keep up with it [26]. Telemedicine is no different. The development and implementation of telemedicine services should not proceed without careful recognition of legislative and policy requirements. A telemedicine service needs to align with national and local legislation, such as legislation in terms of medical care provision, accreditation systems for staff and liability for care provision [24]. Issues associated with privacy and security of medical information when delivering the service also need to be considered and addressed accordingly [7]. This can be particularly tricky as different jurisdictions may have different legislative and policy requirements and are often subject to change. Furthermore, interoperability issues amongst ICT infrastructure also act as a potential barrier when globally accepted standards are absent [21]. With increasing focus on data and cybersecurity, it is imperative that the telemedicine services comply with these requirements and strategies are in place to minimize the risk and misadventure.

1.1.9 Critical factor 9: intersectoral collaboration

As telemedicine draws on the expertise from a number of disciplines and across sectors, intersectoral collaboration is critical to its success. Collaboration between telemedicine initiators and its users is identified as a key characteristic of successful telemedicine models [13]. Acceptability of the new applications and adaptation of the new technology are encouraged through both formal (such as organizing in-house training, communication with government agencies) and informal (such as interaction at local level) collaboration. The stakeholders involved in collaboration can be varied from individuals at management level, researchers and system developers to frontline clinicians and consumers [13]. This is particularly important as these stakeholders can then become advocates for telemedicine and act as ambassadress across sectors. For example, with the move towards patient-centred care and consumer-directed care, consumers are playing an important role in health-care decision-making [27]. By fostering collaboration with consumers, they can help to drive change and promote the uptake of telemedicine. Using consumers to drive change in health care has been trialled and found to be successful in another health field [27]. Furthermore, extensive and effective collaboration across public, private and non-governmental sectors (such as professional associations and networks) has also been emphasized in the literature to promote better uptake of telemedicine [15,28].

1.1.10 Critical factor 10: review and re-focus

As with any new initiative, the development and implementation of telemedicine should be followed by regular evaluation. This is vitally important as evaluation assists to understand what works (and what does not) for whom, when, why and how. A recent literature review identified that *clinical outcomes*, *economics* and *satisfaction* were the three evaluation aspects commonly measured for telemedicine services [12]. A formal evaluation conducted through rigorous research process will help to unpack and understand the impact of the telemedicine service. Using rigorous research process will require formal ethical approval and while this may be seen as superfluous, there are numerous benefits to this. First, the ethics committee will provide independent oversight of the evaluation process in terms of ethical conduct of research as well as methodology utilized. Second, given there is on-going uncertainty regarding the impact of telemedicine services, having ethical approval means, the findings from the evaluation can be disseminated to a wider audience. The onus is on the telemedicine community to share the learnings so that best practice is built on, and inefficient and poor practices are discarded. This can only happen through the open sharing of data.

Literature also suggests that an evaluation framework should be established at the planning stage to warrant an effective evaluation of telemedicine [16]. While there are many quality improvement methods, the plan-do-study-act (PDSA) cycle is a commonly accepted and widely used approach in health-care improvement [29]. The PDSA cycle allows for a structured experimental learning approach to rapid testing of an intervention [30]. In this context, the flexible and adaptable nature of PDSA provides essential features for telemedicine evaluation.

1.2 Conclusion

As telemedicine continues to grow in popularity, driven by its immense potential to offer new and exciting solutions to age-old problems confronting health-care systems around the world, it is also hampered by its 'Achilles heel'. Many telemedicine initiatives do not progress beyond the initial trial stage or lack sustainability over the long term due to being buffeted by multifaceted challenges. For telemedicine to fulfil its full potential, a number of critical factors need to be understood and addressed. The critical factors identified in this chapter are provided in the form of a checklist (Table 1.1) to generate reflection during conceptualizing telemedicine initiatives, streaming efforts and activities and avoiding

Table 1.1 Checklist summarizing the critical factors throughout the lifecycle of telemedicine

Service gap/Purpose	• What is the rationale and/or justification for a telemedicine service model? • Has a needs assessment been conducted to identify local health service gaps? • Has the purpose of and impacts from a telemedicine service model clearly defined? • What outcomes are expected and how will these outcomes be measured? • Has evidence of effective telemedicine delivery within a similar context (e.g. a pilot project) been identified? • Has a business case been developed and scrutinized by, and defended to, appropriate stakeholders?
Organizational structure and governance	• Has the proposed telemedicine initiative received support from senior management? • How will the telemedicine service model be integrated into an existing model of care? • What additional roles and responsibilities (such as a steering committee) are required to provide leadership and governance support? • Is there a sustainable workforce model to meet the demands of the telemedicine initiative? • Have champions been identified to support and promote the telemedicine initiative? • Have administrative and technological supports required for the telemedicine service model considered and catered for?
Change management	• Have regular communications been undertaken to ensure that all stakeholders are well informed about the change process? • Are feedback mechanisms established to capture and respond to any concerns/questions from stakeholders (such as staff who will be at the frontline of telemedicine initiative)? • Have dedicated resources and training sessions for staff been established to ensure adequate competencies in the use of new technology and implementation of the telemedicine service model?
Physical and technological infrastructures	• Is there adequate physical infrastructure (such as appropriate consultation rooms) in place to meet the requirements of the telemedicine service model? • Does technological infrastructure (such as network and equipment) align with the patient and clinical needs?
Financial sustainability	• How will the service be funded? • Have costs and benefits associated with the telemedicine service model thoroughly considered? • Are adequate reimbursements available for health-care professionals to sustainably engage with the telemedicine service model?

Table 1.1 (Continued)

Buy-in from stakeholders	• Have potential stakeholders who are in a position to promote, or hinder, telemedicine service model identified and engaged? • Have health professionals contributed to the development, implementation and evaluation processes that underpin the telemedicine service model? • Have other key stakeholders engaged throughout the lifecycle of the telemedicine initiative?
Intersectoral collaboration	• By recognizing key stakeholders, have opportunities for partnerships been determined? • Have collaborative opportunities within and between sectors considered?
Legislative and policy requirements	• Is the telemedicine initiative aligned with national and local legislative requirements? • Have privacy and security issues (such as security of health records, interoperability amongst ICTs) been considered and addressed?
Review and re-focus	• Has an evaluation framework (such as the plan-do-study-act cycle) been adopted or developed? • Has an evaluation process been established? • What outcomes will be measured and has baseline data been collected? • How will the findings be reported to, and disseminated with, relevant stakeholders?

problems and pitfalls. By reflecting on these factors and using them to inform their own initiatives, we believe health-care stakeholders can successfully develop, implement and evaluate telemedicine services across diverse settings and contexts.

1.3 Future work

Telemedicine in health care has resulted in the emergence of new models of care which ameliorate the tyranny of distance and afforded access to health care for those patients who may have been previously disadvantaged (such as those living in rural and remote regions). While telemedicine may indeed by a safe, efficient and feasible model of care, future work is required to build on this evidence base as there continues to persist the on-going knowledge gaps. From a patient point of view, telemedicine technology may be intimidating to some users (such as the elderly population) and may be perceived as less trustworthy than face to face consultations. Future work could help to map these concerns, from different patient groups, so that enabling strategies can be enacted to allay patient anxieties regarding telemedicine. This will help to understand what works for whom, why and how. From a clinician point of view, telemedicine may pose new challenges such as how best to balance the therapeutic relationship between clinician and patient within technological constraints, upskilling required to effectively engage with and use technology and regular time and resources required to keep up to date with evolving technology. Future work could help understand how, for example, expert clinicians successfully integrate telemedicine as part of routine health-care service, while working within its boundaries, and continue to keep up to date with technological advancements. This can assist in developing the future health workforce which embraces telemedicine and is not sceptical nor fearful of technology. Therefore, unpacking these black boxes through concerted future work is crucial as it will assist in the sustainability of telemedicine initiatives.

References

[1] Zain J. and Clarke M. 'Security in telemedicine: issues in watermarking medical images'. Proceeding of the 3rd International Conference: Sciences of Electronic, Technologies of Information and Telecommunications; Tunisia, March 2005.

[2] Craig J. and Petterson V. 'Introduction to the practice of telemedicine'. *Journal of telemedicine and telecare*. 2005;11(1):3–9.

[3] Moffatt J.J. and Eley D.S. 'The reported benefits of telehealth for rural Australians'. *Australian health review*. 2010;34(3):276–81.

[4] World Health Organization. *Telemedicine: opportunities and developments in member states. Report on the second global survey on eHealth*. Global Observatory for eHealth series – Volume 2. Geneva; 2010.

[5] Bradford N.K., Caffery L.J. and Smith A.C. 'Telehealth services in rural and remote Australia: a systematic review of models of care and factors influencing success and sustainability'. *Rural and remote health*. 2016;16(4):3808.

[6] Young J. and Badowski M. 'Telehealth: increasing access to high quality care by expanding the role of technology in correctional medicine'. *Journal of clinical medicine*. 2017;6(2):20.

[7] Chang H. 'Evaluation framework for telemedicine using the logical framework approach and a fishbone diagram'. *Healthcare informatics research*. 2015;21(4):230–8.

[8] Gagnon M.P., Duplantie J., Fortin J.P. and Landry R. 'Implementing telehealth to support medical practice in rural/remote regions: what are the conditions for success?'. *Implementation science*. 2006;1(1):18.

[9] Van Dyk L. 'A review of telehealth service implementation frameworks'. *International journal of environmental research and public health*. 2014; 11(2):1279–98.

[10] Scott Kruse C., Karem P., Shifflett K., Vegi L., Ravi K. and Brooks M. 'Evaluating barriers to adopting telemedicine worldwide: a systematic review'. *Journal of telemedicine and telecare*. 2018;24(1):4–12.

[11] Turner J.W., Thomas R.J. and Gailiun M. 'Consumer response to virtual service organisations: the case of telemedicine'. *Journal of medical marketing*. 2001;1(4):309–18.

[12] AlDossary S., Martin-Khan M.G., Bradford N.K. and Smith A.C. 'A systematic review of the methodologies used to evaluate telemedicine service initiatives in hospital facilities'. *International journal of medical informatics*. 2017;97:171–94.

[13] Obstfelder A., Engeseth K.H. and Wynn R. 'Characteristics of successfully implemented telemedical applications'. *Implementation science*. 2007;2(1):25.

[14] AlDossary S., Martin-Khan M.G., Bradford N.K., Armfield N.R. and Smith A.C. 'The development of a telemedicine planning framework based on needs assessment'. *Journal of medical systems*. 2017;41(5):74.

[15] Chakraborty C., Gupta B. and Ghosh S.K. 'Mobile telemedicine systems for remote patient's chronic wound monitoring'. *IGI: M-Health innovations for patient-centered care*, Ch. 11, 217–243, 2016.

[16] Department of Health & Human Services (Australia). *Critical success factors: how to establish a successful telehealth service*. Melbourne; 2015.

[17] Agboola S., Hale T.M., Masters C., Kvedar J. and Jethwani K. '"Real-world" practical evaluation strategies: a review of telehealth evaluation'. *JMIR research protocols*. 2014;3(4):e75.

[18] Jennett P.A., Gagnon M.P. and Brandstadt H.K. 'Preparing for success: readiness models for rural telehealth'. *Journal of postgraduate medicine*. 2005;51(4):279.

[19] Al-Abri R. 'Managing change in healthcare'. *Oman medical journal*. 2007;22(3):9.

[20] Blackman D.A., Buick F., O'Donnell M., O'Flynn J.L. and West D. 'Developing high performance: performance management in the Australian Public Service'. *Crawford School Research Paper No. 12-09*. 2012.

[21] Broens T.H., Huis in't Veld R.M., Vollenbroek-Hutten M.M., Hermens H.J., van Halteren A.T. and Nieuwenhuis L.J. 'Determinants of successful telemedicine implementations: a literature study'. *Journal of telemedicine and telecare*. 2007;13(6):303–9.

[22] Australian Medical Association. *Better access to high speed broadband for rural and remote health care – 2016* [online]. 2017. Available from https://ama.com.au/position-statement/better-access-high-speed-broadband-rural-and-remote-health-care-2016 [Accessed 21 June 2019].

[23] Wade V.A., Eliott J.A. and Hiller J.E. 'Clinician acceptance is the key factor for sustainable telehealth services'. *Qualitative health research*. 2014;24(5):682–94.

[24] Kidholm K., Ekeland A.G., Jensen L.K. *et al.* 'A model for assessment of telemedicine applications: mast'. *International journal of technology assessment in health care*. 2012;28(1):44–51.

[25] Armfield N.R., Edirippulige S.K., Bradford N. and Smith A.C. 'Telemedicine–is the cart being put before the horse'. *The medical journal of Australia*. 2014;200(9):530–3.

[26] Moses L.B. 'Recurring dilemmas: the law's race to keep up with technological change'. UNSW Law Research Paper No. 2007-21. Available at SSRN: https://ssrn.com/abstract=979861 or http://dx.doi.org/10.2139/ssrn.979861.

[27] Australian Commission on Safety and Quality in Health Care (Australia). *Patient-centred care: improving quality and safety through partnerships with patients and consumers* [online]. Sydney: ACSQHC; 2011. Available from https://www.safetyandquality.gov.au/sites/default/files/migrated/PCC_Paper_August.pdf [Accessed 30 August 2019].

[28] Chakraborty C., Gupta B. and Ghosh S.K. 'A review on telemedicine-based WBAN framework for patient monitoring'. *International journal of telemedicine and e-health*. Mary Ann Libert Inc., 2013;19(8):619–26.

[29] Taylor M.J., McNicholas C., Nicolay C., Darzi A., Bell D. and Reed J.E. 'Systematic review of the application of the plan–do–study–act method to improve quality in healthcare'. *BMJ quality & safety*. 2014;23(4):290–8.

[30] Reed J.E. and Card A.J. 'The problem with plan-do-study-act cycles'. *BMJ quality & safety*. 2016;25(3):147–52.

Chapter 2

Surgical tele-mentoring

Ramkrishna Mondal[1]

Abbreviations

VC	Video conferencing
WebRTC	Web real-time communication
RCT	Randomized controlled trial
UNN	University Hospital of North Norway
UiT	University of Tromsø – The Arctic University of Norway
NST	Norwegian Centre for Integrated Care and Telemedicine
ICT	Information communication technologies
API	Application programming interface
OSI model	Open systems interconnection model
P2P	Peer-to-peer
SSL/TLS	Secure sockets layer/Transport layer security
HTTP[S]	[Secure] Hypertext transfer protocol
DTLS/SRTP	Datagram transport layer security/Secure real-time transport protocol

Surgical tele-mentoring is a model within the broad discipline of telemedicine that involves the use of information technology to provide real-time guidance and technical assistance for surgical procedures from an expert surgeon at a different location. A way to overcome the logistic obstacles associated with conventional mentoring and can support the distribution of advanced surgical techniques. With its seeming educational benefits, it has the potential to directly impact the patient care by providing immediate access to specialized surgical expertise in areas where there is a lack of qualified surgeons. With advances in technology, surgical tele-mentoring has made significant improvements in the past two decades and many positive experiences have been published in the literature. In spite of this development, questions remain regarding ideal videoconferencing methodology, resolution and latency requirements, security and liability issues, medicolegal issues,

[1]DMS, IQ City Medical College, West Bengal, India

and tele-mentoring in combination with emerging technology. This chapter addresses the history and progression, applications, challenges, limitations, and future directions of surgical tele-mentoring as a means to distribute advanced surgical expertise around the world.

Definitions

Telemedicine: "The practice of medicine or teaching of the medical art, without through physical physician-patient or physician-student contact, via an interactive audio-video system employing tele-electronic devices" [1].

Tele-mentoring: "A real-time and live interactive monitoring of technique[s] or procedure[s] of a candidate seeking privileges, or a surgeon seeking to certify or document his competence in a specific technique or procedure[s]" [1].

Teleproctor: A teleproctor is an experienced surgeon who, through a virtual presence in an operating room, passively observes an on-site surgeon who is perceived to be fully qualified and trained to independently perform the proctored procedures or use of a device. Like a physically present proctor, the teleproctor's interactivity will be limited to the ability to ask questions of the on-site surgeon for clarification. The teleproctor "does not have the ability to physically intervene on-site in the primary activity without the telecommunications interface" [1].

Telestration: A technique enabling the drawing of freehand commands over still image or video. In this research project, telestration is explored as an extra modality for a mentor–mentee communication [2].

Teleobserver: A teleobserver is a less-experienced surgeon seeking education by concurrently observing an experienced surgeon performing a procedure or demonstration of the use of a device. The less-experienced observer will be able to remotely login and view the procedure, interact in the form of questions to the on-site surgeon.

Telementor: A telementor is an experienced surgeon, highly skilled in a particular procedure or use of a device, who, on a remote basis, serves as a resource for an on-site surgeon, already fully trained in his field but may or not be fully trained in performing a particular procedure or using a particular device.

However, the term "telementor" can be further broken down into either "Telementor Advisor" or "Telementor Preceptor" based on the amount of interactivity the telementor may have relating to the level of intervention in patient care during the procedure or use of the device.

Telementor advisor: A telementor advisor is an experienced surgeon, highly skilled in a particular procedure or use of a device, who, on a remote basis, serves as a resource for an on-site surgeon, already fully trained in his field and in performing that procedure or device use. The telementor advisor interacts but typically would not have the authority to intervene in the procedure.

Telementor preceptor: A telementor preceptor, who might also be called a "telesupervisor", observes and mentors but also has the right and responsibility to intervene and direct the individual that is performing the procedure. This potentially involves the actual participation in patient care through the remote direction. This allows for the teaching of new procedures and the use of new devices in a safe and secure environment.

2.1 Introduction

Despite significant advances in surgical techniques and technology in recent decades, disparities in access to necessary surgical care have dramatically increased. Currently, 5 billion people do not have access to safe and affordable basic surgical care, with an estimated 143 million additional surgical procedures needed annually in developing countries to provide life-saving treatment and prevent disability [3]. Developing effective solutions in order to meet this need is imperative to mitigate the increased mortality and morbidity that individuals requiring surgical care face in these regions. The surgical care is dependent on two factors, the accessibility of surgical centers and the availability of qualified healthcare professionals. One of the most promising strategies to achieve these goals derives from an advanced application of telemedicine, known as surgical tele-mentoring. Surgical tele-mentoring involves the use of information technology to provide real-time guidance and technical assistance in performing surgical procedures from an expert physician in a different geographical location. Similar to traditional mentoring, it plays a dual role in educating and providing care at the same time. However, it obviates many of the logistic obstacles associated with traditional mentoring, such as distance, time constraints, and cost. Previous studies have demonstrated no difference in knowledge and skill acquisition when comparing tele-mentoring and onsite mentoring of novice surgeons [4,5]. Studies reinforce this strategy and have demonstrated its reliability, efficiency, and cost-effectiveness as an educational tool and model for mentorship [6,7]. These reports suggest tele-mentoring to be a suitable replacement for onsite mentors and particularly useful for overcoming geographic barriers to distribute surgical knowledge. Numerous reports have suggested that tele-mentoring is a safe and feasible method of providing access to surgical expertise for patients requiring specialized procedures in areas lacking surgeons with significant experience [6–8]. Some studies have even suggested that a remote surgeon may successfully guide an onsite surgeon with extremely limited experience for the procedure at hand [9]. A comprehensive review reported that as of 2010, 433 surgical procedures spanning 11 subspecialties have been documented in the literature [10]. Tele-mentoring systems benefit surgeons and medicos by providing assistance from experienced mentors who are geographically separated [11–15]. The most rudimentary way to implement such a system is by using phones as a connection bridge to have the mentor verbally instruct the mentee [16]. The main limitation of using only verbal communication is that such a system limits the ability of the mentor and the mentee to share visual information. This remote instruction is commonly used in training and educational environments [17–19]. Research has shown the benefits of the visual access to and of the remote proctoring of surgeries [11–13] as well as the potential for tele-mentoring to improve minimally invasive surgery through remote video-assisted instruction [14,15]. A newer branch for tele-mentoring in surgery regards the utilization of visual assistance. Dixon *et al.* [20] looked at the effects of augmented reality on tele-mentoring success with regard to visual attention. This discovery showed that introducing annotations such as anatomical contours to endoscopic surgeons improved accuracy, albeit at a cost to cognitive attentional resources. Augmented reality as defined by Augestad *et al.* [21] to describe "the addition of comments to a viewport to augment the viewer's visual information".

Every one of us is witnessing the rapid technological progress shaping our daily lives in a form never seen before. These introduce a new medium for transforming healthcare services, moving them one step closer to users [22]. This creates a fertile ground for the rapid development of telemedicine, moving medical practices to cyberspace and interactive audio video communication channels, minimizing the need for a physical clinician–patient meeting [1]. Increasing the availability and accessibility of healthcare services and minimizing travelling costs and time consumption are only a few of the potential advantages these technologies bring. More focus is being directed towards the use of certain technologies instead of clinical matters [23]. The limited supply of surgical personnel highlights the growing threat of delayed treatment due to a lack of resources [24,25]. Such a scenario may happen even sooner than expected—a shortage of specialized surgeons in the USA is predicted for the year 2020 [26]. Given the timeframe and costs of training a surgeon, prolonged waiting lists in surgical departments are inevitable. Tele-mentoring has been described as a "surgical tool of the future", with its application ranging from providing guidance during a live surgery to remote training [27]. The outcomes of the approach are comparable to the standard practice of handling such cases—on-site supervision [28]. The number of case reports in tele-mentoring is increasing. The common features describing such systems are an orientation towards client–server software architecture, preconfigured end hardware, and planned supervisions. Such configurations work well for research purposes, but they do not reach the maturity for integration into clinical workflows as tools for daily use [29]. Regardless of the distinction between communication modules and surgery-influencing equipment, tele-mentoring systems fall within the category of Class II medical devices. The same conclusion was made by Intouch Health4, a major vendor of remote presence systems while developing its tele-mentoring solution [30–32]. All development and investigation have to follow the regulations, starting from preclinical testing and being approved as a medical device, to progress to the clinical investigation [33].

Inter- and intra-hospital communication is an important part of healthcare workers' duties [34]. While the actual scale of the interactions is highly dependent on the analyzed workflow, the knowledge of the communication patterns in clinical settings seems to be insufficient [35,36]. Tele-mentoring adds an extra communication channel, emphasizing the visual component, to the existing stack. It also requires more sophisticated end-user hardware than the well-established pager infrastructure [37]. Tele-mentoring is considered to be a "surgical tool of the future" [27]. This is a perfect definition of the expectations of the surgical personnel towards the technology. Tele-mentoring must be easy to use, highly available, and reliable if it is to become a common practice. On the other hand, tele-mentoring is not a complete solution. According to Coiera [38], social and technical system needs are inseparable; thus, the improvement of a simple telephone-based communication link should not be over-engineered; rather, it should maintain the features that made the approach attractive to clinicians in the first place while improving the drawbacks. The benefits of the visual component in surgical decision-making should be a sufficient impetus encouraging more extensive use. Tele-mentoring has the potential to offer more than on-site mentoring, and in the words of Hollan and Stornetta, to go "beyond being there" [39]. Modalities not available in the operating room come into play, enhancing collaborative efforts. Live telestration, overlay of 3D models, navigation, and image analysis are just a few techniques that could make tele-mentoring preferable to on-site and verbal guidance [40–43].

2.2 History of tele-mentoring

The rise of telecommunications subsequent to the invention of the telephone in 1876 has had a great influence on medicine, allowing for communication over long distances and even leading to the development of an entirely new branch of medicine, telemedicine. The first allusions of telemedicine in the literature appeared in 1950 in an article that described the transmission of radiologic images a distance of 24 miles, from Westchester to Philadelphia, Pennsylvania via telephone [44]. The first known report on the medical uses of video communication in the United States occurred in 1959 at the University of Nebraska where clinicians used two-way interactive television as an education tool to convey information to students [45]. This concept was then translated to the clinical setting to assist in the care of patients in remote locations in Nebraska. Throughout the succeeding decade, applications of telemedicine continued to expand and reports of its use included psychiatric group therapy, radiotelemetry, electrocardiography (ECG) rhythm transmissions from first responders, and ship to shore and transoceanic transmission of radiographs and ECG rhythms [46–50]. Also in the 1960s, the first video conference demonstration of open heart surgery was transmitted oversees via satellite [51].

Surgical tele-mentoring is a more forward-thinking telemedical application. It differs from old-fashioned methods of telemedicine in that it accomplishes a dual role of educating and providing care at the same time. Its emergence dates back to some of the earliest reported cases using tele-mentoring in the mid-1990s. Moore *et al.* assessed the feasibility of a tele-mentoring system using a remote surgeon located in a control room [>1,000 ft from the operating room] that controlled an inexperienced surgeon in 23 urologic laparoscopic procedures [4]. Mentoring was accomplished with real-time video images, two-way audio message, a robotic arm used to control the video endoscope, and a telestrator. They stated a 95.6% procedure success rate with no statistical difference in patient outcome. Shortly after,

Schulam *et al.* [52] evaluated a tele-mentoring system using a single T1 line [1.54 megabits per second] point to point communications link that allowed a remotely knowledgeable surgeon to guide a primary laparoscopic surgeon from 3.5 miles away. In a similar study, Rosser *et al.* compared the outcomes of four laparoscopic colonic resections and two laparoscopic Nissen fundoplications performed by surgeons inexperienced with the laparoscopic approach [5]. They reported no differences in performances of the surgeons or outcomes of the patients between those that received tele-mentoring guidance and those with mentors in the operating room. Lee *et al.* established a tele-mentoring system using a PC-based unit utilizing a single high-bandwidth public telecommunication line [53]. They reported no complications and an average of a 1 s transmission time delay that they contributed to the large distance and limitations in hardware and bandwidth. Another early example was reported by Camara and Rodriguez, who successfully telementored an endoscopic laser-assisted dacryocystorhinostomy procedure using an integrated systems digital network (ISDN) line to transmit information in real time from Honolulu, Hawaii, more than 5,000 miles to ophthalmologists at the Makati Medical Center in Manila, Philippines [54].

Application of long distance surgical tele-mentoring proved to be advantageous by the USS Abraham Lincoln, who formed the Battlegroup Telemedicine (BGTM) system in order to connect the Air-Craft Carrier Battleship cruising the Pacific Ocean with locations in California and Maryland [55].

In 1998, Rosser *et al.* applied tele-mentoring to monitor a laparoscopic cholecystectomy using significantly lower bandwidth to support a mobile operating room that provided access to impoverished citizens of rural Ecuador [6]. Although the slow connection speed did create some "pixelation" of the distant images, the telementors were able to properly identify the cystic duct and artery and guide the operating surgeon through the procedure.

In 1996, a group from Johns Hopkins Hospital, USA, successfully used an experienced mentor to supervise an inexperienced surgeon 300 m away. A robotic arm was used to control the video endoscope, and a telestrator was used to indicate important features on the surgeon's screen [4]. Tele-mentoring was successful in 22 out of 23 cases, and the investigators concluded that operative time of basic procedures did not statistically differ between tele-mentored and traditionally mentored procedures. Around the same time as the Johns Hopkins experiment, another experiment compared locally mentored training with tele-mentored training of surgeons in laparoscopic colonic resections and Nissen fundoplication. Performance outcomes did not differ between groups [5]. A collaboration between the John Hopkins group and an Italian group resulted in successful tele-mentoring of geographically remote surgeons in procedures as advanced as laparoscopic nephrectomy [56]. Recently, a renal transplant surgeon who was a relative novice at laparoscopy was able to initiate independent hand-assisted laparoscopic donor nephrectomy by means of international tele-mentoring. There were no adverse events and graft function was excellent. The mean operative time was 240 min, the mean warm-ischemic time was 189 s, and the mean length of hospital stay was 3 days. Early results seemed to show that tele-mentoring can significantly shorten the time taken to learn complex laparoscopic procedures and facilitate independent practice [14]. Following the success of earlier experience with tele-mentoring, the John Hopkins group increased the distance to their remote site to approximately 5.6 km, while incorporating controls to a robotic arm that manipulated the laparoscope and access to electrocautery devices for tissue cutting or hemostasis during the tele-mentored cases. They named this technique "telesurgical mentoring" [52]. Using a similar set-up to the group at John Hopkins, the first international telesurgical mentoring procedure was performed in Baltimore, US and Innsbruck, Austria [laparoscopic adrenalectomy] and subsequently in Baltimore and Singapore [laparoscopic varicocelectomy], using three ISDN lines and a bandwidth of 384 kb/s, and adapting for an approximate 1 s delay [53].

The next logical progression from telesurgical tele-mentoring, where the mentor is not the primary surgeon, was to true telesurgery that is entirely controlled by a surgeon at a remote site. The first published example of the use of this technique was a transrectal ultrasound-guided prostate biopsy performed by Rovetta in 1995. With the introduction of the Da Vinci® and Zeus® robots [Intuitive Surgical, Mountain View, CA] the possibility of true telesurgery arrived. When using these master–slave systems, the surgeon sits at a console several feet away from the robotic arms. As a result, some have used the term "telerobotic" when describing these devices.

The first true [remote] telesurgical operation, however, was the Lindbergh procedure [a laparoscopic cholecystectomy] which was successfully carried out using the Zeus® robot with the surgeon in New York, US, and the patient in Strasbourg, France. In 2002, a collaboration between a group at Johns Hopkins Hospital and one at Guy's Hospital, London, UK resulted in the first randomized, controlled trial of telerobotic surgery.

2.3 Applications of tele-mentoring systems

Modern technology has allowed for numerous advances in the utilization of tele-mentoring. Early tele-mentoring systems were limited by low transmission rates, raising concerns of the deleterious effects that a time delay may have on surgical performance [57]. Current telecommunication systems allow for dramatically increased transmission speeds, permitting a considerably decreased time delay [58]. These different strategies to perform tele-mentoring have numerous advantages and disadvantages as discussed below.

2.3.1 Videoconferencing techniques

Out of several common, free, commercially available software applications, Skype™ (Microsoft, Redmond, WA) is the most common application that has been reported in the literature. Previous studies have successfully used it as a method to connect video feeds from the operating room to a telementor in a remote location [59,60]. Its benefits include its wide availability, easy usability, and cost-effectiveness. Limitations include its lack of interactive abilities, such as camera control or telestration, thus preventing the remote surgeon's ability to control the visual field or draw visual aids on the video stream in order to point out anatomic structures to the on-site surgeon. Further, Skype™ does not establish a secure peer to peer connection and lacks Health Insurance Portability and Accountability Act (HIPAA) compliance [60]. Videoconferencing applications, such as Skype™ and FaceTime (Apple, Cupertino, CA) can be used on a variety of devices.

However, the literature related to the feasibility of these devices as tele-mentoring tools is extremely limited and questions regarding their efficacy exist. In an effort to evaluate the differences between these devices and their efficacy in tele-mentoring, Budrionis *et al.* [61] conducted a randomized cross-over study that streamed video of a laparoscopic procedure to a mentor surgeon through three different devices. Overall, portable tablet and smartphone technology may play a significant role in modern global tele-mentoring due to convenience, accessibility, and low cost but further research is required in order to demonstrate their efficacy to encourage their use [62].

2.3.2 Wearable technology

Google Glass is a wearable computer resembling conventional glasses that includes an integrated display screen, high-definition camera, microphone, bone-conduction sound transducer, and wireless connectivity. It has previously been used on rounds, and in the clinic and operating room to document a variety of conditions [63,64]. Picture and video quality have been reported to be high and definitively sufficient to document relevant clinical findings [64]. In an effort to assess its safety as a means to capture video to be used in a tele-mentoring session, Hashimoto *et al.* surveyed 34 surgeons who blindly compared video captured with Google Glass versus an Apple iPhone 5 (Apple, Cupertino, CA) during the open cholecystectomy portion of a Whipple procedure [65]. A significantly greater proportion of respondents felt that the Google Glass had poorer video quality [$P < 0.001$] and was inadequate for tele-mentoring as compared to the Apple iPhone 5 [82.4% vs. 26.5 %, $P < 0.0001$]. However, Datta *et al.* used Google Glass to stream live intra-operative video from 4 hernia repairs in Paraguay and Brazil, permitting real-time observation and proctoring by mentoring surgeons in the United States and Germany [66]. Further research is required to determine appropriate indications for using wearable technology for surgical tele-mentoring.

2.3.3 Robotic tele-mentoring platforms

To date, several robotic platforms have been implemented as methods of tele-mentoring. The VisitOR1 from Karl Storz Endoscopy-America, Inc. is a tele-mentoring robot that has been documented in the literature as an effective means of tele-mentoring [60,67]. It is a Food and Drug Administration-cleared Class II medical device, that connects to the remote surgeon's laptop providing the mentoring surgeon with internal views via direct connection to endoscopic images and external views of the operation captured from built in high-definition cameras. It allows the remote surgeon to control the external view camera and it provides telestration and laser pointing abilities. Additionally, it is HIPAA-compliant and has a 256-bit, military-grade encryption [67].

The RemotePresence-7 [RP-7] robot from InTouch Health, Inc. has also been used as a means of tele-mentoring while additionally establishing an increased remote presence in the operating room by the remote surgeon [68,69]. Despite the advantages robotic platforms may provide, their limitations are primarily related to their relatively high cost which raises questions about the cost/benefit ratio of these strategies as compared to simpler tele-mentoring methods, particularly for low and middle income countries.

2.3.4 Augmented reality

Augmented reality is well-defined as the integration of digital information with the user's environment in real time. Vera *et al.* developed and evaluated an augmented reality platform in order to assess its value in training laparoscopic skills [70]. Similarly, Andersen *et al.* developed a system for tele-mentoring and augmented reality [STAR] that provided visual instruction to a monitor that the students used to visualize their operating field in order to evaluate its effectiveness in training tasks including a port placement and abdominal incision [71]. Although the data related to augmented reality and tele-mentoring is limited to a small number of experimental studies, this early data suggests that augmented reality may provide certain benefits as a teaching aid.

2.4 Challenges

The main challenges addressed by the tele-mentoring service are discussed below.

1. *Standardization of infrastructure*. The reuse of the core functionality to develop VC services ensures the comparability of the produced research results in contrast to the fragmented current reporting of the studies. It equilibriums the service provider-controlled core technology and gives freedom to third-party API users to customize the interfaces based on the project needs.
2. *Usability*. The disruptive features of the suggested VC service void the need for dedicated mentoring hardware. A low usability threshold for the contributors ensures seamless person-to-person connections regardless of the underlying technical infrastructure.
3. *Connectivity*. Forming VC links crossing the boundaries of the secure networks in hospitals is a major challenge when implementing large-scale clinical services. Specifically, configure firewalls, proxies, and other advanced equipment that ensure a high level of network security create a bottleneck in increasing the availability of the services and enabling them to cross organizational barriers.
4. *Legal regulations*. Studies often ignore regulatory frameworks issued by the European Commission and FDA [discussed earlier], leading to unapproved tele-mentoring systems being tested in clinical settings [72,73]. Due to the

missing legislation explicitly targeting tele-mentoring, patients might face unnecessary risks.

5. *Large-scale service.* Regardless of the potential of the technique, tele-mentoring in a surgical department scope is a luxury. It is unlikely to have one of a few available domain experts on call for mentoring instead of performing surgeries. A large-scale service that crosses institutional barriers is required to succeed. The same on-call expert covering tele-mentoring demand in a country scope is no longer an unaffordable luxury.
6. *Incorporation into current medical systems and clinical workflows.* The number of ICT systems in hospitals is constantly increasing. Interoperability is often limited, increasing support and maintenance costs. Service orientation ensures the easy integration of tele-mentoring into web-based clinical systems without introducing additional software solely dedicated to remote supervision. Moreover, the end-users are not supplied by another device for mentoring purposes in addition to the ones they already have and carry around. However, the increased quality of the mentor–mentee interaction component in the tele-mentoring sessions and the positive feedback from the participants encourages supporting the feature as part of surgical tele-mentoring functionality.

2.5 Limitations

The safety-critical scenario and international regulations [30,74] limited the experiments to a number of test setups instead of the actual clinical assessment, which is the main limitation of the findings. The demo environments were tailored to resemble the actual deployments; however, the attitude of the participants may have been biased by the selected approach. Contribution in the trial had to compete with participants' regular duties in the surgical department in RCT1, setting a lower priority for the study. It is likely that mentoring an actual case would deliver more representative results; however, dramatic differences in the observed trends are not expected.

Both RCTs used videos and images recorded during a regular laparoscopic procedure at UNN. Due to the varying complexity of the case, fluctuations in the observed measures were expected. The trials were targeting a procedure of average complexity to provide quantitative estimates. The reported results may need to be adjusted to encompass either extremely difficult or extremely easy scenarios. The sample size is another weakness of both RCTs, making the results balance between proof and demonstration of effect. The use of language in the trials may have influenced the performance of non-native English speakers and may have introduced additional bias. Further studies are planned to add more subjects and provide solid evidence supporting the findings. The technological literacy of the participants and awareness of the telemedical techniques may have shaped the qualitative results of the study. VC is highly utilized in many care-over distance techniques at UNN, possibly resulting in a more optimistic evaluation of the proposed solution.

2.6 Conclusion and future directions

As the technology required to implement surgical tele-mentoring is currently readily available to many physicians, the advancement of tele-mentoring is now dependent happening several other hurdles limiting its expansion. For example, licensure issues exist due to the fact that tele-mentoring often occurs across directorial borders. Financial models have yet to be determined regarding tele-presence in surgery and questions exist regarding who will pay for the associated costs. Furthermore, the distribution of liability of on-site surgeon and mentor remains unclear, and disclosure to patients is subject to scrutiny as well. The issue of patient privacy is also a significant concern for the clinical application of tele-mentoring and secure HIPPA compliant transmission methods must be appropriately utilized. All of these issues need to be addressed before surgical tele-mentoring can become a routinely used educational tool.

Additionally, despite numerous studies representing the utility and safety of tele-mentoring, the literature is limited by small sample sizes, variation in tele-mentoring platforms, procedure, and the experience of the onsite surgeon. These limitations provide some confusion regarding the optimal use of tele-mentoring. Future studies evaluating clinical and educational outcomes with large sample sizes that span numerous procedures may be necessary to validate its utility and appropriate indications for use. However, some studies have begun investigating its potential to be used in "worst-case scenarios", in which the mentored onsite healthcare professionals have very limited experience or training in the procedure they are required to perform [62].

Future studies are needed in order to determine the feasibility of tele-mentoring in guiding inexperienced healthcare professionals. As discussed in this review, numerous emerging technologies have been developed that may facilitate the advancement of tele-mentoring as an educational tool. Early studies show at new devices such as augmented reality, wearable technology, and telerobotic platforms may enhance the tele-mentoring experience [66,69,71]. The full utility of these approaches as well as the cost/benefit ratio have yet to be determined and need to be further investigated. In order to fit this mold, emerging technologies must maintain an appropriate cost/benefit ratio and demonstrate educational or clinical benefits as compared to current tele-mentoring methodologies to justify their implementation.

The field of international tele-mentoring has steadily expanded, over recent years. This slow expansion is probably the result of financial, ethical and medico legal considerations, and of differences in software and hardware capabilities and specifications between individual countries. Unless these issues are resolved, perhaps by direction from an international body, telemedicine will fail to comprehend its full potential. The risks of security and liability need to be balanced by medicine itself, by proving that patient care is improved as a result of telementoring and telesurgery successes. At present, telemedicine is ideally suited to use in developed countries with remote communities and tele-mentoring will allow the dissemination of knowledge and skills, both nationally and internationally.

References

[1] Guidelines for the Surgical Practice of Telemedicine. Society of American Gastrointestinal and Endoscopic Surgeons, October 2010.

[2] Budrionis A, Augested KM, Patel HR and Bellika JG. *Towards Requirements for Tele-mentoring Software*, 2012 (Linkoping, Sweden: Scandinavian Conference on Health Informatics).

[3] Meara JG, Leather AJ, Hagander L *et al. Global Surgery 2030: evidence and solutions for achieving health, welfare and economic development* Int J Obstet Anesth, 2016, Vol. 25, 75–8.

[4] Moore RG, Adams JB, Partin AW *et al. Telementoring of laparoscopic procedures: initial clinical experience* Surg Endosc, 1996, Vol. 10, 107–10.

[5] Rosser JC, Wood M, Payne JH *et al. Tele-mentoring. A practical option in surgical training* Surg Endosc, 1997, Vol. 11, 852–5.

[6] Rosser JC Jr, Bell RL, Harnett B *et al. Use of mobile low bandwidth tele-medical techniques for extreme telemedicine applications* J Am Coll Surg, 1999, Vol. 189, 397–404.

[7] Chakraborty C. *Mobile Health (m-Health) for Tele-wound Monitoring, IGI: Mobile Health Applications for Quality Healthcare Delivery*, 2019, Chapter 5, 98–116.

[8] Sebajang H, Trudeau P, Dougall A *et al. Tele-mentoring: an important enabling tool for the community surgeon* Surg Innov, 2005, Vol. 12, 327–31.

[9] Ereso AQ, Garcia P, Tseng E *et al. Live transference of surgical sub-speciality skills using telerobotic proctoring to remote general surgeons* J Am Coll Surg, 2010, Vol. 211, 400–11.

[10] Augestad KM, Bellika JG, Budrionis A *et al. Surgical tele-mentoring in knowledge translation - clinical outcomes and educational benefits: a comprehensive review* Surg Innov, 2013, Vol. 20, 273–81.

[11] Ereso AQ, Garcia P, Tseng E *et al. Live transference of surgical subspecialty skills using telerobotic proctoring to remote general surgeons* J Am College Surg, 2010, Vol. 211, 400–11.

[12] Wood D. *No surgeon should operate alone: How telementoring could change operation* Telemedicine and e-Health, 2011, Vol. 17, 150–2.

[13] Ballantyne GH. *Robotic surgery, telerobotic surgery, telepresence and telementoring* Surg Endosc, 2002, Vol. 16, 1389–402.

[14] Challacombe B, Kasvoussi L, Patriciu A, Stoianovici D and Dasgupta P. *Technology insight: tele-mentoring and telesurgery in urology* Nat Clin Pract Urol, 2006, Vol. 3, 611–17.

[15] Moore R and Lee BR. *International tele-mentoring: a feasible method of instruction* World J Urol, 2000, Vol. 18, 296–8.

[16] Eadie LH, Seifalian AM and Davidson BR. *Telemedicine in surgery* Br J Surg, 2003, Vol. 90, 647–58.

[17] Jones G and Harris JB. *A descriptive study of tele-mentoring among students, subject matter experts and teachers: message flow and function patterns* J Res Comp Educ, 1999, Vol. 32, 35–53.

[18] Chen H-H and Price MA. *Promises and challengers: exploring a collaborative tele-mentoring programme in a preservice teacher education programme* Ment Tutor, 2003, Vol. 11, 105–17.
[19] Kasprisin CA, Single PB, Single RM and Muller CB. *Building a better bridge: testing e-training to improve e-mentoring programmes in higher education* Ment Tutor, 2003, Vol. 11, 67–78.
[20] Dixon BJ, Daly MJ, Chan H, Vescan AD, Witterick IJ and Irish JC. *Surgeons binded by enhance navigation: the effect of augmented reality on attention* Surgical Endosc, 2013, Vol. 27, 67–78.
[21] Augestad KM, Chomutare T, Bellika JG, Budrionis A, Lindsetmo R-O and Delaney CP. 'Clinical and educational benefits of surgical tele-mentoring,' in *Simulation Training in Laparoscopy and Robotic Surgery*, Patel HRH and Joseph JV (eds.), London: Springer, 2013, pp. 75–89.
[22] Ontario, Health Quality. *Electronic tools for health information exchange: an evidence based analysis* Ont Health Technol Assess Ser, 2013, Vol. 13, 1–76.
[23] Budrionis A, Hasvold P, Hartvigsen G and Bellika JG. *Video Conferencing Services in Healthcare: One Communication Platform to Support All* 2015 (Sao Paulo, Brazil: Medinfo).
[24] Ellison EC and Williams TE. *Population analysis predicts a future critical shortage of general surgeons* Surgery, 2008, Vol. 144, 548–56.
[25] Satiani B, Williams TE and Go MR. *Predicted shortage of vascular surgeons in the United States: population and workload analysis* J Vasc Surg, 2009, Vol. 50, 946–52.
[26] Grover A, Gorman K, Dall TM *et al. Shortage of cardiothoracic surgeons is likely by 2020* Circulation, 2009, Vol. 120, 488–94.
[27] Ponsky TA, Schwachter M, Parry J, Rothenberg S and Augestad KM. *Telementoring: the surgical tool of the future* Eur Pediatr Surg, 2014, Vol. 24, 287–94.
[28] Panait V, Rafiq A, Tomulescu V *et al. Tele-mentoring versus on site mentoring in virtual reality based surgical training* Surg Endosc Interv Tech, 2006, Vol. 20, 113–18.
[29] Budrionis A, Hasvold P, Hartvigsen G and Bellika JG. *Moving Telementoring to the web* Int J Comput Assist Radiol Surg, 2014, Vol. 9, 279–80.
[30] [FDA], Food and Drug Administration. *Code of Federal Regulations Title 21, Sec. 880.6310 Medical device data system*. June 2015.
[31] [FDA], Food and Drug Administration. *Code of Federal Regulations Title 21, Sec. 890.3710 Powered communication system*. May 2015.
[32] Directorate of Health, Norway. *Guidelines on Notification for Clinical Investigation of Medical Devices in Norway*. October 2010.
[33] Coiera EW, Jayasuriya RA, Hardy J, Bannan A and Thorpe MEC. *Communication loads on clinical staff in the emergency department* Med J Aust, 2002, Vol. 176, 415–18.
[34] Coiera E and Alvarez G. *Interruptive communication patterns in the intensive care unit ward round* Int J Med Inf, 2005, Vol. 74, 791–6.

[35] Solvoll T. *From being interrupted by mobile devices to Call Me Smart: A context-sensitive communication system for mobile communication in hospital*. UiT The Arctic University of Norway.
[36] Coiera E. *Communication systems in healthcare* Clin Biochem Rev, 2006, Vol. 27, 89–98.
[37] Coiera E. *Four rules for the reinvention of healthcare* Br Med J, 2004, Vol. 328, 1197–9.
[38] Stornetta S and Hollan. *Beyond Being There* 1992 (New York, NY, USA: Proceedings of the SIGCHI Conference on Human factors in Computing Systems), 119–25.
[39] Visentini-Scarzanella M, Merrifield R, Stoyanov D and Yang G-Z. *Tracking of irregular graphical structures for tissue deformation recovery in minimally invasive surgery* Med Image Comput. Comput-Assist Interv, 2010, Vol. 13, 261–8.
[40] Mountney P, Stoyanov D and Yang G-Z. *Three dimensional tissue deformation recovery and tracking* IEEE Signal Process Mag, 2010, Vol. 27, 14–24.
[41] Su L-M, Vagvolgyi BP, Agarwal R, Reiley CE, Taylor RH and Hager GD. *Augmented reality during robot assisted laparoscopic partial nephrectomy: toward real-time 3D-CT to stereoscopic video registration* Urology, 2009, Vol. 73, 896–900.
[42] Wolf R, Duchateau J, Cinquin P and Vros S. *3D tracking of laparoscopic instruments using statistical and geometric modeling* Int Conf Med Image Comput Comput-Assist Interv MICCAI, 2011, Vol. 14, 203–10.
[43] Gershon-Cohen J and Cooley AG. *Telognosis* Radiology, 1950, Vol. 55, 582–7.
[44] Benschoter RA, Garetz C and Smith P. *The use of closed circuit TV and videotape in the training of social group workers* Soc Work Educ Rep, 1967, Vol. 15, 18–20.
[45] Wittson CL and Benschoter R. *Two-way television: helping the medical center reach out* Am J Psychiatry, 1972, Vol. 129, 624–7.
[46] Jutras A. *Teleroentgen diagnosis by means of video-tape recording* Am J Roentgenol Radium Ther Nucl Med, 1959, Vol. 82, 1099–102.
[47] Nagel EL, Hirschman JC, Mayer PW *et al. Telemetry of physiologic data: an aid to free-rescue personnel in a metropolitan area* South Med J, 1968, Vol. 61, 598–601.
[48] Monnier AJ, Wright IS, Lenegre J *et al. Ship to shore radio transmission of electrocardiograms and X-ray images* J Am Med Assoc, 1965, Vol. 193, 1060–1.
[49] Hirschman JC, Baker TJ and Schiff AF. *Transoceanic radio transmission of electrodiograms* Dis Chest, 1967, Vol. 52, 186–90.
[50] Debakey ME. *Telemedicine has now come of age* Telemed J, 1995, Vol. 11, 3–4.
[51] Schulam PG, Docimo SG, Saleh W *et al. Telesurgical mentoring. Initial clinical experience* Surg Endosc, 1997, Vol. 11, 1001–5.

[52] Lee Br, Bishooff JT, Janetschek G *et al. A novel method of surgical instruction: international tele-mentoring* World J Urol, 1998, Vol. 16, 367–70.

[53] Camara JG and Rodriguez RE. *Real time tele-mentoring in ophthalmology* Telemed J, 1998, Vol. 4, 375–7.

[54] Cubano M, Poulose BK, Talamini MA *et al. Long distance tele-mentoring. A novel tool for laparoscopy abroad the USS Abraham Lincoln* Surg Endosc, 1999, Vol. 13, 673–8.

[55] Micali S, Virgili G, Vannozzi E *et al. Feasibility of tele-mentoring between Baltimore [USA] and Rome [Italy]: the first five cases* J Endourol, 2000, Vol. 14, 493–6.

[56] Fabrizio MD, LEE BR, Chan DY *et al. Effect of time delay on surgical performance during telesurgical manipulation* J Endourol, 2000, Vol. 14, 133–8.

[57] Antoniou SA, Antoniou GA, Franzen J *et al. A comprehensive review of tele-mentoring applications in laparoscopic general surgery* Surg Endosc, 2012, Vol. 26, 2111–16.

[58] Miller JA, Kwon DS, Dkeidek A *et al. Safe introduction of a new surgical technique: remote tele-mentoring for posterior retroperitoneoscopic adrenalectomy* ANZ J Surg, 2012, Vol. 82, 813–16.

[59] Ponsky TA, Bobanga ID, Schwachter M *et al. Transcontinental tele-mentoring with pediatric surgeons: proof of concept and technical considerations* J Laparoendosc Adv Surg Tech A, 2014, Vol. 24, 892–6.

[60] Budrionis A, Hartvigsen G, Lindsetmo RO *et al. What device should be used for tele-mentoring? Randomized controlled trial* Int J Med Inform, 2015, Vol. 84, 715–23.

[61] Mitrasinovic S, Caamacho E, Trivedi N *et al. Clinical and surgical applications of smart glasses* Technol Health Care, 2015, Vol. 23, 381–401.

[62] Chakraborty C, Gupta B and Ghosh SK *Tele-wound Monitoring through Smartphone, IEEE: Int. Conf. on Medical Imaging, m-Health and Emerging Comm. Syst. (MedCom)*, 2014, 197–201.

[63] Muensterer OJ, Lacher M, Zoeller C *et al. Google glass in pediatric surgery: an exploratory study* Int J Surg, 2014, Vol. 12, 281–9.

[64] Hasimoto DA, Phitayakorn R, Fernandez-del Castillo C *et al. A blinded assessment of video quality in wearable technology for tele-mentoring in open surgery: the Google glass experience* Surg Endosc, 2016, Vol. 30, 372–8.

[65] Datta N, MacQueen IT, Schroeder AD *et al. Wearable technology for global surgical teleproctoring* J Surg Educ, 2015, Vol. 72, 1290–5.

[66] Ponsky TA, Schwachter M, Parry J *et al. Tele-mentoring: the surgical tool of the future* Eur J Pediatr Sur, 2014, Vol. 24, 287–94.

[67] Rothenberg SS, Yoder S, Kay S *et al. Initial experience with surgical tele-mentoring in pediatric laparoscopic surgery using remote presence technology* J Laparoendosc Adv Surg Tech A, 2009, Vol. 1, 219–22.

[68] Agarwal R, Levinson AW, Allaf M *et al. The RoboConsultant: tele-mentoring and remote presence in the operating room during minimally*

invasive urologic surgeries using a novel mobile robotic interface Urology, 2007, Vol. 70, 970–4.

[69] Vera AM, Russo M, Mohsin A *et al. Augmented reality tele-mentoring [ART] platform: a randomized controlled trial to assess the efficacy of a new surgical education technology* Surg Endosc, 2014, Vol. 28, 3467–72.

[70] Andersen D, Popescu V, Cabrera ME *et al. Medical tele-mentoring using an augmented reality transparent display* Surgery, 2016, Vol. 159, 1646–53.

[71] Bogen EM, Augestad KM, Patel HR and Lindsetmo R-O. *Tele-mentoring in education of laparoscopic surgeons: an emerging technology* World J Gastrointest Endosc, 2014, Vol. 6, 148–55.

[72] Miller JA, Kwon DS, Dkeidek A *et al. Safe introduction of a new surgical technique: remote tele-mentoring for posterior retroperitoneoscopic adrenalectomy* ANZJ Surg, 2012, Vol. 82, 813–16.

[73] Kirkpatrick AW, Tien H, Laporta AT *et al. The marriage of surgical simulation and tele-mentoring for damage-control surgical training of operational first responders: a pilot study* J Trauma Acute Care Surg, 2015, Vol. 79, 741–7.

[74] *Guidelines on the qualification of stand alone software used in healthcare within the regulatory framework of medical devices*. Commission, European. s.l.: MEDDEV 2.1/6, January 2012.

Chapter 3

Technologies in medical information processing

Hoger Mahmud[1], Mokhtar Mohammadi[2], Nabeel Ali Khan[3], Tarik Ahmed Rashid[4], Nawzad K. Al-Salihi[4], Rebaz Mohammed Dler Omer[4] and Joan Lu[5]

Providing healthcare is a multidisciplinary effort where Information plays a life-saving role. Advances in health technologies have diversified the sources of information that can be analyzed and used for correct diagnostics and decision-making. Researchers and system developers in the field of telemedicine are consciously inventing and improving data generation, collection, and processing methods with a view to improving the quality of care and possibly reduce cost and effort need in providing care. Bringing newly developed technologies specific to information processing to the attention of healthcare providers (individuals or healthcare institutes) is vitally important to improve the quality of care. With this in mind, in this chapter the authors explain the importance of a number of health indicators that can be measured for data collection purposes such as temperature, heart rate, blood pressure, and respiration rate. This chapter also presents several latest technologies that capture data and process it to produce meaningful and visual information that can be used for diagnostics and treatment purposes such as X-ray, computerized tomography (CT) scan, magnetic resonance imaging (MRI) and ultrasound.

The chapter highlights the importance of data mining techniques in retrieving the required information from an information-pool in providing the right healthcare. The authors emphasize the fact that retrieving the required information may not be enough to provide the right healthcare service since the retrieved information needs to be interpreted by healthcare professionals to resolve a healthcare case.

[1]Department of Computer Science, College of Science and Technology, University of Human Development, Sulaymaniyah, Iraq, and Department of Computer Science, School of Computing and Engineering, University of Huddersfield, Huddersfield, United Kingdom
[2]Department of Information Technology, College of Science and Technology, University of Human Development, Sulaymaniyah, Iraq
[3]Department of Electrical Engineering, Foundation University, Islamabad, Pakistan
[4]Computer Science and Engineering Department, School of Science and Engineering, University of Kurdistan Hewler, Kurdistan, Iraq
[5]Department of Computer Science, School of Computing and Engineering, University of Huddersfield, United Kingdom

On many occasions, all the needed healthcare professionals are not available at one location and they need to be found and contacted to interpret the produced information. Finding and recruiting the right healthcare professional is a difficult challenge especially if the healthcare professionals are not located in one location. To tackle the challenge, the authors propose an interpretation virtual collaboration framework that has the potential to locate the right healthcare professional in a timely manner for a temporary need-base virtual collaboration to deal with a specific interpretation request. The framework contribution is demonstrated through applying it to a simple healthcare service scenario which provides a convincing case for the effectiveness of the framework. To summaries, this chapter explains the importance of several advanced data collection and processing technologies as well as proposing new technologies to improve the current practices.

3.1 Introduction

Governments and organizations around the world are investing a lot of time and resource in healthcare with the aim to improving the service quality and reduce provision time. Researches in the field of healthcare indicate that one of the most invested areas of healthcare is in bringing in new information technologies to facilitate care provision [1]. Quality of healthcare service is one of the attributes that the development of a country is measured against, and this is due to its vital role in raising the quality of life. Information and communication technologies have been utilized in many areas of healthcare for data processing and storage, as well as providing the medium for healthcare providers to collaborate and work together. One of the most widely used technologies in the healthcare sector is known as telemedicine.

Telemedicine is a remote medical practice, which employs information and communication technology to provide healthcare and exchange of health information for distance places [2]. Telemedicine plays a vital role in saving lives in today's healthcare environments, facilitating arrange of services from first aid operations to complicated surgical operations [3]. Telemedicine generates important digital data and information that supports decision-making during healthcare provisions [4]. Electronic devices installed to capture data for different aspects of specific care generate different types of data that each can be processed to provide more insights for diagnosis and treatment purposes. Wireless body area networks (WBAN) can facilitate capturing data [5]. Generated data can be used for research purposes to advance medical science. Recording data can be categorized into time series or image data. The time series data can be analyzed using signal processing methods in time, frequency, or time–frequency domains [6–8]. Image processing techniques can be used to enhance and analyze image data [9,10]. Data generated by telemedicine devices have to be sent to designated processing locations within a system in order to produce meaningful results. The process of sending data involves wide variety of technologies that span from signal process to multimedia. Besides processing data, telemedicine facilitates data and information storage for future uses and referral purpose. Information storage can be used as medical history records that serve both patients and healthcare providers during care provision. In these regards, internet of things (IoT) is very beneficial [11]. Stored data can also serve healthcare researchers for case study, statistical analysis and planning to provide better healthcare services and develop more effective delivery mechanisms.

The data produced and processed through telemedicine technologies cannot provide all answers as they need to be analyzed and examined by healthcare professionals. Due to the complex nature of healthcare provision and the need for multidisciplinary healthcare professionals, healthcare providers are moving away from relying on just local resources to more broad and external resources to provide the needed care [12], and this is where the concept to virtual collaboration can serve. To over time and space barriers in bring closer external resources, the concept of virtual collaboration in healthcare is gaining momentum. During the virtual collaboration, collaborators use information and communication technologists work together and share resources in order to achieve a common goal. However, regulating and managing collaboration and resource sharing is a challenge that researches have been working on for some time. Recently the concept of virtual breeding environment (VBE) [13] and virtual organization (VO) [14] have been developed by researchers to tackle the challenge. The concepts are claimed to create the platform capable of regulating the collaborations between virtual collaborators and facilitate resource sharing in an organized manner [15,16]. VBE is a virtual environment operated and managed by a number of permanent individuals, organizations, and companies that can facilitate and organize temporary goal-based collaborations known as VO. Requests can be sent to the VBE for creating VOs based on the needs and requirements of the requester for a specific period. When the goal of the VO is accomplished, the VO is dissolved. In this chapter, we outline an information interpretation framework in Section 3.5 based on VBE and VO concepts. This chapter contributes towards the ongoing search for capturing, processing and managing information in the field of healthcare.

The structure of the chapter is as follows: in the following section, we discus different methods for collecting, analyzing, and transmitting medical data, then in the next section, we provide data mining and knowledge management topics. Finally, we introduce a virtual collaboration framework for information interpretation.

3.2 Data collection

Due to the complex nature of human health, capturing all health-related measurable data is a mighty task that presents many technical, ethical, and scientific challenges. For the purpose of this book chapter, we concentrate on some basic attributes of human health to demonstrate medical information processing.

The attributes are the ones that are known to be vital signs of human health such as breathing and heartbeats. These signs can be influenced directly by any healthcare issued, the body may experience and they can be used as an indicator of human health. In the next few sections, we shall explain how data relating to these health attributes are captured using telemedicine technologies.

3.2.1 Temperature

Body temperature is the most common attribute of human health that is widely used as an indication for health issues such as hyperthermia and hypothermia. Body temperature can be affected easily by any alteration in the body; it is so sensitive that [17] states the mean body temperature can is different for different genders.

Measuring body temperature accurately is vital in analyzing human health as extreme high body temperature may result in irreversible organ damage if left untreated. The methods and techniques to measure body temperature vary each with specific time requirements and level of precision. The common points of the human body used for temperature reading are armpit, ear, rectum, and mouth. The normal body temperature is known to be 37.6–38.0 °C.

Reference [18] outlines some factors that affect body temperature readings such as the age of the subject, the environment and the device used to take the reading. For instance, the temperature taken from the mouth can be influenced by drinking hot or cold drinks prior to measurement and armpit temperature can be affected by whether the subject is sweating or not.

Advances in medical devices have provided more reliable methods for measuring temperature, for example, an infrared thermometer can measure body temperature based on infrared energy radiation.

Hypothalamus is the body temperature regulator of the body and it is very close eardrums, for this reason, body temperature taken from the ear is deemed accurate and the time require producing the measurement is very short (0.1 s to be more precise). The measurement is fast to obtain and can be sent to designated processing locations for processing and update purposes using network technologies (e.g. wireless technology).

3.2.2 Heart rate

Heart rate is another commonly measured health indicator that is used to assess body fitness to fatal conditions such as heart failure. Heart beats also vary like body temperature and affected by body activity and physiological conditions. The human heart beats 30% more during the day compared to the night and average heartbeat rate is 70 beats/min. Gender affects the rate of heartbeat as well; in general, female heartbeat is 5% faster than that of a male. To eliminate sudden rise and fall heartbeat-reading readings are normally taken in time intervals (e.g. every 2 h). Heartbeats can be recorded and sent to appropriate processing location for further analysis and health examination.

Heartbeats measurements are known to have fewer errors compared to body temperature; therefore, they more reliable to medical professionals. Reading points in the human body for heartbeat reading can be anywhere that an artery near the skin can be located such as the radial and carotid arteries in the wrist and neck. The number of beats is counted in 1 min to determine state of heart conditions. Heartbeat sensors can be fitted to equipment used for exercises and record the ratio that can be transferred to other locations for analyzing. This method is widely used and it is easy to measure and record heartbeats ratios. Another way to record, heartbeat is using wearable counter that is capable of reading the electrical signal produced as a result of heart muscle construction. Each reading is sent to a signal receiver where it is counted and recorded.

Telemedicine is used to monitor health status and the process that goes on within it has to be based on carefully tuned techniques and algorithms to produce reliable results. For example, it has to be smart enough to the age of the individual into account as heartbeat decreases as aging progress [19]. Telemedicine aids abnormal heartbeat detection that may happen suddenly such as hypothyroidism and is able to alert the relevant party to examine the abnormality.

3.2.3 Blood pressure

Blood pressure is one of the most common health indicators that is measured regularly. It is described as the amount of pressure put on artery walls [20]. Blood pressure drives blood around the body carrying oxygen and food to all parts of a body. High or low blood pressure leads to health status changes in the body and it can be affected by many factors such as lifestyle and exercise. Blood pressure measurement, which is referred to as systolic pressure, is measuring the amount of pressure exerted on blood vessel walls when the heart pumps blood through the body. There is traditional measuring method using sphygmomanometer and modern methods that uses digital pressure reader. In most cases, the pressure that is exerted on the vessel walls when the heart is at rest between beats is also measured and it is known as diastolic pressure.

Telemonitoring devices are also used to monitor blood pressure for patients that are in serious condition. The device takes readings throughout the specified time (every day for example) and sends the data to a center for the data to be examined by medical professionals. Digital blood pressure reader devices are available over the counter at different prices and capabilities. Modern telemedicine devices do more than just reading blood pressure; they can perform tasks such as data analysis to provide diagrams for data visualization and alert medical professionals about the suitability of a particular measuring method for a patient. For example, telemedicine devices can establish links with central databases to retrieve patient medical history so that healthcare personnel take into consideration the patient medical history during measurement capture and analysis.

3.2.4 Respiration rate

Respiratory rate measuring is more challenging compared to other health attributes simply because it is very unstable can change in a short time. The deepness of a single breath has a direct effect on the rate of respiration. If a deep breath is taken the amount of taken in provides more oxygen to the body which means the next breath would come longer and consequently slows the rate of respiration [21]. The rate also varies in different ages; the average breathing of a healthy adult is 12–24 times per minute where as newborns normally breathe 40 times per minute. Respiratory rate is normally measured for patients that suffer from lung diseases, breathlessness or other medical conditions that affect respiration. Measuring respiration rate is quite easy and can be done simply by counting the number of breathes an individual takes per minute. Respiratory rate becomes useful when measured and combined with other health indicators since they are closely linked. For example, there is a strong link with heartbeat and breathing, more heartbeat requires more oxygen and hence more breathing.

3.2.5 Blood oxygen saturation

Blood gets its supplies of oxygen from lungs and depending on the health condition of individuals, the ability of lungs to supply required oxygen differs. Blood oxygen saturation measurement refers the efficiency level of lungs in supplying oxygen to blood.

The measurement is performed to find out the level of oxygenation and saturation of blood hemoglobin. During the measurement, blood attributes such as partial pressure of oxygen in arterial blood (PaO_2) and blood oxygen saturation level (SaO_2, SpO_2) are used. To measure the blood attributes pulse oximetry and blood gas sampling are two common methods. These blood measurements are affected by certain factors like other measures; anticoagulant medications, for example, affects arterial blood gas sampling. The measurements can be done using small portable devices such as Pulse oximeters that can measure the arterial oxygen saturation (SaO_2); however, the measurement is less reliable than the ones taken by oximeter that uses red and infrared LEDs as they are more accurate [22]. The common point in human body to measure blood oxygen saturation are fingers or ear lobes and the way the measurement works is by passing light through blood vessels and measuring the unabsorbed lights that come out on the other sides of a vessel using light detectors. Fully saturated blood in terms of SpO_2 normally allows 0.5% of lights through.

To ensure the accuracy of the measurement it is recommended that sufficient time is allowed (at least the time taken for two sequential heartbeat) before the blood sample is taken for measurement. This is because the amount of arterial blood flow differs according to heartbeat rates. However, it is worth pointing out that there are certain situations that oximeter does not work accurately, for example in case of carbon monoxide poisoning it is not capable to distinguish carboxy hemoglobin from normal oxygen carrying hemoglobin [22].

3.3 Bio-signal transmission and processing

Remotely providing medical services is the main responsibility of telemedicine. To this aim, data should be transferred from one point to another. Besides that, data should be preprocessed before extracting information for analysis and storage.

For collecting and processing any kind of data biosensors are required to capture data, then analog-to-digital converter converts the analog data into digital domain, finally transmitter transmits the digital data.

At the receiving point, the data will be processed and/or stored to be retrieved for analysis at any time.

The maximum amount of data that can be transferred across a given communication channel can be measured based on the Shannon entropy. The theory essentially describes the capacity of a given channel based on a statistical model of the channel under the influence of additive noise during the transmission process.

3.3.1 Medical imaging

Vast medical devices such as anatomy, body scan, X-ray, accident recovery, and remote surgery use medical imaging technology. Medical images can be captured for instant analysis whereas immediate attention will be given once the image is obtained in case of an emergency or for later referral for archive purpose.

3.3.1.1 X-ray

X-ray image creates a picture of the inside of the body using electromagnetic wave radiation [23] which is usually taken for diagnosis purposes. Figure 3.1 shows the X-ray of a hand. X-ray incurs energy that is sufficient to ionize atoms resulting in positively charged ions that may damage human tissue [23]. X-ray is electromagnetic radiation of the same nature as light, but with a much shorter wavelength which gives the rays their ability to penetrate things light cannot. Due to their high energy, they can break chemical bonds in the living tissues they penetrate. Repeating this process can lead to altered structures or functions of cells [24]. There is a compromise between producing a clear image and patient's safety.

To provide efficient transmission of silver-based films, the conversion of images into digital format is necessary. Thus, maintaining of tiny but essential details requires digital imaging techniques that provide sufficient resolution and bit-depth that can distinguish any tumor from the background. Transmission loss or

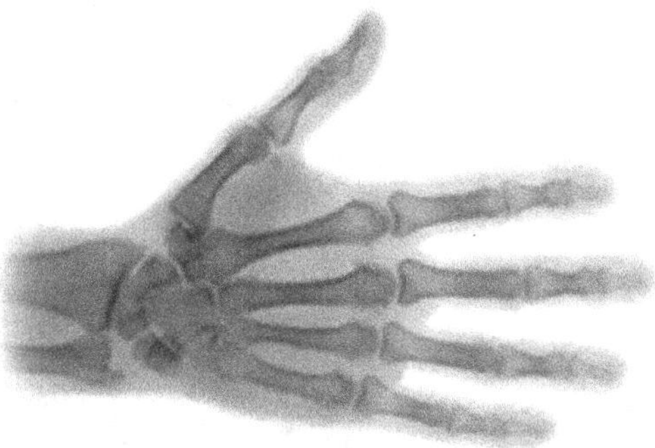

Figure 3.1 X-ray of the hand

additive noise imposed on the image may completely deteriorate the usefulness of a radiograph.

3.3.1.2 CT scan

A CT scan is a combination of a series of X-ray images taken from different angles around your body and uses computer processing to generate a cross-sectional image based on the X-ray images. CT scan images provide more detailed information than plain X-rays do [25]. A CT scan has many uses, but it is particularly well suited to quickly examine people who may have internal injuries from car accidents or other types of trauma. A CT scan can be used to visualize nearly all parts of the body and is used to diagnose disease or injury as well as to plan medical, surgical, or radiation treatment. Figure 3.2 shows a brain CT scan of a human. During a CT scan, you're briefly exposed to ionizing radiation. The amount of radiation is greater than you would get during a plain X-ray because the CT scan gathers more detailed information. The low doses of radiation used in CT scans have not been shown to cause long-term harm, although, at much higher doses, there may be a small increase in your potential risk of cancer [26].

3.3.1.3 Magnetic resonance imaging

Magnetic resonance imaging (MRI) works in a similar way as nuclear magnetic resonance (NMR) used in chemical analysis which uses magnetic moments of nuclei to capture images of organs in the body. The device used to capture MRI is a scanner that is designed to cover the human body in a long tube-like shape. The scanner is made of large circular magnet and RF coil that generates strong magnetic

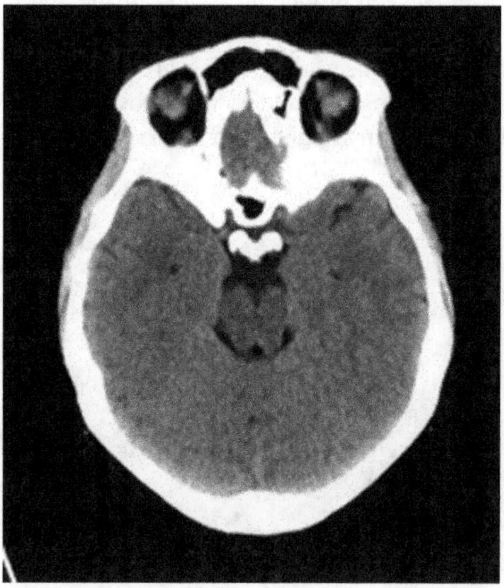

Figure 3.2 Brain CT scan of a human

fields to excite protons in hydrogen atoms. The short waves produced by the RF coil displace protons from their original position in human body. When the scanner stops operating, protons return to their natural and compositions and, in the process, radio signals with various lengths are emitted from different body tissues.

Across sectional image of the body, organs will be produced by the scanner using installed techniques such as spectrometer that can read the different radio signals. Figure 3.3 shows the brain MRI of a patient.

Both of these are vastly more efficient and detailed than X-rays and provide a much more detailed view of the human body, thus, making it easier for doctors to assess the ailment. The difference in the techniques becomes the biggest factor when choosing a particular scan and one or the others suggested by the doctor depending on the scan requirements. MRI scans usually provide a far more detailed image of the soft tissues and internal organs such as the brain, skeletal system, reproductive system and other organ systems than that provided by a CT scan, however, they are more expensive than CT scans.

3.3.1.4 Ultrasound

Ultrasound measurement relies on several different properties of sound propagation; these include propagating velocity, attenuation, phase shift, and acoustic impedance mismatch. With variation of these properties while propagating through different substances, tissue structure characteristics can be analyzed [27]. It is a high frequency sonic signal above the audible frequency range that propagates through fluid and soft tissues. The ultrasonic signal is then reflected back as "echo" to form an image. The denser the tissue it strikes the more is reflected back producing a lighter image. Images of organs and structures with different shades of gray can therefore be created.

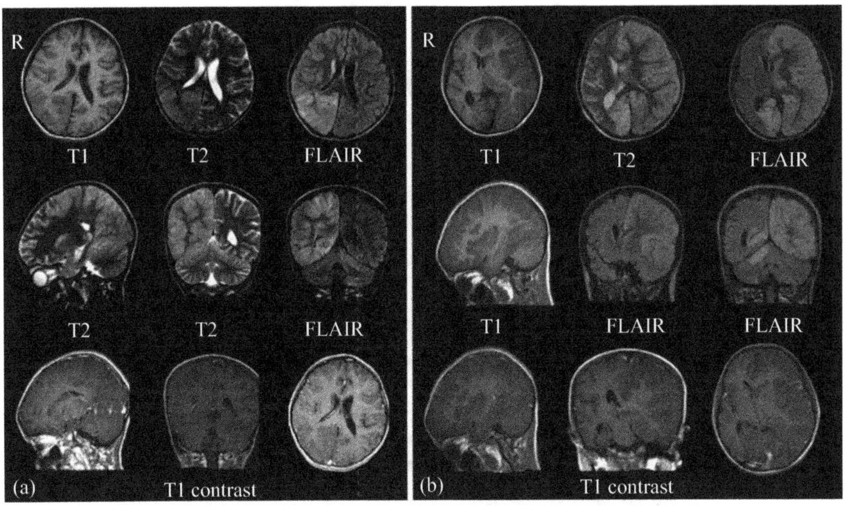

Figure 3.3 Brain MRI of a patient

An image is formed by scanning a probe across the area of interest, this probe does not have to enter the body and the entire process is carried out on the skin. The probe emits pulses of ultrasound and picks up the echo as the ultrasound signal is reflected back. We first take a look at how an image is generated by using an example of a heart scan that generates an "echocardiogram". The ultrasound signal penetrates through blood in the heart chamber and is reflected back when it strikes the solid valve. The presence and absence of tissue reflecting the signal produce a black and white image with varying contrast as in Figure 3.4. A monochrome image that shows a healthy heart is formed. This is particularly useful in detecting any abnormalities that may lead to heart problems. Very similar techniques can be used in different areas such as detection of breast tumor and renal calculi (kidney stones) for cancer and hydronephrosis diagnosis at early stages so that early treatment can be provided before the condition deteriorates.

In addition to providing early treatment, an ultrasound scan is also very widely used on pregnant women to constantly monitor the development of their unborn babies in the womb.

3.3.2 Medical image transmission and analysis

Four main types of medical image acquisition approaches were studied above. Next, these medical images will be processed without switching to other alternatives such ascot and PET, as these methods demonstrate numerous relationships when related to the image types that have been covered to do image processing algorithms.

Techniques, which transfer medical images from one place to another, might be identical to those used for common purpose photo transfers, such as uploading a digital image to the web and taking a picture with a 3G mobile phone with a camera

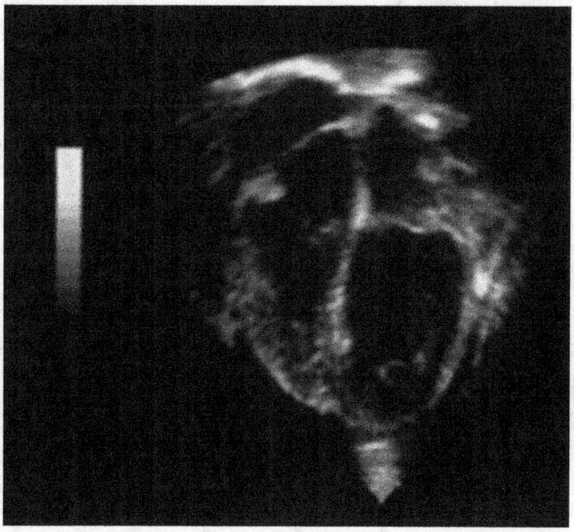

Figure 3.4 Ultrasound image of a beating heart

and the processes might be alike, nonetheless, the desires vary greatly in the sense that cloning is the key to the benefit of the image because the primary goal of a medical image is likely to first determine any exact details included in the image. A tumor may be unseen somewhere in a restricted zone of the image that needs to be recognized.

Furthermore, several of these images are monochromatic with the purpose of unlike shades of gray be able to grasp the analytical key of the image.

The visual world consists of comparable images. This decision is logical because the images we perceive in the real world are sets of the nonstop spectrum of colors with unbounded details. It is not possible to transmit any picture with unlimited detail. Therefore, digitizing an image will reduce its size to a limited extent so that transmission or storage becomes possible. Effective image transfer requires bandwidth for the available channel due to a large amount of data.

3.3.3 Image compression

The pressure is adjusted when storage or a picture of the transmission is reduced to save space or increase transmission competence. The issue is that numerous data compression procedures are lossless; in other words, the original image's detail cannot be retained so that the image treated by uncompressing does not precisely match the original image before compression. While with undamaged pressure, the original image can be transformed into its correct form after decompression without damage of detail or precision. This means that no variance should be detected when relating both images before and after pressure and succeeding compression.

Compression works through discovering spaces in a picture of the same color, then being marked as this space is the same color. Compression is fundamentally the course of removing openings and unfilled fields and duplicating an image. The key issue with medical image compression is that it typically comprises a huge amount of fine and significant detail, constructing lossy compression commonly inappropriate [28].

These details are preventing the spaces to have the same color or gray shade, and intrinsically, the details will certainly be disappeared because of pressure. In various medical images, details or specifics represent slight color variations and gray shades that might be so slight that they cannot be distinguished by the human eye despite the fact that containing vigorous facts about the patient's health. This comprises conditions, for example, the initial growth of the malignant tumor or the fetus that is malfunctioning. Corrupt image compression techniques may ignore dimmed details. The term "quality factor" is usually used to refer to the deterioration of image quality.

Unlike the lost compression, uncompressed image compression sets the original information to a series of data bits to reduce the file so that the original image can be restored entirely from the encrypted bit stream. Uncompressed pressure does not achieve a high compression ratio such as loss methods, so the compressed file size for the same image will be larger.

Uncompressed image compression sets the original information to a series of data bits to shrink the file to facilitate the original image to be repaired completely from the encrypted bit stream. Lossless compression does not attain a great compression ratio, for example, lossy methods, as a result, the size of the compacted file for the same picture will get greater.

3.3.4 Biopotential electrode sensing

Electrical actions, for example, EEG, ECG, and EMG require measurement of the behavior of the brain, heart, and muscles [6,29,30]. These electrical properties are typically measured on the external of the appropriate tissues, which are compatible with nerve impulses, and muscle shrinkage during the duration of the measurement. These are graphical images or signs of a medical wave form that was created through plotting electrical current amplitude over time. Our discussion will be focused on data processing of ECG where other parameters show very comparable characteristics.

Heart electrical movement is recorded via ECG. It can be said that the body will not receive electricity in the entire measurement course. The electrical impulses that made during the heartbeat are plotted with the aim of any irregular activity can be identified with the rhythm of the heartbeat. A set of possible reasons can also be deduced from the plot.

ECG is tremendously beneficial to sense and observing complications such as coronary artery disease, the spread of left ventricular hypertrophy, heart attacks, and carotid artery wideness. Many noise sources can weaken the measured signal, including ablation, fibrillation, electrophoresis, and speed. Any drive noise, excessive amplitude, and minor duration might strongly affect the discovery of the distortions in the signal. Some measurement processes may also have an impact on the ECG measurement efficiency.

A doctor usually does an ECG chart manually. If the graphic is presented or kept electronically, there must be also quality as in the case of processing the images discussed in the aforementioned section. ECG patterns should be regenerated with such clarity to keep all valuable properties. The signal must be noticeably separated from the back grid, this process of scanning might be problematic. That is why; the pure black and white colors are not appropriate although the plot signifying the signal is a monochromatic line. Occasionally, splitting the image into three distinct primary color channels supports to remove the signal from the background grid. The pink grid, which appears only in the red channel, can be removed easily from the ground simply by removing the red component from the ground.

3.4 Data mining and knowledge management

A record of physician visits to the patient has been recorded practically providing medical science initiated centuries ago. Old paper card records are still broadly perceived in numerous clinics to record details of each patient's visit. Certainly, there is a decent object to store all these records.

First, the conditions of the patient can be followed over time. You can also notify your doctor to cases, for example, sensitivities to some elements or medications. In addition, the frequent presence of assured signs might specify that a little serious is existing. The clinical associate will by hand delete the patient's record and make it accessible to the clinician beforehand the appointment or visit.

The clinician informs the record through a letter at the end of the visit and the assistant deposits it to the book stand. The procedure looks simple, nonetheless, there are many key complications. First, the doctor or patient possibly will change or move, once the doctor discontinues functioning for the reasons for retirement or for other reasons, then the records will be leftover due. A wide question people possibly will ask is whether inscription on these cards is legitimate.

If a first-hand doctor came and could not read the information on the cards, then it would be useless. The additional key issue is that records possess adding. A number of patients might have a dense block of registry cards, and subsequently, it is difficult for identifying people who are no longer in the clinic, there might be a number of records stay on the rack forever. The record will remain unnecessary and there will be no prior medical record accessible to the first-hand family doctor if the patient migrates. If we just contemplate by keeping medical records related to each patient separately since the birth, counting all test outcomes, decisions, treatments, and each visit details, then, what amount of data is shared. Thus, data mining technology emanates to address this issue. It is important to mention that informal data cannot be repossessed to analyze disease outbreaks and spread among data collected daily except through data mining technology.

Data mining depends on statistical models for rapid information retrieval from a large database. Data mining includes mining of patterns through scrutinizing and classifying records in large-scale relational databases of different dimensions. With increased computing capacity and disk storage, it is possible to conduct a further robust statistical analysis program to search in very large amounts of information over a portion of a second.

Electronic patient history is maintained in numerous countries for reasons such as patient care, statistical analysis of health risks, insurance claims, etc. The actions of how to search for data were described in [31], which suggested that examining for text across a huge amount of material is still a common practice among doctors. Based on this statement, an approach is needed to be found to deal effectively with the preservation and storage of medical information because it will contain much more data than patient information alone. Knowledge-based clinical applications extend through parts of management to clinical and clinic practice.

The main features of knowledge management are producing, relocating, and recognizing useful information. The process of knowledge transformation is a continuous process of change and improvement consisting of maintaining and strengthening knowledge. Knowledge transfer can also be seen as the construction, transference, and distribution of knowledge in order to improve access to knowledge.

The output can be fed by input for the next operation for continuous enhancement. In the medical setting, knowledge management accomplishments are primarily aimed at establishing and retaining processes to increase healthcare facilities with the intention of the public is in good health and living with less demand for medical amenities. Therefore, the diagnostic process to deliver the best conduct depends largely on the effectiveness of knowledge management.

3.5 Virtual collaboration framework for information interpretation

The healthcare industry is seeking new computer platforms continuously and healthcare professionals are encouraged to collaborate and deliver their services using information and communication technologies [32]. Healthcare provision, in general, is highly collaborative in nature. According to [33] "integrated care across disciplines" is gaining interest and the use of collaboration technologies is the mechanism that has fueled the interest. With the growing interest in integrated care across disciplines and organizations, collaboration technologies are increasingly seen as solutions for robust communication within healthcare environments [34].

In healthcare environments, sharing both explicit knowledge and tacit knowledge is important especially for situations such as diagnoses and consultation. Sharing knowledge in the healthcare environment poses many challenges especially when it comes to sharing tacit knowledge since it is communicated in narrative forms and requires real-time collaboration that is close to face-to-face meetings [35]. ICT advances have addressed some of the challenges and have made it possible for individuals and organizations to work together and collaborate in real-time virtual settings anywhere in the world [16].

Virtual collaboration has facilitated better access to specialized knowledge sharing in many scientific and professional fields that have led to better outcomes at a lower cost [36]. The authors of [16] state that due to globalization "collaboration in virtual settings is occurring on a regular and increasing basis" and in healthcare, the increase is going to be even greater [37]. Collaboration with others in any task-oriented settings only adds value if the task cannot be accomplished by oneself, and healthcare is a field that is known to require constant collaboration due to its complex nature.

The information generated as a result of incoming processed medical data requires expert interpretation for diagnoses and decision-making purposes. To diagnose a patient with a particular health issue, healthcare professionals need to make medical interpretation of data and assess the case in all aspects. In many medical cases, the information available cannot be interpreted by a single healthcare professional and requires a collective view and interpretation of a team of professionals. Knowledge interpretation has been researched in telemedicine by researchers, for example [38] refers to it as tele-evaluation where information is interpreted and transferred between care providers and they have provided a number of examples of tele-evaluation such as teledermatology, and telepathology.

Healthcare service is valuable when it can be provided on time and, any relevant knowledge that can facilitate the provision of the service has to be available when needed and, in the form, that is needed [16].

In such cases, a collaboration mechanism that can recruit and connect the right and required healthcare professionals in a timely manner becomes vitally important. The concept of utilizing virtual collaboration technologies to provide the medium for healthcare professionals to collaborate and work together to interpret produced medical information in real-time contributes towards the outcome greatly. This adds a new layer to medical information processing layers whereby healthcare stakeholder scan interprets and draws conclusions more efficiently. In this section, we propose a virtual collaboration framework for information interpretation and decision-making based on VBE and VO concepts. VBE is a permanent environment organized and managed by a number of collaborators (i.e. medical professional and healthcare authorities) using ICT that facilitate the creation of temporary request-based services known as VO to provide services (e.g. healthcare service) [39–42].

3.5.1 The interpretation framework

The concept of teleconsultation is explained in [38] where healthcare providers seek each other's advice in dealing with a healthcare case. The framework we present in this section facilities collaboration in healthcare for the purpose of consultation and information interpretation.

Healthcare generates a great amount of tacit knowledge that is difficult to share without a face to face like communication. This is due to the intangible nature of healthcare, which is known as the "art of care" [43]. Currently, the common way of using ICT for consultation and collaboration is using tools such as e-mail, for example, images produced digitally can be e-mailed to a radiologist to explain and send the explanation back to where needed.

VBE concept takes collaboration and consultation one step further by providing a real-time virtual environment where healthcare professionals can collaborate face to face without the need for being in the same location. The concept of VBE supports the exchange of narratives, stories, emotions, and human intuitions since collaborating parties can see and communicate with each other in real time. Facilitation of face to face like collaboration is vital in effective knowledge sharing generally and in healthcare virtual collaboration especially [16]. Collaboration facilitates information sharing and knowledge transfer to participants in need [32], VBE and VO concepts is developed to perform the same task but in an organized and managed environment. The framework we present is specific to healthcare professionals that are in need of collaboration with other healthcare professionals to interpret medical data for diagnostic and treatment purposes.

We have followed the direction of others such as [44] to focus on "tele-expertise" where healthcare experts use ICT to collaborate and communicate about a particular patient diagnoses or treatment. The authors of [44] claim that the use of such collaboration tools encourages healthcare providers to share and adapt their skills, knowledge, and way of treatments with each other with the aim to provide better and faster healthcare services. There are a number of similar proposals for example [32] presents a web-based application whereby physicians can collaborate and share resources; they have tested the system by asking a number of physicians to use the system and their feedbacks were positive.

The authors of [45] have proposed a system for image interpretation. The system allows a healthcare professional to share images provided by a patient with other healthcare professionals for diagnostic and treatment purposes.

The framework for medical information interpretation adds an extra layer to the traditional healthcare system processing layers. Healthcare systems normally have two layers to collect and process data, and they usually operate on a local level (within a healthcare institute or specific health authority). Figure 3.5 shows the framework position that sits on the existing traditional healthcare systems processing layers. Let us look at each layer separately and see how the new layer can serve its purpose.

Data collection layer: This layer collects data from various sources and prepares it for processing in the next layer. Data sources could be a patient electronic record that contains patient's medical history and personal details, information

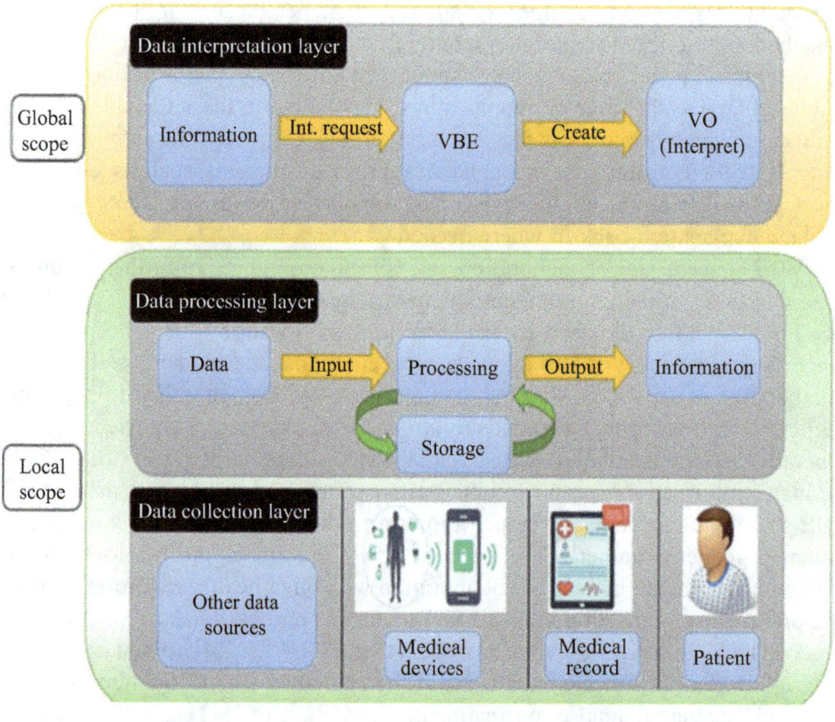

Figure 3.5 Framework processing layer

provided directly from a patient during a visit or/and medical devices such as heart rate monitoring devices.

Processing layer: This layer, process the collected data sent in by the previous layer. The collected data goes through the normal data processing cycle (input, process, and output). The processed result depends on the required outcome and processing techniques used to process the data. However, it is important to point out that at this stage it may occur that not all the information outputted by the processing layer is interpretable by local and available healthcare professionals and they may need to seek other healthcare professionals help. This is where the third layer plays a role.

Data interpretation layer: This layer can work on a global scope and it is based on VBE and VO concept. The layer consists of a healthcare VBE that is ready to receive information interpretation requests from healthcare professionals that cannot interpret the information on their own. The layer created a VO for each data interpretation request that is received and recruits the right participants to collaborate in a real-time virtual setting to interpret the information and make appropriate decisions. We explain how the framework works in Section 3.5.3.

3.5.2 Components of interpretation layer

The interpretation framework is a virtual environment which is composed of a number of integrated services that are provided by dependent components, in this section we provide a brief description of the components:

Request checker: This component is at the forefront of the framework and works as a gate keeper for the incoming interpretation requests that are sent in from healthcare professionals or healthcare institutions to recruit other healthcare professionals to interpret information. Requests are normally sent in a form of a filled in request form that should contain several vital information to trigger the subsequent component. Depending on the interpretation case the request information could be the names of the healthcare professional or institution, their contact details, the date and time of the interpretation request and the number of other healthcare professionals needed to be recruited. The information is checked by the component for validity and completeness, if any information is missing the request will be sent back to the requester to provide the missing information.

Request processor: This component is responsible for processing the request by parsing the information contained within it and passing it through to the relevant component for further processing. For example, interpretation requester may have requested a radiologist and a physician, these will have to be found in relevant tables in a database. The function of this component is to make sure the requested healthcare professionals are queried correctly.

Recruiter: The identified healthcare professionals will be contacted though the functions of this component for permission to be recruited to provide an information interpretation service. The component gathers all relevant information about the request, packages it, and sends it to the identified healthcare professional. If the healthcare professional agrees to the request, this component will trigger the next

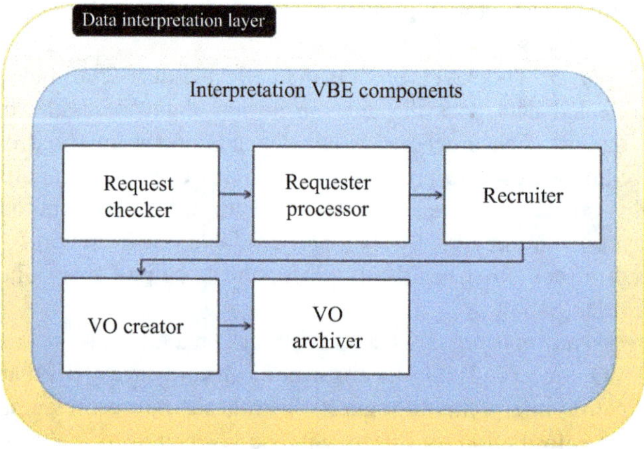

Figure 3.6 Information interpretation framework components

component to create a virtual room which we call VO for the interpretation collaboration to begin.

VO creator: The job of this component is to facilitate the virtual collaboration and connect all relevant healthcare professionals in a dedicated virtual setting for the duration the collaborators have agreed. Facilitation could include video conferencing technologies and text chart channels.

VO archiver: When the collaboration time has expired and the objectives of the VO has been achieved or it has been terminated for whatever reason. This component is responsible for archive the details of healthcare professionals, services requested and any other relevant information for future use and references. Figure 3.6 depicts the above-mentioned components.

3.5.3 How the framework works

In this section, we explain how the framework works systematically to create temporary interpretation VOs. Figure 3.7 shows the major processing stages in the framework.

Step 1: A healthcare professional creates a request for data interpretation collaboration and sends it to the VBE. In the request, the healthcare professional specifies some basic scope of the collaboration such as how many other healthcare professionals are required, for how long and when.

Step 2: Once the request is received, the VBE will process the request by checking for required information and parse the request to separate the basic elements of the request as mentioned in the previous step.

Step 3: In this step, the VBE recruits the required participants for the interpretation collaboration. Recruited participants could be from local healthcare pool or from an external global pool. In both cases, only those

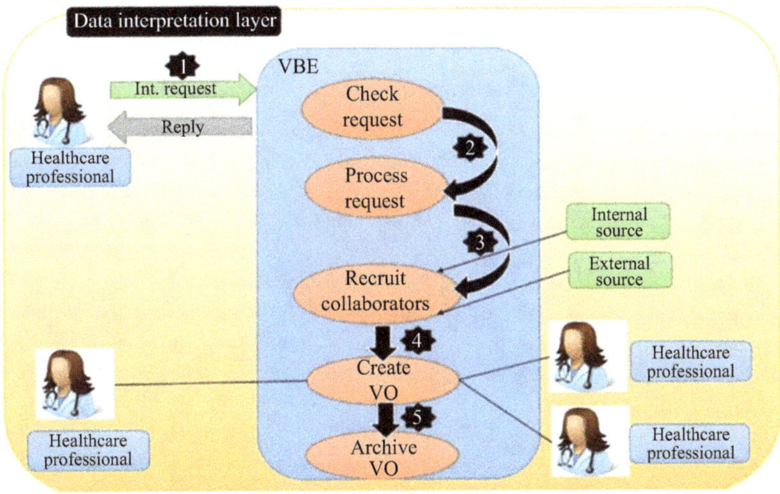

Figure 3.7 Framework working steps

healthcare professionals are recruited that are specified in the request sent to the VBE.

Step 4: After the right participants are recruited, the VBE creates a temporary VO where the participants can collaborate in real-time to interpret the information. The VO concept created is similar to the one in step 4 of Figure 3.7 which shows three healthcare professionals collaborating. It is important to point out that many different VOs can be in operation in parallel at the same time. Participants of VOs only have access to the VO they are assigned to and they don't have access to other VOs. This is for privacy and data protection purposes.

Step 5: This is the final step where the documentation and archiving of the VO takes place for future use and referral when needed.

3.5.4 Case study example

Multidisciplinary teams have been researched by [46] as an example of collaboration. According to [33] multidisciplinary cancer team consists of a surgeon, a pathologist, a medical oncologist, and a social worker and their main task is to review patient cases. In this section, we try to demonstrate how the framework serves collaboration between healthcare professionals in such multidisciplinary teams.

Mr Ali has been diagnosed with lung cancer. His health has been deteriorating, his local doctor who is also a surgeon has sent him to take some tests and the results are back. The doctor needs to understand and interpret the test results to find out what has caused the health deterioration.

He has concluded that he needs to consult with a pathologist and a medical oncologist, but the specialists are not available in his local hospital.

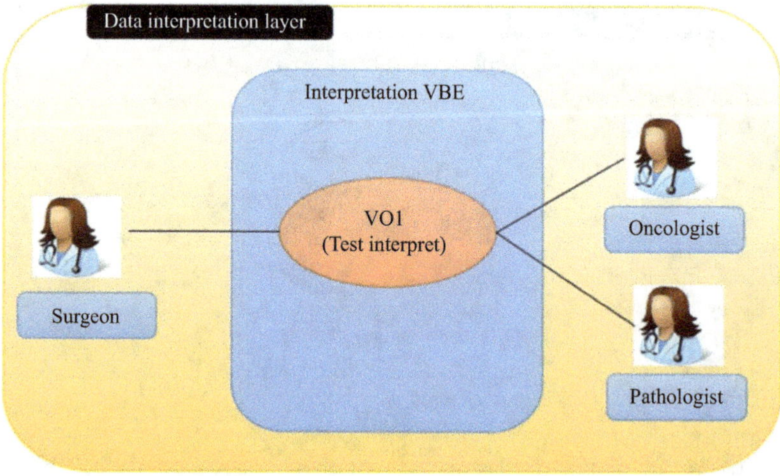

Figure 3.8 Cancer case study collaboration

He sends a request to the Interpretation VBE for collaboration with the two required specialists. Once the request is received, the VBE checks the content of the request and recruits the required specialist using the steps outlined in the previous section. Once the virtual collaboration is created all specialists can collaborate and share information to interpret the test results in a virtual setting where they can speak to each other in real time. Once the service need is fulfilled, the VO will be terminated and archived for future references by the VBE. Figure 3.8 illustrates the case study collaboration.

3.6 Conclusions and future work

The amount of medical data produced by healthcare information systems is growing rapidly as healthcare technologies advances. Processing and mining the generated data efficiently are vitally important to produce effective healthcare outcomes. This chapter explains in detail some of the main obvious but crucial sources of medical data such as temperature and heart rate and provides the current state of the art in processing and mining technologies that can capture, analyze, and present meaningful information, which can be used by healthcare professionals for diagnostics, treatment, and research purposes. The authors emphasize that due to the complex nature of healthcare information collaboration between healthcare professionals are needed to interpret it. To facilitate collaboration for the purpose of medical information interpretation, a healthcare virtual collaboration interpretation framework has been proposed by the authors. The framework is developed with the aim to bring healthcare professionals together in virtual settings to provide interpretation of information produced by medical information systems regardless of time and space.

Facilitating virtual collaboration between healthcare professionals comes with a number of challenges that require the attention of researchers. Bearing in mind that virtual collaboration takes place between individuals who may not know each other, on management level, finding a mechanism to recruit the right healthcare professional from a pool of professionals is a challenge. Verifying and validating the credentials of healthcare professionals before recruiting them to provide an interpretation service is another challenge to be addressed, without which, the validity of medical information interpretation conclusions would be questionable. The contractual aspect of virtual collaboration between healthcare professionals that come together to provide an interpretation service is another important area that requires research. The authors intend to research the challenges identified in a near future with the aim to transfer the interpretation framework from concept into practicality and ultimately implement and validate the proposed framework.

References

[1] Barzdins J, Barzdins J, Rencis E *et al.* Graphical modeling and query language for hospitals. Health Information Science and Systems. 2013;1(1):14.

[2] Sasikala S, Indhira K and Chandrasekaran VM. Performance prediction of interactive telemedicine. Informatics in Medicine Unlocked. 2018;11:87– 94.

[3] Cerrato P and Halamka J. Chapter Eight - Telemedicine: Is It Good Patient Care? In: Cerrato P, Halamka J (editors). The Transformative Power of Mobile Medicine. Cambridge, MA: Academic Press; 2019. pp. 145–68.

[4] Rezaeibagha F and Mu Y. Practical and secure telemedicine systems for user mobility. Journal of Biomedical Informatics. 2018;78:24–32.

[5] Chakraborty C, Gupta B and Ghosh S. A review on telemedicine-based WBAN framework for patient monitoring. Telemedicine journal and e-health: the official journal of the American Telemedicine Association. 2013;19(8):619–26.

[6] Mohammadi M, Ali Khan N and Pouyan AA. Automatic seizure detection using a highly adaptive directional time–frequency distribution. Multidimensional Systems and Signal Processing. 2018;29(4):1661–78.

[7] Mohammadi M, Pouyan AA, Abolghasemi V *et al.* Enhancement of the spikes attributes in the time-frequency representations of real EEG signals. In: 2017 IEEE 4th International Conference on Knowledge-Based Engineering and Innovation (KBEI); 2017. pp. 768–72.

[8] Mohammadi M, Pouyan AA, Abolghasemi V *et al.* Radon transform for adaptive directional time-frequency distributions: Application to seizure detection in EEG signals. In: 2017 3rd Iranian Conference on Intelligent Systems and Signal Processing (ICSPIS); 2017. pp. 5–10.

[9] Hossain MF, Alsharif MR and Yamashita K. Medical image enhancement based on nonlinear technique and logarithmic transform coefficient histogram matching. In: IEEE/ICME International Conference on Complex Medical Engineering; 2010. pp. 58–62.

[10] Senthilkumaran N and Thimmiaraja J. Histogram Equalization for Image Enhancement Using MRI Brain Images. In: 2014 World Congress on Computing and Communication Technologies, IEEE; 2014. pp. 80–3.
[11] Gupta A, Chakraborty C and Gupta B. In: Mittal M, Tanwar S, Agarwal B *et al.* (editors). Medical Information Processing Using Smartphone Under IoT Framework. Singapore: Springer; 2019. pp. 283–308.
[12] Benyoucef M, Kuziemsky C, Afrasiabi Rad A *et al.* Modeling healthcare processes as service orchestrations and choreographies. Business Process Management Journal. 2011;17(4):568–97.
[13] Ermilova E and Afsarmanesh H. Modeling and management of profiles and competencies in VBEs. Journal of Intelligent Manufacturing. 2007;18(5): 561–86.
[14] Zirpins C and Emmerich W. Virtual Organisation by Service Virtualisation: Conceptual Model and e-Science Application. Research Notes RN/07/07, University College London, Dept of Computer Science. 2007.
[15] Walker H. The virtual organisation: a new organisational form? International Journal of Networking and Virtual Organisations. 2006;3(1):25–41.
[16] Paul DL. Collaborative activities in virtual settings: A knowledge management perspective of telemedicine. Journal of Management Information Systems. 2006;22(4):143–76.
[17] Mackowiak P, Wasserman SS and Levine MM. A critical appraisal of 98.6 F, the upper limit of the normal body temperature, and other legacies of Carl Reinhold August Wunderlich. JAMA: the journal of the American Medical Association. 199209;268(12):1578–80.
[18] Sandsund M, Geving IH, Reinertsen RE *et al.* Body temperature measurements in the clinic; evaluation of practice in a Norwegian hospital. Journal of Thermal Biology. 2004;29(7):877–80. International Thermal Physiology Symposium: Physiology and Pharmacology of Temperature Regulation.
[19] Londeree BR and Moeschberger ML. Effect of age and other factors on maximal heart rate. Research Quarterly for Exercise and Sport. 2013; 53(4):297–304.
[20] Dary P. 0032: Analysis of blood pressure variability in the systolic hypertension with telemonitoring: feasibility and results on 108 patients. Archives of Cardiovascular Diseases Supplements. 2015;7(1):79–80. 25es Journées Européennes de la Société Française de Cardiologie, 14–17 Janvier 2015, Palais des Congrès, Paris.
[21] Mimoz O, Benard T, Gaucher A *et al.* Accuracy of respiratory rate monitoring using a non-invasive acoustic method after general anaesthesia. British Journal of Anaesthesia. 2012;108(5):872–5. Available from: http://www.sciencedirect.com/science/arti cle/pii/S0007091217322390.
[22] Toffaletti JG and Rackley CR. Chapter 3 - Monitoring Oxygen Status. vol. 77 of Advances in Clinical Chemistry. Cambridge, MA: Elsevier; 2016. pp. 103–24.
[23] Hessenbruch A. A brief history of X-rays. Endeavour. 2002;26(4):137–41.
[24] Reed AB. The history of radiation use in medicine. Journal of Vascular Surgery. 2011;53(1, Supplement):3S–5S. Radiation Safety in Vascular Surgery.

[25] Olegário TMM, Amato MBP and Lima RG. Modifications on CT-Scans for the computation of an anatomical atlas of the human chest. IFAC-Papers Online. 2018;51(27):253–57. 10th IFAC Symposium on Biological and Medical Systems BMS 2018.
[26] Sulieman A, Serhan O, Al-Mohammed HI *et al.* Estimation of cancer risks during mammography procedure in Saudi Arabia. Saudi Journal of Biological Sciences. 2019;26(6):1107–11.
[27] Ackland TR and Müller W. In: Hume PA, Kerr DA, Ackland TR (editors). Imaging Method: Ultrasound. Singapore: Springer Singapore; 2018. pp. 131–41.
[28] Devaraj SJ. Chapter 2 - Emerging Paradigms in Transform-Based Medical Image Compression for Telemedicine Environment. In: Jude HD, Balas VE, (editors). Telemedicine Technologies. Cambridge, MA: Academic Press; 2019. pp. 15–29.
[29] Wang W, Zhang G, Yang L *et al.* Revisiting signal processing with spectrogram analysis on EEG, ECG and speech signals. Future Generation Computer Systems. 2019;98:227–32.
[30] Bi L, Feleke AG and Guan C. A review on EMG-based motor intention prediction of continuous human upper limb motion for human-robot collaboration. Biomedical Signal Processing and Control. 2019;51:113–27.
[31] Dawes M and Sampson U. Knowledge management in clinical practice: a systematic review of information seeking behavior in physicians. International Journal of Medical Informatics. 2003;71(1):9–15.
[32] Maglogiannis I, Constantinos D and Kazatzopoulos L. Enabling collaborative medical diagnosis over the Internet via peer-to-peer distribution of electronic health records. Journal of Medical Systems. 2006;30(2):107–16.
[33] Li J and Robertson T. Physical space and information space: studies of collaboration in distributed multi-disciplinary medical team meetings. Behaviour & Information Technology. 2011;30(4):443–54.
[34] Winthereik BR and Vikkelsø S. ICT and integrated care: some dilemmas of standardising inter-organisational communication. Computer Supported Cooperative Work (CSCW). 2005;14(1):43–67.
[35] Tiwana A and Mclean ER. Expertise integration and creativity in information systems development. Journal of Management Information Systems. 2005;22(1):13–43.
[36] Te'eni D. A cognitive-affective model of organizational communication for designing IT. MIS Quarterly. 2001;25(2):251–312.
[37] Alavi M and Tiwana A. Knowledge integration in virtual teams: The potential role of KMS. Journal of the American Society for Information Science and Technology. 2002;53(12):1029–37.
[38] Field MJ. Telemedicine: A guide to assessing telecommunications for health care. Washington, DC: National Academies Press; 1996.
[39] Afsarmanesh H and Camarinha-Matos LM. On the classification and management of virtual organisation breeding environments. International Journal of Information Technology and Management. 2009;8(3):234–59.

[40] Grootveld M, Swaak J, Brussee R *et al.* Virtual Organisations in Healthcare: Organisation, People and Technology. Telematica Instituut; 2004.

[41] Reinicke BA. Virtual Organizations: A Definitional Framework. Washington, DC: Proc CONISAR; 2009.

[42] Camarinha-Matos LM and Afsarmanesh H. A framework for virtual organization creation in a breeding environment. Annual Reviews in Control. 2007;31(1):119–35.

[43] Stroehlein M. Caring Concept. SOJ Nursing & Health Care. 2016;1(2):1–3.

[44] Doumbouya MB, Kamsu-Foguem B, Kenfack H *et al.* A framework for decision making on teleexpertise with traceability of the reasoning. IRBM. 2015;36(1):40–51.

[45] Okuyama F, Hirano T, Nakabayasi Y *et al.* Telemedicine imaging collaboration system with virtual common information space. In: The Sixth IEEE International Conference on Computer and Information Technology (CIT'06). IEEE; 2006. pp. 214–214.

[46] Kane B and Luz S. Information sharing at multidisciplinary medical team meetings. Group Decision and Negotiation. 2011;20(4):437–64.

Chapter 4

A comparative note on recent advances of signal/ image processing techniques in healthcare

Bala Subramanian Chockalingam[1], Hemalatha Jeyaprakash[2] and Geetha Subbiah[3]

Of late, there has been a great deal of exploration and scope in the development of computer-oriented visuals and image processing in healthcare sectors. Despite timely expansions in this technological arena over the years, there is a lack of progress in explorations, which requires revived concentration. Based on this need, healthcare diagnosis through image processing and computer-oriented visuals with the help of sensors is promoted [48]. This approach involves integration of cues and modalities of images and visuals, which enhances the performance of processing the visuals and images. This chapter deals with the latest and the recent advancements in signal/image processing techniques, and network design in healthcare applications. Further, the study aims at academic and scientific contributions to the fellow researchers of this emerging area of technology. Also, the viability/ compatibility among electrophysiological signals such as ECG, EMG, EEG along image processional functionalities have been identified. In addition, some real case studies such as neuroscience, cardiovascular system have been discussed.

4.1 Introduction

Developments in image processing and computer-based visuals in healthcare sectors need to be explored to a greater extent. Though this amphitheater has been in academic studies for a long time in few decades, the evolutions have not met the requirements of healthcare investigations. Therefore, this study is mooted on exploring the suitability of image processing and computer-oriented visuals in healthcare. Though sensor-based activity is also an identical key extent, amalgamation of several nods and modalities can enrich the enactment of image-based or vision-based analysis.

[1]Department of Computer Science & Engineering, Kalasalingam Academy of Research and Education, Krishnankoil, Tamil Nadu, India
[2]Department of Computer Science & Engineering, Sri Vidya College of Engineering and Technology, Viruthunagar, Tamil Nadu, India
[3]Department of Computer Science, Vellore Institute of Technology, Chennai, Tamil Nadu, India

Simultaneously, biomedical signals have been used to design the system of both bio-mechanical and bio-electrical devices. Professionals involved in human service and medical physicians are familiarizing the advanced diagnosis related to health issues. The images and visuals extracted by the diagnosis experts adduce the health status and fitness of a patient. In bio-medical signals, event-related potential and action potential are dominant under which many processes are undertaken. EGG (electrogastogram), CP (carotid pulse), speech signal, VAG (vibro arthrogram), PCG (phono cardiogram), signals from catheter-tip sensors, vibro myogram (VMG), otoacoustic emission signals are classified under event-related potential. Similarly, ECG (electro cardiogram), EEG (electro encephalogram), ENG (electro neurogram), EMG (electromyogram) are classified under action potential. Under the domain of biomedical signals, image modalities such as CT (computed tomography), fMRI (functional magnetic resonance imaging) and PET (positron emission tomography) play a vital role in biomedical turf [1]. Of these modalities, fMRI provides necessary functional data during the diagnosis. This functional data accounts for spatial resolution data, and a reasonably low temporal resolution, through which the function of the brain at active mode and idle mode is examined [2]. Another role played by functional data is categorizing the epileptic seizures by applying cassette quiescent state [3]. Yet another major contribution from functional data is identifying the modified activities of brain [4]. Similar to fMRI, CT presents the temporal and spatial resolution data. The multi-detector CT, known for its high-resolution process, is considered as the latest technological tool in cardiac anatomy [5]. In the case of estimating the plaque morphology, ultrasound imaging process is employed on two-dimensional methods. It is to be noted that two-dimensional ultrasound process is prone to affect the precise accounting of morphological plaque variation. This may also occur due to discrepancy and deficiency of image resolution. Hence, to cope hardship in diagnosing pathology and complex anatomy [6], three dimensional techniques have been applied. In the case of nerve and fetal measurements [7], both two-dimensional and the three-dimensional techniques are put into action along with the cross correlation [8]. For nerve identification, Hadjerci *et al.* [9] proposed the application of UGRA (ultrasound guided regional anesthesia) by using despeckling filter in their filtering technique. CT and fMRI are highly reliant in detecting Rhabdoid tumors [10] and breast cancer [11,12].

The bio-medical field is related to detecting, analyzing and observing the diseases by employing advanced medical processes [13,14]. Of these processes, image processing has certain key methods, which are preprocessing of an image, denoising, image enhancement, image segmentation, ROI detection, filtering technique, thresholding and morphological analysis. Preprocessing is an essential step carried out prior to specific processing, which is resizing, rescaling and rotation. Under denoising unwanted noise is removed from an image thereby enhancing the results of the same. Segmentation is done to remove the image complex procedures, using information such as texture shape and contour.

It is feasible to dignify the forms of biomedical signals and images by means sensors. The dispensation of biomedical analysis is described with common steps as follows:

(a) Obtaining the germane biomedical data via sensors.
(b) Preprocessing after an image acquisition.
(c) Effecting the biomedical process by feature extraction under denoising.
(d) Later, classification can be done based on that diagnosis carried over, in which the results are extracted from both normal and abnormal samples.

4.2 Data-driven cardiac gating signal extraction method for PET

The authors Tao Feng, Jizhe Wang, Yun Dong, Jun Zhao and Hongdi Li presented Data driven cardiac gating signal extraction method for PET [15]. CARDIAC PET scanning is primarily a process that exhibits pictures and images of the heart of human beings thus derived. This enables the medical field, especially cardiology, by which the physicians can easily diagnose the nature of diseases. These physicians highly rely on this scanning to track some of the sensitive diseases, for example, coronary artery disease [16,17]. The peculiar feature of PET scanning under cardiac gating is the minimized blurring of images. In addition, it facilitates tracing of abnormal cardiac movements [18] and secures reliable information related to the stress and strain of the affected heart [19,20]. In spite of these possibilities, there is another method which can enhance the quality of scanned images and can provide authentic and accurate level of diagnosis, such as the ejection and fraction of the heart [21]. This method is the combination of techniques involved in cardiac gating and correction of motion [22]. However, this advanced method works upon the accurate results derived from cardiac gating, since cardiac gating demands data and information about the cardiac motion. Based on this information, the PET data are divided or distributed to requisite gates in accordance with the defined number of cardiac phases. Over the years, the clinical diagnosis depends electrocardiography (ECG) for deriving the information related to cardiac gating from PET data. The same ECG illustrates the live monitoring of the cardiac signals transmitted during the diagnosis. For this reason, the medical field has recognized ECG monitoring under PET scanning as the standard imaging protocol [23]. So far, ECG has been utilized for cardiac monitoring as the chief reliable process, in the place of scanning.

The scanning process faces a hindrance by way of external scanning devices, so that complications may arise. In addition, the medical analysts encounter more labor to undertake the diagnosis. By analyzing these practical difficulties, a new method involving data-driven gating is proposed in this paper. This method is already in use for diagnosing respiratory motion and has become a viable one. However, focusing this method on the cardiac gating is still at its primary level and only less satisfactory results have come in this area [24,25].

Buther *et al.* [24] proposed three approaches in analyzing the data-driven respiratory and cardiac gating. Among these three approaches, the first one is concerned with the geometric sensitivity, as the second approach deals with the center-of-mass (COM) and, the third approach bases its analysis on Standard Deviation (SD). The authors justified their attempt by claiming that these approaches are worth in generating cardiac signals out of PET data list mode. They made the justification that the approaches, along with the application of the Fourier transform, can provide the peak rating of respiration and cardiac signal. Generally, the cardiac signal is measured in the ranges surrounding spectrum signal frequencies. Physiologically, the peak respiratory range is higher than that of the cardiac signal.

Thielemans *et al.* [25] while dealing with the data driven gating, proposed the Principal Component Analysis (PCA), which is an integral part of the sinogram series. This scheme is much akin to that of COM-based approach and the geometric sensitivity approach. PCA is capable of generating a spectrum of frequency, wherein both the respiratory and cardiac peaks could be identified, when the range of cardiac peak is high. There had been a practice to make use of a band-pass filter to wipe out the components of respiratory segment.

However, Thielemans came out with the method involving a two-step procedure by which the cardiac signals are derived. Of these two procedures, by employing the first one, the sinogram is compensated by making use of respiratory motion. To be more precise, this is carried out by getting the estimate of respiratory signal from the first PCA, followed by extraction through the second PSA-based signal. The authors have extracted the cardiac signal along with the respiratory signal, by way of utilizing the typical signal extraction algorithm. Nevertheless, this algorithm excludes the usage of the salient features of cardiac motion in the scenario.

Another method on the lines of data-driven cardiac gating meant for small-animals called PET system is there in practice [26]. This method is unique in a way that it makes use of the change arrived at the sum of weighted counts identified in the inner portions of the cardiac region, taken for analysis. This sum is deemed as the cardiac signal. In tune with the advancements of technology, there have been developments in data-driven cardiac gating methods. Such imaging modalities have been recognized and duly validated for practice, as in the case of MRI [27,28]. However, beyond all these proposals and procedures, the PET imaging faces a lack of feasibility when these methods are translated directly for processing. This is the cause of variations in the acquisition of images and the qualities of such images.

As a remedy and the novel approach, the present paper proposes an innovative method based on dedicated data-driven cardiac gating. This model works upon incorporating the pattern of the heart motion, such as the expansion/the contraction. In addition, in order to enhance the signal quality, an automatic parameter optimization approach, which was proposed in the previous study is also employed. 4D XCAT phantom was utilized for simulation so that the outcome of the results on different situations can be proved for better performance. Also, for demonstrating the efficiency of the proposed method, datasets derived from the corresponding clinical environments have been included.

4.2.1 Discussion

In this proposed study, the focus is made on employing the data-driven cardiac gating method exclusively for detection of the expansion/the contraction of myocardium. In its approach, the proposed method is similar to the SD method proposed by Buther *et al.* [24], justifying the involvement signal extraction under the second order moment of tracer distribution. However, the proposed method has comparatively better results and more accuracy in terms of model regarding heart expansion and contraction. Same is the case with the signal optimization, where more accuracy could be noticed. As mentioned in the previous context, the proposed method is modeled as an exclusive pattern for cardiac gating. In addition, the better performance of the proposed method is validated under simulations derived from the exact clinical data.

During the simulation, the examination was carried out by fixing the calculation time for signal optimization of 15 seconds scan time as ~7.5 seconds. MATLAB® is used by implementing a PC having a 3.6 GHz CPU and avoiding parallel computation. It is to be noted that in terms of signal computation, the location of the reference point is to be given due importance. This reference point for expansion/contraction of the heart can be determined on the basis of segmentation. Also, the empirical knowledge of the corresponding heart-lung position is to be determined, while keeping the variation in the patient mode at bay. Quite interestingly, the simulation results of the proposed study exhibit that the accuracy factor of the reference point does not play crucial role in defining the accuracy of the data-driven signal. Perhaps, in studies that may come in future, more enhanced approaches on segmentation can be employed, so that still more accuracy with regard to the estimation of the reference point can be achieved. Such an improved accuracy can enable the reliability and robust application of cardiac data-driven gating method. As mentioned earlier, the reference point proposed in this study was calculated on the basis of sufficient data about the patients involved.

The previous study on data-driven respiratory gating method calculated the image domain signal by making use of estimation under the so-called Maximum Likelihood Annihilation (MLA) point estimation, which was based on Time of flight (TOF) information [22]. However, the current study aims at estimating the cardiac signal by involving the projection domain and leaving the TOF information. This is because, quite differently, TOF information is ideal for calculating the cardiac signal under the image domain. Yet, in terms of theoretical definition, utilizing the TOF information is sure to enhance the performance of the proposed method. Still, this could be possible when the photons are kept away from the background region, which may not ally with the cardiac motion. The proposed method is validated, and the performance of the method is proven by simulation results. The simulation included cardiac PET data by placing them with various parameters, thereby each parameter factor got isolated. Further, the influence of myocardium uptakes, respiratory motion, time/duration of scanning, rate of counting, and the variation in the heart rate could be fully comprehended for this method. Yet, out of the considered parameters, two of them affected the accuracy of the proposed study, namely the ratio of myocardium/body uptake and the level of count rate. While the ratio of myocardium/body uptake is the factor contributing to the signal strength, the noise level is determined by the level of count rate.

In fact, this proposed study involved data sets of 18F-FDG and is not constrained to any viability studies for a specific purpose. The simulation results are compatible with tracking of other kinds, even to the extent of myocardium uptakes of 13N-NH3 or 82Rb. It is to be noted down that in this study, the perfusion defects were not simulated, based on the assumption that the influence of defect over myocardium perfusion images and the reduced myocardium/body uptake ratio would be identical. This is due to the fact that the amalgamation of various activities of the myocardium plays a role in calculating the signal. The proposed method is certain to function well if the range of myocardium uptake arising out of defects is reduced and the minimum level of count rate both matches the fixed region. The proposed method has a limitation in the simulation study, in the form of single phantom and a single normal cardiac motion model.

In the case of the patient being bigger, there is a possibility of increase in the ratio of the required myocardium/body uptake. This increase is the outcome of possible increased attenuation, scatter and maximized ratio counts from the body of the patient. For proving the better performance of the proposed method, datasets of nineteen high cardiac uptakes were employed, under proper clinical environments and situations. Comparatively, the performance of the quantitative evaluation of the dataset with ECG signal and those of simulation studies is found to be similar. For more validation and the robustness of the method, in future, comprehensive sets of data with ECG may be employed.

4.3 3-D subject-specific shape and density estimation of the lumbar spine

Mirella *et al.* [29] have presented novel density estimation of the lumbar spine. The definition of OSTEOPOROSIS goes thus, “a systemic skeletal disease characterized by low bone mass and micro architectural deterioration of bone tissue with a consequent increase in bone fragility and susceptibility to fracture” [9]. In medical field, this term indicates the commonest prevailing bone disease. According to the report declared by the European Union, an approximated 22 million women and 5.5 million men who are in their age of more than 50 years are affected by this disease [30]. The lack of proper identification of early symptoms precipitates the case as millions of people have not undergone any diagnosis and/or not treated thereof. Such a lack is prone to end up with bone fracture. Another survey report indicates that among the global population, every woman out of 3 women and 1 man out of 5 men at their age of 50+ face the criticalities of osteoporotic fractures [31,32]. The World Health Organization, for its part, is initiating the diagnosis of osteoporosis, based on the assessment of Bone Mineral Density [33,34]. The BMD is crucial in calculating the T-score, which is derived from the division of the difference between the patient's BMD and the mean BMD of a reference young healthy population, and the standard deviation of the reference population.

The assessment of BMD is made at postmenopausal women and men age 50 years and older. They underwent a diagnosis with osteoporosis whereby the T-score was calculated at the critical bone segments. The T-score was calculated at their lumbar spine, total hip, or femoral neck and it was measured as 2.5 [35].

The recent medical field has started employing Dual Energy X-ray Absorptiometry (DXA) for evaluating the BMD, due to its less radiation, painless and cost-efficient method. The areal bone mineral density (aBMD, g/cm^2), a unique measurement, is measured by using 2D images facilitated by DXA. The medical field is already familiar with the direction issued by the International Society for Clinical Densitometry (ISCD) in this regard. According to this recommendation, the projected density along the anteroposterior (AP) direction is utilized for diagnosing osteoporosis at the lumbar spine. It is a well-known fact that the vertebral body is prone to face vertebral fractures [36]. Yet, in case of scans made on the lumbar spine using AP DXA, there occurs a superimpose of the posterior part of the vertebrate (informally known as pedicles, spinous processes and facets). This supports the claim that there is no possibility of estimating the vertebral body BMD in AP DXA scans, by excluding the posterior part of the vertebra. Nevertheless, this is a major shortcoming in the case of DXA-based diagnosis of osteoporosis at the lumbar spine. The medical field makes it known that the risks related to the strength and the fracture of the bone are not directly allied to BMD. The bone quality too endorses the casualties to the bone condition [37]. Yet, the level of aBMD decides the strength of the bone and the fracture risks [38] and the condition may vary for different sorts of bones. That is to say, osteoporotic fractures are possible to occur irrespective of BMD [39]. As per the laboratory conditions, low aBMD count stands at 60%–80% range of bone strength [40], with 50% postmenopausal women having a T-score of less than −2.5 face osteoporotic fractures [41]. In fact, bone quality is determined by two constituent elements such as Trabecular bone architecture and cortical bone thickness [42]. The bones of osteoporotic conditions face decrease of trabecular and cortical volumetric BMD (vBMD) (with varied rates). This decrease is the result of decrease of cortical bone thickness and the trabecular bone becoming more porous [43]. However, cortical and trabecular bones are subjected to different processes of metabolism and they exhibit differed response to the medication [44]. Again, it is important that in a DXA scan, it is difficult to assess either trabeculars or the cortical tissues separately.

Of late, there has been an alternative technique in the process of measuring BMD, which is known as quantitative computed tomography (QCT). This QCT employs a common and standard CT scanner aided with a calibration phantom. This is done for converting the Hounsfield Units of the CT image to BMD values. This technology helps in performing a 3D analysis of the bone structure, in measuring the vertebral body vBMD individually of the posterior part of the vertebra. Using this technique, individual evaluation of trabecular or cortical structure can be done. Nevertheless, compared to DXA, in spite of these advantages, QCT results are prone to expose easily at higher range of radiation dosage and is a costly process as well. Further, as known by the medical field, the cortical thickness, for instance at the vertebral body, elicits spatial dimension ranges of clinical QCT scans. This supports the view that more advanced techniques are required for accurate measurement of thin cortices [45]. Hence, in practice, there have been a rare usage of QCT in osteoporosis management. As seen from the above discussion, it is evident that there are limitations with regard to DXA and QCT, seeking fresh and refined proposals. Thus, use of statistical models and registration algorithms has been proposed in estimating the 3D shape and thickness of bone, by availing few DXA scans. As such, Cootes [46] proposed statistical shape models (SSM), to capture variable statistical shape structures anatomically by taking the stipulated population out of a trained dataset. The Statistical Appearance Models (SAM) [47] involve capturing the gray-level appearance, facilitating the characterization of the inner structure of the desired objects. Next, the SSM and the SAM are registered and fixed by Active Shape and Appearance Models, thereby similar structures are characterized and interpreted in new data. The 3D shape of the proximal femur out of certain amounts of radiographs is recovered by SSMs which are generated from CT images [48–50]. Similarly, the estimation of 3D subject-specific scoliotic spines from posterior anterior and lateral radiograph is done by way of using SSMs of individual vertebral kind [51,52]. To say more concrete, the referred methods aim at estimation of 3D bone shape out of 2D images, while there are other methods which involve in estimation the BMD distribution, in addition to the bone shape [53–55].

Despite the nature of activation in these methods, there has been no exclusive algorithm for quantitative estimation of the cortical and the trabecular bone. As a result, Väänänen *et al.* [56] put in their dependency upon 3D–2D modeling method, for estimating the thickness of cortical bone, for which they used thresholding and morphological operations. Yet, thresholding techniques proved to yield less accuracy when thin cortices are estimated [57]. Humbert *et al.* [58] proposed a method by which the macrostructure of the cortex and trabecular proximal femurin 3D out of an AP DXA scan can be estimated. The estimation of the cortical thickness and density and accurate measurements of thin cortices by way of a model-based approach is proposed [59]. However, it is to be asserted that such application of methodologies for the sake of deriving 3D subject-specific shape and density estimation of the lumbar spine out of DXA scans has not been treated as a straightforward approach. This is due to the fact that, in general, the images derived out of DXA spine are noisier compared to the DXA scan subjected to hip region. The reason for this noisier atmosphere is the penetration effected at the biological tissues by way of rays. Another reason is the complexity of the spine than the femur and the final reason is the existence of several anatomical structures, probably 4 lumbar vertebrae, which necessitates modeling of inter-object allegiance in addition to shape and density.

Yet another factor to be kept in mind is that the cortex of the vertebral body has a thin range, from 180 to 600 μm with a mean thickness of 380 μm [60,61]. Such thinness evokes the challenge during the segmentation of the cortical bone and the trabecular bone. Whitmarsh *et al.* [62] made use of a method using two DXA images, namely AP and lateral views, in a bid to secure a 3D subject-specific estimation of the lumbar spine, from L2 to L4. They involved in generating an individual statistical shape and density model for each of the vertebrae. By simultaneous registration of these three models in to the AP and lateral DXA scans, they generated a 3D model of the lumbar spine. They performed the measurements of trabecular compartment, there was no exclusive algorithm meant for the quantitative assessment of cortical bone.

In addition, there has been a practice in clinical analysis in evaluating the existence of vertebral fractures. For this purpose, the medical field has been using lateral spine imaging with densitometric Vertebral Fracture Assessment (VFA). This VFA uses single-energy X-rays which could not measure BMD. Also, lateral DXA which has double-energy is not suited for osteoporosis screening, as there is a possibility of high precision occurrence. From the analysis of all the literature analyzed and reviewed for this proposed paper, it is found that there has been no reference to the 3D modeling methods of the shape and density of the lumbar spine using a single AP DXA scan. The same is the case with the cortical and trabecular bone assessment.

A novel method in estimating the shape and vBMD at the lumbar spine (from vertebra L1 to L4) using a single AP DXA image is proposed [29]. The method is modeled on a 3D statistical shape and density, which is designed by having a training set of 90 QCT scans. The proposed model aims at elaborating the chief variations in the statistical data of shape and density, derived from the training database. The AP DXA image is registered and fitted with a statistical model to secure the 3D shape and density estimation of the lumbar spine. Also, the cortical layer is segmented by a model-based algorithm; an exclusive estimation of the trabecular and cortical bone at the vertebral body is proposed using the same algorithm. The clinical observations for measuring the data are done at various vertebral regions and compartments occupied by bones. The comparative results, in terms of accuracy, are evaluated by having both DXA-derived and QCT-derived 3D subject-specific models. A comparison is also carried out for clinical measurements for a validation set of 180 subjects.

4.3.1 Discussion

This paper discusses the proposed method for estimating the 3D shape and vBMD distribution of the lumbar spine (L1–L4 segment) from a single AP DXA image [29]. Also, the method is utilized for assessing the cortical and trabecular bone. The proposed method is of fully automated nature; by which it is freed of any user iteration. In general, 3D modeling methods of state-of-the-art nature demand a stipulated landmark for positioning amidst the DXA image [63]. As a result, in this proposed attempt, the processing of AP DXA scans and obtaining of 3D subject-specific models were carried out by using an Intel Core i7-4790K CPU 3.60 GHz. From the simulation results, the mean (SD) number of iterations was observed to be

1,628,218, whereby a mean computing time of 3 min 28 s could be achieved. The range of computing time is in direct proportion to the size of the region meant for scans under 3D–2D registration procedure. This proves that there could be higher computing time if there is a corresponding higher or wider region, L1–L4 segment. However, clinical practice seeks lesser computation time. In this regard, various approaches have been proposed in yielding low computation time. In case of femur, Humbert *et al.* could achieve the lowest possible computing of 1 min 30 s, for which they used an Intel Core i7-4790K CPU 4.0 GHz. Similarly, Väänänen *et al.* achieved a low computation time of 40 h when they used an Intel Sandy Bridge 2.6 GHz.

Another instance of low computing time achievement is from Whitmarsh *et al.*, who yielded 1 h by making use of an Intel Core i7 CPU 920 2.67 GHz. There is another method developed by Whitmarsh *et al.* wherein they used an Intel Core i7 CPU 920 2.67 GHz to generate a 3D subject-specific estimation of the L2–L4 segment but at the computation time of more than 4 h. Having analyzed all these methods, low computation time is achieved in the proposed method in this study by using C++, ITK and multi-core system techniques.

In practice, the geometry of the spine is viewed as complex compared to the one of femur. It is to be observed that the current study had 20,428 nodes, against 5,546 for; similar is the case with the bone structures, wherein four were assessed in place of one, which leads to increased computing time. Again, in clinical practice, the average computing time of less than 5 min is treated as low. As for the shape accuracy, in this paper, the mean unsigned distances between DXA- and QCT-derived surfaces have been arrived at, which are in the range between 1.37 and 1.72 mm at the total vertebra and between 0.63 and 0.68 mm at the vertebral body.

Whitmarsh *et al.* came out with their estimation of lower errors counted at the net vertebra, i.e. between 1.00 and 1.34 mm, while there had been larger errors at the vertebral body i.e. between 0.73 and 1.12 mm. The proposed study also encountered similar correlation coefficients (R) in the case of vBMD. In case of total vertebra, the range of R-values has been between 0.90 and 0.92 for the integral vBMD which is against 0.86 and 0.93 in [62]. In case of vertebral body, the current study could achieve R-values in the range between 0.82 and 0.85 (integral vBMD) and between 0.79 and 0.83 (trabecular vBMD) compared to 0.80 and 0.89 (integral vBMD) and 0.82 and 0.90 (trabecular vBMD) in [19].

When the comparative analysis of the lower errors in modeling the shape of the posterior processes and the current study are considered, the latter shows low errors. These results are outlined by demonstrating both AP and lateral DXA projections. Yet, there has been a slight reduction in terms of accuracy for modeling the vertebral body shape. The utility of the lateral DXA scans is in vogue in clinical practice and this is the lone limitation with regard to the method proposed. In addition, there has been no exclusive algorithm for quantifying the cortical bone. Further, there has been no assessment of L1. Similar approach to the one proposed in this current study is found in Humbert *et al.* for the proximal femur. The authors came out with their results of R-values as 0.95, 0.85 and 0.94 (integral, trabecular and cortical vBMD, respectively) at the total femur. This is in contrast to the current study, which derived the corresponding results as 0.85, 0.83 and 0.84 at the L1–L4 segment vertebral bodies.

As for CTh, Humbert *et al.* [62] could achieve an R-value of 0.92, compared to the one illustrated in this current study, 0.83. There has been a slight low accuracy in the proposed study which is the outcome of the fact that the geometry of the spine is more complex compared to one of the femurs. Another factor is that the average thinner of the cortex is in the vertebral body, which is, again, compared to the one found in the net region of the femur.

In all, 180 subjects were included for this proposed study. As such, there have been accurate bone masks and landmarks at L1–L4 segment, duly enabled by the software of the DXA manufacturers. This accuracy is sufficient to exhibit the proper form of the "L1–L4 Mask". This "L1–L4 Mask" is ideal for initializing the statistical model and carry out the registration. Yet, it should be remembered that the process is prone to encounter failure if pathologies of as severe scoliosis or severe osteoarthritis existed. This sort of hindrance would invoke the manual input of data, even modification of data already provided by the software of the DXA manufacturer. Such a modification, manually, has to be done well in advance to the process of 2D/3D modeling.

It should be noted that the outer and inner surfaces of the cortical shell underwent modeling was carried out in the vertebral body alone. Further, as mentioned earlier, the complexity of the geometry of the back processes invoke challenging task of segmenting the cortical bone in the region of desire. From the simulation studies it was observed that the bone density, caused by osteoporosis, alone was not the affecting factor towards the lumbar vertebrae included in the training and validation databases. In addition, the lumbar vertebrae got affected by several other factors such as shape deformation, occurring out of degenerative osteoarthritis, compression. Still more factors affecting in such a manner are the deposits of accumulated local bone mineral, otherwise known as calcification in the peripheral region of the vertebrae.

A survey illustrates that Osteoarthritis [64] is viewed as the most common among bone diseases, which could be noticed in 40% women of 50 years and 60% among the women of 70 years. However, the proposed shape and density model has been designed typically to cover the global variations, which indicates that no local variations, such as bone spurs, or osteophytes, are considered. Also, osteophytes are rare to be witnessed in AP DXA scans. These factors form a limitation in the present study, wherein, a model for local defects was not included. The significance of this limitation is that it has a direct impact on measuring the accuracy of the cortical bone volume and CTh. Hence, it is recommended that in future studies, attempt shall be made on developing the statistical models for the lumbar spine. Under such considerations, articulate and/or multi-level model shall be included, thereby better accuracy could be projected in models meant for deformations and the posterior regions of the vertebrae.

The diagnosis of the disease could yield wrong results if osteoarthritis is present, which is prone to affect the accurate estimation of the aBMD. The accumulation of local bone mineral at the periosteal surface is possible to end up with the overestimation of vBMD under the computation done by DXA and higher T-score. Under these conditions, an alternative measurement could be derived by the vertebral body when the trabecular bone is measured by DXA-derived 3D. In this way, bone spurs, local deformations at the periosteal surface or in the back processes can be wiped out. As the existence of fracture has been an exclusion factor in considering the statistical model, the proposed algorithm has conveniently left modeling the fractured vertebrae. The alternative for this is manual or automatic hiding of the fractured vertebra(e) in the 2D Mask at the time of registration process. Thus, there has been a provision for the excluded region of interest, such as L3, to have the estimation on the lines of already included regions, such as L1, L2, L4. However, there is a possibility for this region to be discarded subsequently, during shell modeling and measurements made at clinics. Based on the observations made under this study, it is recommended that future studies can focus on measuring other regions of the vertebrae, especially the lumbar spine. Hence, there is a possibility to cover the regions of the intervertebral space, the lumbar curvature (so-called lordosis) and vertebral body heights, which are parameters associated to fracture risk.

4.4 Abnormality detection based on ECG signal preprocessing in remote healthcare application

In the present world scenario, the diagnosis of heart-related diseases based on electrocardiogram (ECG) is more fashionable and significant. In an ECG, each and every heartbeat in the cardiac cycle is defined by the waveform. The time evolution of the heart's electrical bustle made by electrical depolarization-repolarization is described by the ECG waveform. ECG waveform [65] will be continuously recorded, wherein if there is any uncertainty in heartbeat or deviation in a morphological pattern, then it is a significant alarm or warning of arrhythmia.

In the medicinal sphere, basically, two types of heart diseases are reported. They are myocardial ischemia and cardiac arrhythmias. Owing to the blood supply reduction to myocardium there is a resultant of myocardial ischemia which sternly rehabilitated the morphology (2) of ECG signal. Cardiac arrhythmias are specified due to cardiovascular problems such as chest pain, cardiac arrest (3) and cardiac death. Since the two decades, ECG signal-based examination has been given more attention, where the variation of every heart beat in specified timing is analyzed. This type of analysis is called heart rate variability (HRV) (4). Hence this is a vital feature extracted from ECG signal variations and it is very helpful in detecting cardiac disorders and its related ailments.

Generally, while extracting the features from an image or a signal it should be completely free from the noise. To remove such a noise, in signal processing, preprocessing is an important artifact. While recording the original ECG signal (6), base line wander, motion artifacts and other disruptions should be removed. In order to do this, the ECG signal should be preprocessed. In a transmission of ECG signal on a wireless channel, those signals should be pretentious by a white

Gaussian noise [56,66,67]. To remove such a noise, researchers are suggesting voluminous filterings and noise removals techniques, such as mean filtering, adaptive filtering, curvelet denoising [68], etc. Removing Gaussian noise with the help of wiener filtering is more traditional. This filter is more supportive when the noise and input signal's power spectrum is non-detachable by the obsolete low pass filter. The ensuing choice of confiscating Gaussian noise with the aid of adaptive filter is functioned [69] to obtain the ECG data. Delayed error normalized LMS adaptive filter has been used to remove noise from ECG signal with less computation. And then, Heart Rate Variability is analyzed by extracting the R-peaks from the denoised version of ECG signal. While discussing the researcher's wavelet-based feature, extraction occasioned the best results, whereas selecting the mother wavelet plays a major role [70]. On the other hand, the performance purely influenced the number of levels of decomposition and number of coefficients. In this HRV-ECG feature extraction [69], coiflets wavelet is used. Coiflet is a symmetric and linear phase wavelet molded from Daubechies wavelet. While comparing spline [71] and basic Daubechies filter, the performance of coiflet is more flexible, better and more fashioned. To reduce the computation cost, the authors have chosen R-peak detection methods which can calculate the RR interval on the heart rate function. For the given ECG signal, RR interval is calculated as follows (4.1).

$$\text{RR interval} = \frac{1\ (\text{minute})}{\text{rapid heart rate}} \tag{4.1}$$

Sequential RR intervals are considered from the initial interval of the heart rate function. The authors have mentioned that among the several wavelets, coiflets gave successful results for QRS complex in detecting ECG.

HRV feature extraction based on frequency domain analysis provides highly crucial information which enables to find the undertakings of both sympathetic and parasympathetic. While monitoring the HRV signal on a human, researchers list out the frequency regions as follows: (i) VLF (very low frequency) which ranges below 0.04 Hz, (ii) LF (low frequency) which ranges amid (0.04–0.15 Hz), (iii) HF (high frequency) which ranges amid (0.15–0.5 Hz). Here, sympathetic could affect the LF spectrum and parasympathetic could affect the HF spectrum. The computed features and extracted features have been classified into abnormal or normal via machine learning classification algorithms.

4.4.1 Preprocessing using DENLMS algorithm

DENLMS [69] is an algorithm used to preprocess the ECG signal. Due to low computational cost, the LMS algorithm is more famous among the adaptive filters. FIR filter coefficients in a standard LMS algorithm are modified depending upon weight updating. Its weight updating equation is given in (4.2).

$$\text{weigh}(n+1) = \text{weigh}(n) + \mu x(n)e(n) \tag{4.2}$$

where n is a time step, $\text{weigh}(n)$ is a current weight and $\text{weigh}(n+1)$ is a new updated weight. Step size is represented as μ, $e(n)$ denoted the error signal and $x(n)$

denotes the filter input. Update of weight for the corresponding filter coefficients are fully controlled by the error signal. The adaptive filter output is calculated as follows (4.3).

$$y(n) = w^t(n)x(n) \tag{4.3}$$

whereas $w^t(n)$ is the updation of weight.

The structure of an adaptive filter is like a feedback structure and hence pipelining of this adaptive filter is very difficult. Once the filter is pipelined, it is very important to ensure that the filter has the same number of coefficients used for the non-pipelined filter.

The authors evaluated the ANFIS based on the following criterion.

1. ECG signal has collected from MIT-BIH signal.
2. With the help of an adaptive filter ECG signal has been preprocessed.
3. Detection of R-peak signal.
4. From the HRV signal, frequency domain feature has been extracted such as VLF power HF and LF power, HR and LF norm and final HF/LF ratio.
5. Using the SVM classifier, it is classified into abnormal or normal.

The features used for classification are a totally 14 HRV features from both time and frequency domain. Frequency domain features used were: LF power, HF power, VLF, LF norm, ratio of LF/HF and HF norm. And the time domain features used were: are RR mean, RR Std, HR mean, HR Std, RMSSD, NN50, pNN50, RR Triangular Index, TINN.

4.5 Breast cancer classification using histology images

In the present era, breast cancer is the hot research topic in health care because it is said to be the second major reason for cancerous death among women. From a woman a sample tissue can be taken, studied and observed using microscopy called biopsy. Based on the findings and observation of histopathology, diagnosis results will be analyzed. Diagnosis leads to identification of the problem in patients if the histopathologist is not well-trained. With the aid of pattern recognition, machine learning and image processing advancements, researchers are paying interest to improve the quality of diagnosis. A deconvolution-based classic for modulation transfer function (MTF) enhancement in CT is employed to attain uniform spatial resolution. The authors deliberated eleven sub-band regions which can diminish the noise and enrich the spatial resolution. Soft tissue region has been well explored through manipulating the estimated blurring point spread function (PSF) kernel.

Dalal *et al.* [72] compared the two famous machine learning algorithms in classifying the breast cancer histology images into the benign, malignant group and its subclasses. Two machine learning algorithms used here are Support vector machine (SVM) and Convolutional Neural Networks (CNN). The input to the SVM is the handcrafted extracted features encoded by bag of words and liner coding locality constrained.

The dataset used for this experiment is BreakHis [73]. This dataset consists of a totally of 7,909 images, fully biopsy microscopic images for benign and malignant breast tumors. Whereas, every breast tumor slide is stained with eosin and hematoxylin. Also, eight different categories of benign and malignant tumors images got settled in this dataset. Ductal carcinoma, mucinous carcinoma, lobular carcinoma, papillary carcinoma belongs to a category called malignant tumor. Phyllodes tumors, tabular adenoma, adenosis, broadenoma belong to a category called benign tumor. With the help of four magnification factors such as 40, 100, 200, 400 all the images were acquired.

4.5.1 CNN architecture

A convolutional neural network is a recent fashionable and successive machine algorithm, where there is an absence of handcrafted features. CNN topology using Caffe was proposed by the authors [74]. Designing of Caffe is a very easy modular and the interfaces are similar to that of both python and MATLAB. It supports both GPY and CPU. CNN, proposed by the authors are, convolutional layers followed by the two fully connected layers. Filter size and hidden units used are as follows:

1. Convolution layer 1 with filter size 3×3 and feature maps – 63.
2. Convolution layer 2 with filter size 3×3 and feature maps – 96.
3. Convolution layer 3 with filter size 3×3 and feature maps – 128.
4. Convolution layer 4 with filter size 3×3 and feature maps – 256.
5. Convolution layer 5 with filter size 3×3 and feature maps – 256.
6. Fully connected layer with hidden units – 2,000.
7. No hidden units on fully connected layers are equal to total class numbers.
8. Softmax layer.

To familiarize the non-linearity and to hustle the convergence learning, the RELU layer has been applied to all convolutional and fully connected layers. The purpose of RELU layer is, for a given input it will change all the negative activation values making to zero by applying the function as $f(x) = \max(0, x)$. For the first, second and fifth convolutional layers, max pooling has been used. To diminish the filter size of 3×3 and stride of length 2, max pooling layer has been smeared by following the RELU layer. Consuming the Gaussian distribution with low distribution network weight has been initialized as 0.01 for all the layers.

With the above CNN setup, the images were trained for 20,000 iterations. And the images were trained in Tesla K40m GPU. Accuracies, Confusion matrix, precision, recall measures were taken for the comparison. The accuracy obtained was approximately 94.56% of the image with 40× magnification. Once the training dataset was augmented, flipped and rotated for 20,000 iterations the accuracy attained was 96.96%. Thus, it implies that, with the help of applying augmentation, the accuracy factor can be improved for all the images with various magnification factors.

4.6 Conclusion

This chapter delivered the most up-to-date and recent advancements in signal/image processing techniques of system and network design of healthcare applications. In detail, a study has explained about the abnormality detection of ECG, signal processing played a major role, where coiflets given the successful results for QRS complex in detecting ECG and HRV feature extraction based on frequency domain analysis offered highly crucial information which enabled to found the undertakings of both sympathetic and parasympathetic. Later the study has discussed the successful findings in results of 3-D subject-specific shape and density estimation of the lumbar spine and data-driven cardiac gating signal extraction method for PET. Later, this continuation classification of breast cancer has discussed with the help of histology images using two famous machine learning algorithms names: SVM, CNN. Further, the study served environment researchers in both academia and industries working in this fascinating and emerging area who share their experiences and findings with the readers. In addition, some real case studies such as neuroscience, cardiovascular system had been discussed.

4.7 Future work

As we are as researchers, the study will be taken place about the functions of the brain as:

1. To implement the wiring maps of neural links in the brain, which may assist surgeons in brain tumor removals.
2. To measure biochemical changes in the brain, in the presence of tumors.
3. To study Alzheimer's, Parkinson's and ADHD while using MRI Diffusion Imaging methods.
4. To study and determine the activeness of the brain parts while a person tells a lie.

References

[1] Kayvan N. and Robert S. *Biomedical signal and Image processing*. 2nd edition. New York: CRC Press; 2012

[2] Sakoglu U. and Calhoun V.D. 'Temporal dynamics of functional network connectivity at rest: a comparison of schizophrenia patients and healthy controls'. in *Proceedings of the 15th annual meeting of the organization for human brain mapping*. San Francisco: CA; 2009

[3] Zhang C.H., Lu Y., Brinkmann B., Welker K., Worrell G. and He B. 'Lateralization and localization of epilepsy related hemodynamic foci using presurgical fMRI'. *Clin. Neurophysiol.* 2015, vol. 126(1), pp. 27–8

[4] Darbari D.S., Hampson J.P., Ichesco E. *et al.* 'Frequency of hospitalizations for pain and association with altered brain network connectivity in sickle cell disease'. *J. Pain.* 2015, vol. 16(11), pp. 1077–86

[5] Zidan S.H. and Shetata S.M. 'Value of multi-detector computed tomography in delineation of the normal cardiac conduction system and related anatomic structures'. *Egypt J. Radiol. Nuclear Med.* 2016, vol. 14(4), pp. 13–33

[6] Hemalatha R., Santhiyakumari N., Madheswaran M. and Suresh S. 'Segmentation of 2D and 3D images of carotid artery on unified technology learning platform'. *Procedia in Global Colloquium in Recent Advancement and Effectual Researches in Engineering, Science and Technology (RAEREST 2016).* 2016, vol. 25(1), pp. 12–19

[7] Yu J., Wang Y., Chen P. and Shen Y. 'Fetal abdominal contour extraction and measurement in ultrasound images'. *Ultrasound Med. Biol.* 2008, vol. 34(2), pp. 169–82

[8] Kasehagen B., Ellis R., Mawston G., Allen S. and Hing W. 'Assessing the reliability of ultrasound imaging to examine radial nerve excursion'. *Ultrasound Med. Biol.* 2016, vol. 42(7), pp. 1651–9

[9] Consensus Development Conference. 'Diagnosis, prophylaxis and treatment of osteoporosis'. *Amer. J. Med.* 1993, vol. 94(6), pp. 646–50

[10] Nguyen H., Stelling A., Kuramoto A., Patel C. and Keller J. 'Malignant rhabdoid tumor of the liver: findings at US, CT, and MRI, with histopathologic correlation'. *Radiol. Case Rep.* 2014, vol. 9(1), pp. 1–3

[11] Chou C.P., Peng N.J., Chang T.H. *et al.* 'Clinical roles of breast 3T MRI, FDG PET/CT, and breast ultrasound for asymptomatic women with an abnormal screening mammogram'. *J. Chin. Med. Assoc.* 2015, vol. 78(12), pp. 719–25

[12] Aswathy M.A. and Jagannath M. 'Detection of breast cancer on digital histopathology images: present status and future possibilities'. *Inform. Med. Unlocked.* 2017, vol. 8, pp. 74–9

[13] Chakraborty C. 'Performance analysis of compression techniques for chronic wound image transmission under smartphone-enabled tele-wound network'. *Int. J. E-Health Med. Commun (IJEHMC).* 2019, vol. 10(2), pp. 1–15

[14] Chakraborty C. 'Chronic wound image analysis by particle swarm optimization technique for tele-wound network'. *Wireless Pers. Commun.* 2017, vol. 96(3), pp. 3655–71

[15] Feng T., Wang J., Dong Y., Zhao J. and Li H. 'A novel data-driven cardiac gating signal extraction method for PET'. *IEEE Trans. Med. Imag.* 2019, vol. 38(2), pp. 629–37

[16] Schindler T.H., Schelbert H.R., Quercioli A. and Dilsizian V. 'Cardiac PET imaging for the detection and monitoring of coronary artery disease and microvascular health'. *JACC Cardiovasc. Imag.* 2010, vol. 3(6), pp. 623–40

[17] Di Carli M.F., Dorbala S., Meserve J., El Fakhri G., Sitek A. and Moore S.C. 'Clinical myocardial perfusion PET/CT'. *J. Nucl. Med.* 2007, vol. 48(5), pp. 783–93

[18] Tsui B.M.W., Feng T., Wang J. *et al.* 'Advances in 4D gated cardiac PET imaging for image quality improvement and cardiac motion and contractility estimation'. *Perspectives on Nuclear Medicine for Molecular Diagnosis and Integrated Therapy*. Tokyo: Springer; 2016, pp. 3–16

[19] Wang J., Fung G.S.K., Feng T. and Tsui B.M.W. 'A papillary muscle guided motion estimation method for gated cardiac imaging'. *Proc. SPIE*. 2013, vol. 8668, pp. 86682G

[20] Xu J., Wang J., Lee T-S. *et al.* 'Cardiac strain analysis using clinical myocardial perfusion PET images'. *J. Nucl. Med.* 2017, vol. 58(1), pp. 580

[21] Tang J., Wang X., Gao X., Segars W.P., Lodge M.A. and Rahmim A. 'Enhancing ejection fraction measurement through 4D respiratory motion compensation in cardiac PET imaging'. *Phys. Med. Biol.* 2017, vol. 62(11), pp. 4496

[22] Feng T., Wang J. and Tsui B.M.W. 'Dual respiratory and cardiac motion estimation in PET imaging: methods design and quantitative evaluation'. *Med. Phys.* 2018, vol. 45(4), pp. 1481–90

[23] Klein G.J., Reutter B.W., Ho M.H., Reed J.H. and Huesman R.H. 'Real-time system for respiratory-cardiac gating in positron tomography'. *IEEE Trans. Nucl. Sci.* 1998, vol. 45(4), pp. 2139–43

[24] Buther F., Dawood M., Stegger L. *et al.* 'List mode-driven cardiac and respiratory gating in PET'. *J. Nucl. Med.* 2009, vol. 50(5), pp. 674–81

[25] Thielemans K., Schleyer P., Marsden P.K. *et al.* 'Data-driven dual-gating for cardiac PET'. in *Proc. IEEE Nucl. Sci. Symp. Med. Imag. Conf. (NSS/MIC)*. 2014, pp. 1–4

[26] Herraiz J.L. 'Automatic cardiac self-gating of small-animal PET data'. *Mol. Imag. Biol.* 2016, vol. 18(1), pp. 109–16

[27] Larson A.C., White R.D., Laub G., McVeigh E.R., Li D. and Simonetti O.P. 'Self-gated cardiac cine MRI'. *Magn. Reson. Med.* 2004, vol. 51(1), pp. 93–102

[28] Lyu J., Nakarmi U., Zhang C. and Ying L. 'Highly accelerated cardiac cine parallel MRI using low-rank matrix completion and partial separability model'. *Proc. SPIE*. 2016, vol. 9857(98570C-1), pp. 98570C

[29] Lopez Picazo M., Magallon Baro A., del Rio Barquero L.M. *et al.* 'Humbert 3-D subject-specific shape and density estimation of the lumbar spine from a single anteroposterior DXA image including assessment of cortical and trabecular bone'. *IEEE Trans. Med. Imag.* 2018, vol. 37(12), pp. 2651–62

[30] Svedbom A., Hernlund E., Ivergard M. *et al.* 'Osteoporosis in the European union: a compendium of country-specific reports'. *Arch. Osteoporos.* 2013, vol. 8(1–2), pp. 137

[31] Melton L.J., Chrischilles E.A., Cooper C., Lane A.W. and Riggs B.L. 'Perspective how many women have osteoporosis?'. *J. Bone Mineral Res.* 1992, vol. 7(9), pp. 1005–10

[32] Melton L.J., Atkinson E.J., O'Connor M.K., O'Fallon W.M. and Riggs B.L., 'Bone density and fracture risk in men'. *J. Bone Mineral Res.* 1998, vol. 13(12), pp. 1915–23

[33] World Health Organization Collaborating Centre for Metabolic Bone Diseases (UK). *Assessment of osteoporosis at the primary healthcare level*. University of Sheffield. 2008

[34] Kanis J.A., Melton L.J., Christiansen C., Johnston C.C. and Khaltaev N. 'The diagnosis of osteoporosis'. *J. Bone Mineral Res.* 1994, vol. 9(8), pp. 1137–41

[35] International Society for Clinical Densitometry. Official Positions—Adult [Online]. Middletown, CT, USA. 2015. Available from https://www.iscd.org/official-positions/2015-iscd-official-positions-adult/ [Accessed June 2015]

[36] Genant H.K., Wu C.Y., Van Kuijk C. and Nevitt M.C. 'Vertebral fracture assessment using a semiquantitative technique'. *J. Bone Mineral Res.* 1993, vol. 8(9), pp. 1137–48

[37] NIH Consensus Development Panel on Osteoporosis Prevention, 'Osteoporosis: prevention, diagnosis, and therapy'. *JAMA*. 2001, vol. 285(6), pp. 785–95

[38] Melton L.J., III, Atkinson E.J., O'Fallon W.M., Wahner H.W. and Riggs B.L. 'Long-term fracture prediction by bone mineral assessed at different skeletal site'. *J. Bone Mineral Res.* 1993, vol. 8(10), pp. 1227–33

[39] Siris E.S., Chen Y.T., Abbott T.A. *et al.* 'Bone mineral density thresholds for pharmacological intervention to prevent fractures'. *Arch. Intern. Med.* 2004, vol. 164(10), pp. 1108–12

[40] Silva B.C., Broy S.B., Boutroy S., Schousboe J.T., Shepherd J.A. and Leslie W.D. 'Fracture risk prediction by non-BMD DXA measures: The 2015 ISCD official positions part 2: Trabecular bone score'. *J. Clin. Densitom.* 2015, vol. 18(3), pp. 309–30

[41] Bauer J.S. and Link T.M. 'Advances in osteoporosis imaging'. *Eur. J. Radiol.* 2009, vol. 71(3), pp. 440–9

[42] Bala Y., Zebaze R. and Seeman E. 'Role of cortical bone in bone fragility'. *Curr. Opin. Rheumatol.* 2015, vol. 27(4), pp. 406–13

[43] Engelke K., Adams J.E., Armbrecht G. *et al.* 'Clinical use of quantitative computed tomography and peripheral quantitative computed tomography in the management of osteoporosis in adults: The 2007 ISCD official positions'. *J. Clin. Densitom.* 2008, vol. 11(1), pp. 123–62

[44] Rachner T.D., Khosla S. and Hofbauer L.C. 'Osteoporosis: now and the future'. *Lancet*. 2011, vol. 377(9773), pp. 1276–87

[45] Prevrhal S., Fox J.C., Shepherd J.A. and Genant H.K. 'Accuracy of CT-based thickness measurement of thin structures: modeling of limited spatial resolution in all three dimensions'. *Med. Phys.* 2003, vol. 30, pp. 1–8

[46] Cootes T.F. 'An Introduction to Active Shape Models'. in Baldock R. (ed.). *Introduction to Image Processing and Analysis*. London, U.K.: Oxford Univ. Press. 2000, pp. 223–48

[47] Cootes T.F., Edwards G.J. and Taylor C.J. 'Active appearance models'. *IEEE Trans. Pattern Anal. Mach. Intell.* 1993, vol. 23(6), pp. 681–5

[48] Fleute M. and Lavallee S. 'Nonrigid 3-D/2-D registration of images using statistical models'. in *Proc. Med. Image Comput. Comput. Assist. Intervent (MICCAI)*. 1999, vol. 1679(1), pp. 38–147

[49] Zheng G., Gollmer S., Schumann S., Dong X., Feilkas T. and Ballester M.A.G. 'A 2D/3D correspondence building method for reconstruction of a patient-specific 3D bone surface model using point distribution models and calibrated X-ray images'. *Med. Image Anal.* 2009, vol. 13(6), pp. 883–99

[50] Baka N., Kaptein B.L., de Bruijne M., van Walsum T., Giphart J.E., Niessen W.J. *et al.* '2D-3D shape reconstruction of the distal femur from stereo X-ray imaging using statistical shape models'. *Med. Image Anal.* 2011, vol. 15(6), pp. 840–50

[51] Benameur S., Mignotte M., Parent S., Labelle H., Skalli W. and de Guise J. '3D/2D registration and segmentation of scoliotic vertebrae using statistical models'. *Comput. Med. Imag. Graph.* 2003, vol. 27(5), pp. 321–37

[52] Boisvert J., Cheriet F., Pennec X., Labelle H. and Ayache N. 'Articulated spine models for 3-D reconstruction from partial radiographic data'. *IEEE Trans. Biomed. Eng.* 2008, vol. 55(11), pp. 2565–74

[53] Querol L.B., Buchler P., Rueckert D., Nolte L.P. and Ballester M.A.G. 'Statistical finite element model for bone shape and biomechanical properties'. in *Proc. Med. Image Comput. Comput. Assist. Intervent (MICCAI)*. 2006, vol. 4190(1), pp. 405–11

[54] Ahmad O., Ramamurthi K., Wilson K.E., Engelke K., Prince R.L. and Taylor R.H. 'Volumetric DXA (VXA): A new method to extract 3D information from multiple in vivo DXA images'. *J. Bone Mineral Res.* 2010, vol. 25(12), pp. 2744–51

[55] Whitmarsh T., Humbert L., De Craene M., Del Río Barquero L.M. and Frangi A.F. 'Reconstructing the 3D shape and bone mineral density distribution of the proximal femur from dual-energy X-ray absorptiometry'. *IEEE Trans. Med. Imag.* 2011, vol. 30(12), pp. 101–14

[56] Hemalatha J., Kavitha Devi M.K. and Geetha S. 'Performance Analysis of Image Denoising with Curvelet Transform in Detecting the Stego Noise'. in Saini. H.S. (ed.). *Innovations in Computer Science and Engineering*. Singapore: Springer. 2019, vol. 32, pp. 445–53

[57] Hangartner T.N. 'Thresholding technique for accurate analysis of density and geometry in QCT, pQCT and μCT images'. *J. Musculoskelet. Neuronal. Interact.* 2007, vol. 7(1), pp. 9–16

[58] Humbert L., Martelli Y., Fonolla R. *et al.* '3D-DXA: Assessing the femoral shape, the trabecular macrostructure and the cortex in 3D from DXA images'. *IEEE Trans. Med. Imag.* 2017, vol. 36(1), pp. 27–39

[59] Humbert L., Marangalou J.H., Del Rio Barquero L.M., Van Lenthe G.H. and Van Rietbergen B. 'Technical note: Cortical thickness and density estimation from clinical CT using a prior thickness-density relationship'. *Med. Phys.* 2016, vol. 43(4), pp. 1945–54

[60] Chen H., Zhou X., Fujita H., Onozuka M. and Kubo K.Y. 'Age related changes in trabecular and cortical bone microstructure'. *Int. J. Endocrinol.* 2013, vol. 2013(213234), pp. 213–34

[61] Ritzel H., Amling M., Posl M., Hahn M. and Delling G. 'The thickness of human vertebral cortical bone and its changes in aging and osteoporosis: A histomorphometric analysis of the complete spinal column from thirty-seven autopsy specimens'. *J. Bone Mineral Res.* 1997, vol. 12(1), pp. 89–95

[62] Whitmarsh T., Humbert L., Del Rio Barquero L.M., Di Gregorio S. and Frangi A.F. '3D reconstruction of the lumbar vertebrae from anteroposterior and lateral dual-energy X-ray absorptiometry'. *Med. Image Anal.* 2013, vol. 17(4), pp. 475–87

[63] Vaananen S.P., Grassi L., Flivik G., Jurvelin J.S. and Isaksson H. 'Generation of 3D shape, density, cortical thickness and finite element mesh of proximal femur from a DXA image'. *Med. Image Anal.* 2015, vol. 24(1), pp. 125–34

[64] Chen L., Hoey J., Nugent C.D., Cook D.J. and Yu Z. 'Sensor based activity recognition'. *IEEE Transactions on Systems, Man, and Cybernetics.* 2012, vol. 42(6), pp. 790–808

[65] Gacek A. and Pedrycz W. *ECG Signal Processing, Classification and Interpretation: A Comprehensive Framework of Computational Intelligence.* London: Springer; 2012

[66] Kolbitsch C., Ahlman M.A., Davies-Venn C. *et al.* 'Cardiac and respiratory motion correction for simultaneous cardiac PET/MR'. *J. Nucl. Med.* 2017, vol. 58(5), pp. 846–52

[67] Stolojescu C., Railean I., Moga S. and Isar A. 'Comparison of wavelet families with application to WiMAXtraf_c forecasting'. in *Proc. 12th Int. Conf. Optim. Electr. Electron. Equip.* 2010, pp. 932–7

[68] Hemalatha J., Kavitha Devi M.K. and Geetha S. 'Improving image steganalyser performance through curvelet transform denoising'. *Cluster Comput.* 2019, vol. 22(5), pp. 11821–11839

[69] Venkatesan C., Karthigaikumar P., Paul A., Satheeskumaran S. and Kumar R. 'ECG signal preprocessing and SVM classifier-based abnormality detection in remote healthcare applications. Special section on soft computing techniques for image analysis in the medical industry current trends, challenges and solutions'. *IEEE Access.* 2018, vol. 6, pp. 9767–73

[70] Stolojescu B., Railean I., Moga S. and Isar A. 'Comparison of wavelet families with application to WiMAX traffic forecasting'. in *Proc. 12th Int. Conf. Optim. Electr. Electron. Equip.* 2010, pp. 932–7

[71] Hashim A., Ooi C.Y., Bakhteri R. and Hau Y.W. 'Comparative study of electrocardiogram QRS complex detection algorithm on Field Programmable Gate Array platform'. *Proceedings of IEEE Conf. Biomed. Eng. Sci. (IECBES)*, Dec. 2014, pp. 241–6

[72] Dalal B., Kun Z. and Ahmad S.M. 'Classification of breast cancer based on histology images using convolutional neural networks'. *IEEE Access*. 2018, vol. 6(1), pp. 24680–93
[73] Spanhol F.A., Oliveira L.S., Petitjean C. and Heutte L. 'A dataset for breast cancer histopathological image classification'. *IEEE Trans. Biomed. Eng.* 2016, vol. 63(7), pp. 1455–62
[74] Jia Y., Shelhamer E., Donahue J. *et al.* 'Caffe: Convolutional architecture for fast feature embedding'. in *Proc. 22nd ACM Int. Conf. Multimedia*. 2014, pp. 675–8

Chapter 5

A real-time ECG-processing platform for telemedicine applications

Sandeep Raj[1]

In day-to-day life, the usage of portable and smart monitoring devices performing diagnosis has shown explosive growth in personalized healthcare technology. These devices facilitate increased quality of life, reduced costs, enrich the user's experience, remote monitoring and automatic analysis of long-term biomedical signals such as electrocardiogram (ECG). The advancement in the domain of clinical and telemedicine applications highly demand the automatic analysis of ECG. The necessity of the ECG devices in personalized healthcare is increased due to the fact that cardiovascular diseases are leading causes of mortalities worldwide and will remain 2030 as reported by the World Health Organization (WHO). This chapter focuses on the development of an efficient method for automated classification of ECG which combines the feature extraction and classification algorithms along with its implementation on a microcontroller test platform. The cosine Stockwell transform (CST) is used for extracting the significant amount of information from the corresponding heartbeats. These features resemble each heartbeat and are further classified using particle swarm optimization (PSO) optimized support vector machines (SVMs) into subsequent classes. The proposed method is implemented on a 32-bit advanced RISC machine (ARM) microcontroller platform. The platform is validated by generating real-time ECG signals using benchmark MIT-BIH data and evaluated under category-oriented assessment scheme. The platform is interfaced with a Wi-Fi module that sends the information of classified outputs to a remote microcontroller-based platform. Once an abnormality is detected by the platform, a pop-up message is viewed on the displaying module interfaced with the platform behaving as alarm. The test platform has reported an accuracy of 95.8% in the category-oriented assessment scheme. Such kind of implementation provides an enriched platform capable of performing real-time diagnosis and can be utilized in hospitals for telemedicine applications.

[1]Electronics and Communication Engineering, Indian Institute of Information Technology Bhagalpur, Bhagalpur, India

5.1 Introduction

The study of electrical activities of vital organs has increased in medicine to provide accurate diagnosis or therapy. These electrical characteristics exhibit necessary information on physiological behavior of a human body [1]. The measurement of physiological signals allowed a better understanding of the electrical activities of certain organs, for example the heart by the electrocardiogram (ECG). The heartbeats or ECG signals are graphical representation that reflects the electrical activities occurring within the human heart [1–3]. The human heart undergoes three processes namely atrial depolarization reflecting the P-wave, ventricular depolarization reflecting the QRS wave and ventricular repolarization reflecting the T-wave [1]. All this wave represents one cardiac cycle or heartbeat or ECG [1–3]. These waves convey significant amount of diagnostic information about the functioning of heart. Each wave of an ECG signal has fixed characteristics either in time, amplitude and shape or morphology. Any variation in any of these parameters leads to the generation of an abnormality or arrhythmia within the heart [1–4]. Often, these arrhythmias are not always dangerous but may result in pose a serious threat or cardiac death in near future [1–4]. There are various types of arrhythmia that can occur inside in heart that must be detected on time so that a person can lead a healthy lifestyle. Each class of arrhythmia corresponds to a definite appearance or morphology depends upon which they are being identified among various categories [1–4]. The recognition arrhythmias can be divided into two major classes, i.e., morphological arrhythmia and rhythmic arrhythmias. The morphological arrhythmia is based on the morphology of individual irregular heartbeat [1–4]. While the other rhythmic arrhythmias are a set of irregular heartbeats with varying heart rate. The variation in frequency or morphology or any other changes like absence of waves shall be identified by examining the ECG [1–4]. The analysis of long-term ECG by an expert is a tedious job and thus requires an automated solution for diagnosis. In this work, the arrhythmia classification is performed depending on their morphology.

Several kinds of devices are available in the market targeting mass market that performs different functions towards heartbeat diagnosis. Many researchers have also reported and studied several methods on hardware platforms [1–20]. Some of the devices such as Holter monitors store the data only for a maximum of two day's period [3–6]. The other class of devices performs the storage of data and sends it to the nearest hospital where the data is analyzed in off-line diagnosis. As such, these devices perform remote real-time diagnosis of heartbeats [3–6]. The last class of ECG devices performs some local and intermediate levels of diagnosis at the place of patients based on the heart rate of the subject. Among all the devices available in today's market, none of them deliver a complete solution for diagnosis of ECG [3–6]. All of these devices available bear certain limitations which provide significant room for improvement to be adopted by the subjects. As such, the developed device must be capable of providing signal-by-signal analysis (i.e., individual heartbeat analysis) at the place of data acquisition such that the subject must be aware of their cardiac condition failing may lead to cardiac failure. Such devices can be developed by integrating efficient signal processing and machine learning methods that can automatically [3–6] classify the heartbeats. Such methods should be highly efficient such that they can be prototyped on suitable hardware platforms to perform automated real-time diagnosis of ECG signals.

The domain of ECG signal analysis or arrhythmia classification has been thoroughly studied and experimented with by many researchers across the world. These studies have been performed on different publicly available standard databases while some of them have been validated on the data acquired directly from the subjects. Several methods or techniques [21–32] have been developed serving different tasks. More often, four steps [21–32] are integrated together to perform automated diagnosis of heartbeat. They include the filtering, R-peak detection, feature extraction and classification stages. Various robust filters have been designed to eliminate the noises associated with the heartbeats. However, the main focus of the current study is based on signal processing and machine learning algorithms. The feature extraction step extracts the information and represents the heartbeats while they are being categorized into different classes using the machine learning tools. Several feature extraction algorithms have been reported in literature. Among them include the statistical features [33], time domain [25–27], time-frequency domain [31], spectral domain [28] and various others. In particular, Raj *et al.* [33] used principal component analysis (PCA) and independent component analysis (ICA) to extract the ECG features in lower dimensional space. Raj *et al.* employed the discrete wavelet transform [6] and discrete orthogonal Stockwell transform [23] to extract the time-frequency features from the corresponding ECG signals. In Sharma *et al.* [32] extracted the intrinsic mode functions (IMFs) by implementing the empirical mode decomposition technique and also estimated the instantaneous frequency and phase information of the heartbeats. In [25–27], the authors extracted the time-domain information from different heartbeats intervals, while authors in [28] used the Hermite polynomials for classification. It is to note that each of these techniques has certain pros and cons based on their performance and complexity. These extracted features are applied as input to the classifier mechanisms such as artificial neural networks (ANNs) [6,33], k-NN [34], SVMs [34,35], hidden Markov models (HMMs) [36], deep learning methods [37,38] and many more. These models are trained and tested to determine their classification performance. Among all the classifier mechanisms, the deep learning models are believed as most efficient one, however, the current study has not focused due to higher computational involved in implementing these algorithms on hardware platforms. As such, they will require more memory, high speed processors for their implementation to provide real-time output. Further, the output must be stored and sent to the nearest hospital such that proper medical care can be provided upon any condition for telemedicine applications.

This study focuses on the development of an efficient method by combining the feature extraction and classification methods and their implementation on the microcontroller test platform. The cosine Stockwell transform (CST) is used for extracting the significant amount of information from the corresponding ECG signals in lower dimensions. These features represent each of the ECG signals and are further identified using PSO-tuned twin support vector machines (TSVMs) into their different categories. The proposed method is implemented on the 32-bit advanced RISC machine (ARM) platform. The platform is validated on the benchmark MIT-BIH arrhythmia data [39] generated in real time and evaluated under category-oriented analysis scheme. The platform is integrated with the Wi-Fi module which sends the information of classified outputs to a remote platform. Once an abnormality is detected by the platform, a pop-up message can be viewed on the displaying module interfaced with the platform which behaves as an alarm. The platform reported an accuracy of 95.8% in the category-oriented assessment scheme. Such type of prototyping of proposed method on hardware platforms deliver an assistive diagnostic solution to the users and should be employed in hospitals for cardiovascular disease diagnosis by providing an enriched platform capable of performing real-time diagnosis for telemedicine applications.

The rest of the chapter is organized as follows: the existing methods are summarized in Section 5.2 while the proposed methodology involved in the automated diagnosis of heartbeat is explained in Section 5.3. Section 5.4 presents the hardware implementation of the proposed method and the development of the experimental hardware setup. The results and discussion of the chapter are presented in Section 5.5 and lastly, Section 5.6 concludes the chapter.

5.2 Methods

This section deals with a brief description of existing feature extraction, learning algorithms and optimization techniques used in this study.

5.2.1 Stockwell transform (ST)

The Stockwell transform (ST) [3,30,40] maps a 1-D time domain non-stationary signal into two-dimensional time-frequency (TF) domain [3,30,40]. The ST can be considered as an extension of wavelet transform (WT) or short time Fourier transform (STFT) with a variable window. The ST is a linear transform that fills the gap between the Fourier transform (FT) and WT. The ST [3,30,40] of an input signal $a(t)$ is defined as:

$$S_{(\tau,f)} = \int_{-\infty}^{\infty} a(t)h(t-\tau,f)e^{-2i\pi ft}dt \tag{5.1}$$

where the Gaussian modulation function $h(\tau; f)$ is given by:

$$h(\tau,f) = \frac{|f|}{\sqrt{2\pi}}e^{-(\tau^2/2\sigma^2)} \tag{5.2}$$

Here, t, f and τ represent the time, frequency and the localized Gaussian window, respectively. And, $\tau = 1/|f|$ which is frequency dependent. Therefore, the ST can be rewritten as:

$$S_{(\tau,f)} = \int_{-\infty}^{\infty} a(t)\frac{|f|}{2\pi}e^{-\frac{(t-\tau)^2 f^2}{2}}e^{-2i\pi ft}dt \tag{5.3}$$

The ST provides the frequency dependent resolution using a scalable localizing Gaussian window. However, the ST is redundant and involves higher computational complexity. It generates N2 coefficients for an N-point input signal. An efficient version of ST is reported which is known as discrete orthogonal Stockwell transform (DOST) which generates N-size coefficients for an N-size signal by using an orthogonal transformation. The DOST representation can be defined as the inner product between a time series $h[kT]$ and the basis functions having parameters such as center frequency (υ), frequency resolution (β) and time localization parameter (τ).

5.2.2 Twin support vector machines (TSVMs)

A new machine learning tool, i.e., twin support vector machine (TWSVM) [41,42] is employed for classifying input data. In the beginning, it was used to solve binary classification problems. It uses two non-parallels plane binary classifiers. It generates two nonparallel planes [41,42] around which the data points of the corresponding class get clustered. Each plane is closer to one of the two classes and is as far as possible from the other. In TWSVMs [41,42], all data points are distributed in the sense that the objective function corresponds to a particular class and the constraints are determined by patterns of the other class [41,42]. The algorithm finds two hyperplanes by solving a pair of quadratic programming problems (QPPs) similar to SVM's single QPP, one for each class. The classification of the new point is done according to which hyperplane out of two; a given point is closest to. TWSVM [41,42] is approximately four times faster than the traditional SVM. Figure 5.1 shows a hyperplane separating the two classes of data problems in the

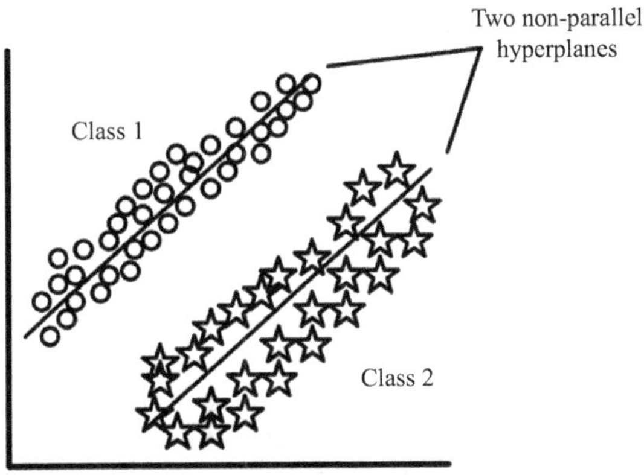

Figure 5.1 Hyperplane separating the two classes in the TSVM classification scheme

higher dimensional space. In k-dimensional real space R_k, the matrix X_1 represents the positive class data samples while X_2 represents the negative class data samples. Further, a pair of the non-parallel hyperplanes [41,42] in the real space can be represented as:

$$x^T w_1 + b_1 = 0 \quad \text{and} \quad x^T w_1 + b_2 = 0$$

Here, symbols b_1 and b_2 represent the bias terms of the hyperplane whereas w_1 and w_2 indicate vectors normalized to hyperplane. The TWSVM developed for performing linear and non-linear classification is reported in [41,42]. Here, the training of pth class is performed with qth class. In the training phase, the positive class is considered as the data samples of pth class whereas negative class is considered as the data samples for the qth class and vice versa [41,42]. This work employs the twin SVM classifier model as such it has computational complexity about four times lesser and achieves comparable accuracy than standard SVM [41,42]. Therefore, the TSVM method is chosen as an alternative for analysis of heartbeats.

5.2.3 Particle swarm optimization (PSO)

PSO [43] technique is inspired by the social behavior of birds and fish, to attend the minimum of quadratic programming problem (QPP). Many particles (variable) participate in finding the global minimum value for QPP by communicating with each other. The position vector and velocity vector are two components associated with each particle. After every iteration, ith particle share its personal minimum value and updates the global minimum if this value is less than the existing global minimum. All particles update its velocity vector using its previous velocity vector (inertia term), the personal minimum value (cognitive component), the global minimum value (social component), and user-defined coefficients. Once the velocity vector updated, each particle computes new position vector and examines its new position for the global minimum. This process repeats until all particles achieve the global minimum. PSO is comparatively faster than other optimization techniques. The steps involved in the PSO algorithm are depicted in the flow chart as in Figure 5.2.

5.3 Proposed method

The proposed method comprises a combination of four significant stages such as preprocessing, R-peak detection, feature extraction, and classification stages as shown in Figure 5.3 to classify different categories of heartbeats. Initially, the raw ECG signals extracted from the human body are preprocessed to improve their quality by removing various noises associated with them during data acquisition. The preprocessing step is followed by the feature extraction approach where significant characteristics from the heartbeats are extracted to represent them into

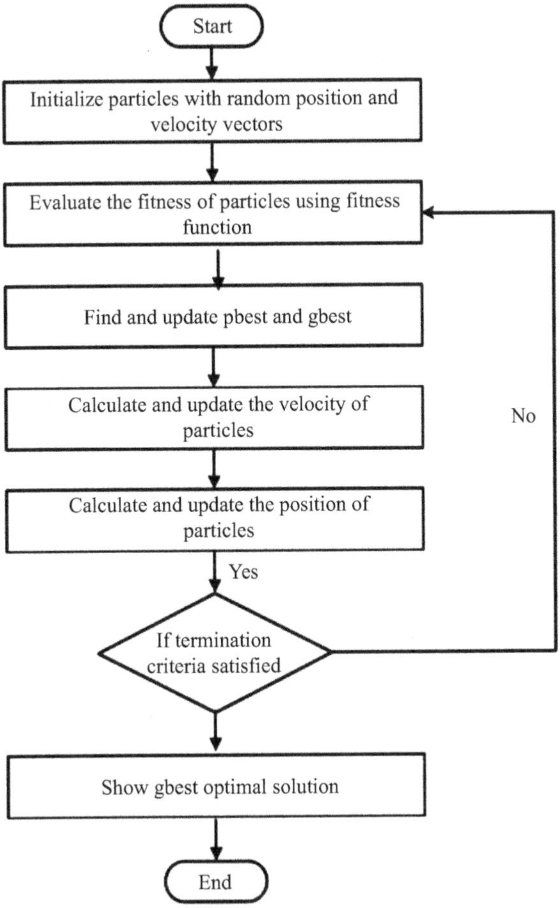

Figure 5.2 Flowchart of the PSO technique

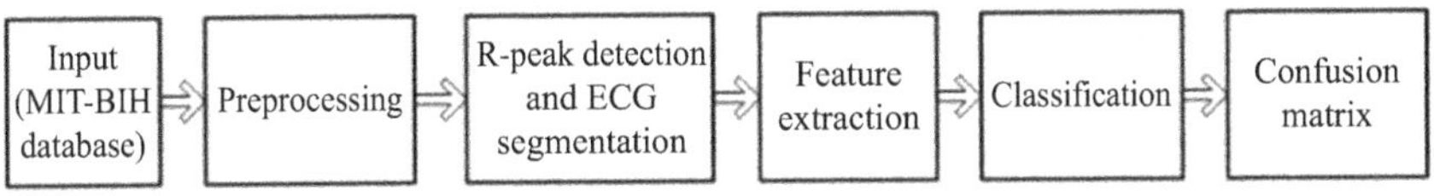

Figure 5.3 Steps involved in the automated classification of cardiac arrhythmias

lower dimensions. Finally, these features are applied to learning algorithms for classification.

5.3.1 MIT-BIH data

In this study, a well-known database, i.e., Massachusetts Institute of Technology-Beth Israel Hospital (MIT-BIH) arrhythmia data [39]. The database contains the

Table 5.1 Training and testing datasets

ECG class	Annotation	Total	Training	Testing
Normal (NOR)	N	75017	12000	63017
Right bundle branch block (RBBB)	R	7255	2600	4655
Unclassifiable beat (UN)	Q	33	16	17
Paced beat (PACE)	P	7024	2500	4524
Ventricular flutter (VF)	!	472	200	272
Nodal (junctional) escape beat	j	229	100	129
Atrial premature contraction (APC)	A	2546	900	1646
Atrial escape beat (AE)	e	16	8	8
The fusion of ventricular and normal beat (VFN)	F	802	400	402
Preventricular contraction (PVC)	V	7129	2500	4629
The fusion of paced and normal beat (FPN)	f	982	450	532
Left bundle branch block (LBBB)	L	8072	2800	5272
Ventricular escape beat (VE)	E	106	50	56
Nodal (junctional) premature beat (NP)	J	83	40	43
Aberrated atrial premature beat (AP)	a	150	70	80
Blocked atrial premature beat (BAP)	x	193	90	103
Total		110109	24724	85385

records of 47 subjects comprising 48 files or records having a total of 110109 heartbeat labels [39]. The data contain the annotations of the signals which is finally used to formulate the results in the supervised learning classifier mechanism. A total of 16 classes of heartbeats including normal is available in the database for experimental purpose. The sampling rate of the database is 360 Hz while the signals are digitized using an ADC having 11-bit resolution within 10 mV range [39]. For performing the experiments all the records comprising different classes of signals are used which is passed through a band-pass filter with a cut-off frequency of 0.1 to 100 Hz [39]. To determine the training and testing datasets, a certain fraction from all the 16 categories of the heartbeats are selected [39]. Table 5.1 summarizes the total number of training and testing signals for all the 16 classes used for performing the experiments. A few different classes of ECG signals are depicted in Figure 5.4.

5.3.2 Preprocessing

The quality of heartbeats greatly affects the performance of any classification system. The noises associated with a heartbeat may contain baseline drift, power line interference, muscle artifacts, contact noise, electrosurgical noise and quantization noise. It is necessary to eliminate these different kinds of noises failing which can lead to false alarms. Further, this step improves the signal-to-noise (SNR) ratio which helps in the accurate detection of the fiducial points within the heartbeats. In order to remove noise, different filters are employed to remove different kinds of noises.

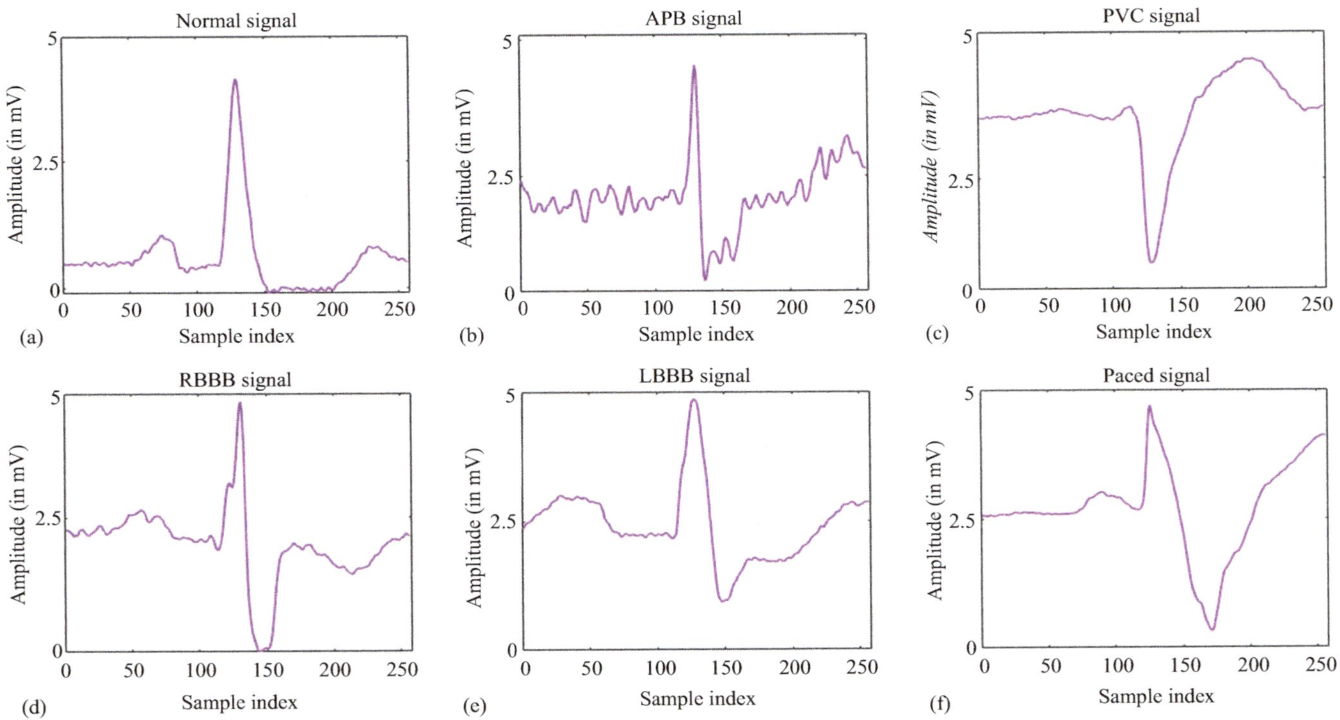

Figure 5.4 Few types of ECG signals

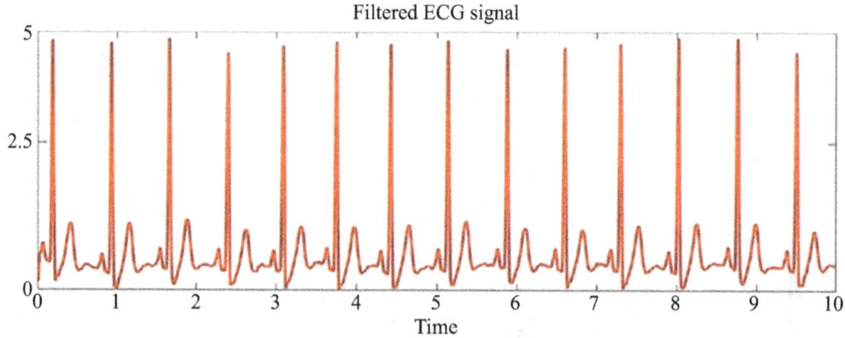

Figure 5.5 Preprocessed ECG signal

A set of two median filters are employed for eliminating the baseline wander [3] within the heartbeats. A 200 ms primary median filter is used to demarcate the QRS wave [3] and P-wave. Whereas, a 600 ms [3] secondary filter demarcates the T-wave within the heartbeat. Finally, the baseline wander is removed by subtracting the output of the secondary filter from the raw ECG data [3]. Then after, the power-line interference and high-frequency noises are removed from the heartbeats by passing the baseline corrected heartbeat through a 12-tap low-pass filter [3]. This filter has a cut-off frequency of 35 Hz with equal ripples in the pass and stops bands. The output of this filter is considered as preprocessed ECG signal which is passed through the R-peak detection and segmentation steps for automatic classification of ECG signals [3]. Figure 5.5 shows the filtered ECG output from record #100 of the database.

5.3.3 R-wave localization and ECG segmentation

In this study, the classification of different types of ECG signals is based on the localization of R-waves of the ECG signals. Prior to segment the ECG signals before feature extraction, it is necessary to determine the locations of R-waves. A lot of research works have been reported in literature for detecting the R-peaks [44] among which this study employs a well-established Pan-Tompkins (PT) algorithm [44]. It is chosen due to its proven lower computational burden, higher performance under noisy environments. The detected R-waves are verified with the positions of annotations of R-peaks provided in the database. Figure 5.6 shows the R-peak detection within the heartbeats of record #100 of the database.

In this study, the segmentation step is a bit different from almost all the works reported. They use a rectangular window of constant time or samples. A new segmentation step is proposed as proportional segmentation in which 35% of anterior RR interval from the left side of the R point and 65% of posterior RR interval after R point is taken as a heartbeat. This ensures that all the information of the ECG from starting P-wave and ending T-wave is contained and no information regarding any wave is lost.

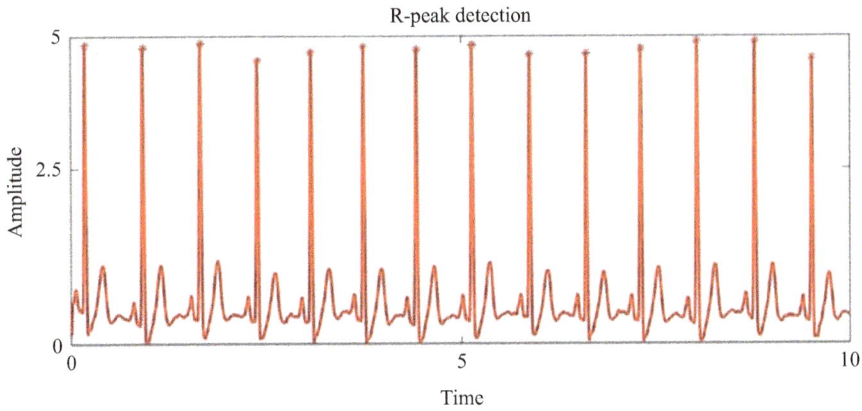

Figure 5.6 R-wave localization within ECG signals

5.3.4 Feature extraction

The feature extraction from an input signal plays a significant role in any classification system. These features represent the characteristics of an input ECG signal. In literature several types of features are extracted from the corresponding ECG signals, such as fiducial points within ECG signals, wavelet features [6], RR interval features [25–27] and high order accumulants [19]. Many of the works concatenated different features together which results in achieving higher accuracy. Rather, concatenation of different types of features results in increased computational complexity of the classification system. This study employs an efficient method, i.e., CST [3] for extracting the features from the corresponding heartbeats. The dataflow of the CST is depicted in Figure 5.7.

In this method, the discrete cosine transform (DCT) kernel [3] is replaced with the conventional fast Fourier transform (FFT) kernel as in DOST to analyze the ECG signal in time-frequency space. The cosine kernel has the advantage of the lack of discontinuities. The application of DCT enables an input signal to attain its original shape while truncating more coefficients. Further, the cosine kernel does not contain negative frequency and computes real coefficients only, thus reducing the overall complexity of the method. As a result, the most significant coefficients are present in the lower frequency components and the energy is gathered together.

In this chapter, the CST is used for capturing the time-frequency characteristics of the heartbeats to detect potential arrhythmias. The output components obtained bears no symmetry in this method as opposition to the coefficients extracted from the classical DOST method. While these CST components are uniformly distributed in the frequency band which is due to the presence of positive frequencies only. The step-by-step procedure employed in the implementation of CST is summarized below [3].

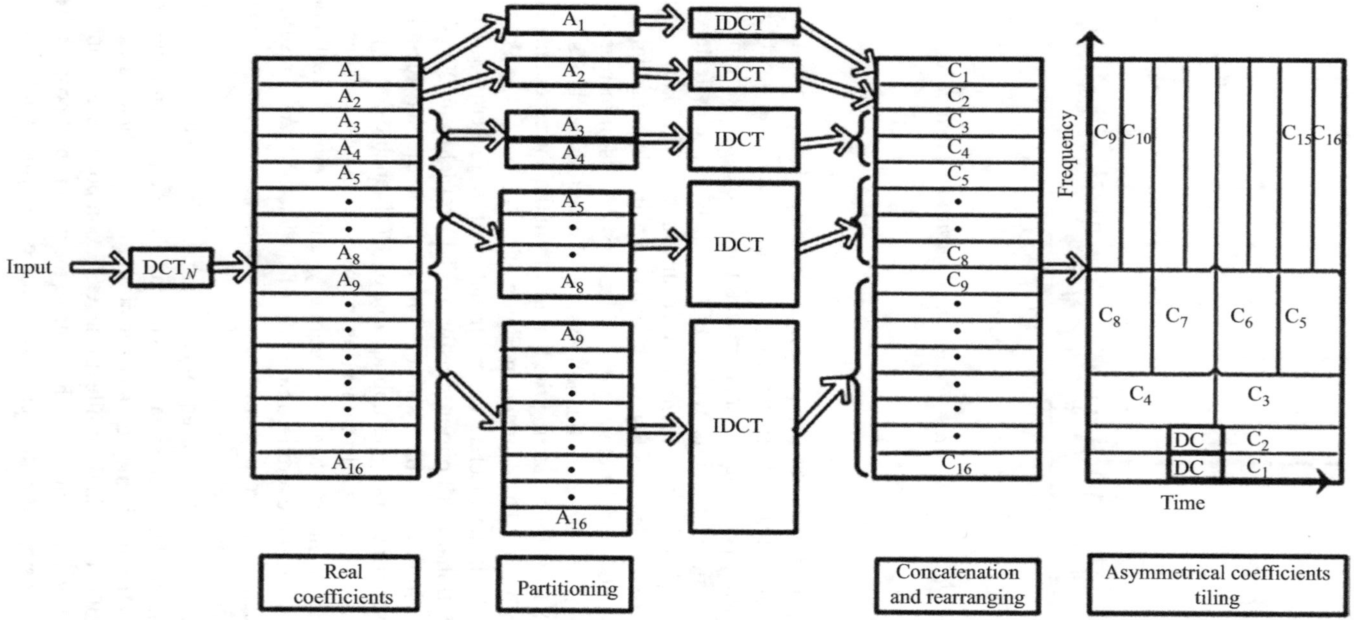

Figure 5.7 Dataflow of the proposed feature extraction approach

(a) Step 1: Apply an N-point DCT: It computes the cosine spectrum of the N-size input heartbeat.
(b) Step 2: The output of first step $z[n + p]$ is multiplied with a rectangular window $[-\beta/2, \beta/2 - 1](n)$.
(c) Step 3: For every central frequency a β-point inverse DCT is applied to $V[p]$ $z[n + p]$ which ensures that the decomposition to be orthogonal.
(d) Step 4: A β-point DCT is applied to $s[q, p]$ with respect to time index q to obtain the windowed cosine spectrum $V[p]z[n + p]$ for each central frequency $m = 0, 1, 3, \ldots, 3\beta/2, \ldots$.

Figure 5.8 depicts the output of Normal, PVC and RBBB signals when passed through the CST-based feature extraction stage.

5.3.5 CST feature recognition using TSVMs

In this work, a TSVM classifier model [41,42] is used for recognition of extracted CST features representing each heartbeat into 16 classes. Initially, the TSVMs were designed for a binary class recognition problem. In this study, the multi-class classification problem is addressed by using the one-against-one (OAO) model [41,42] is studied. Under this scheme, the selection of the kernel argument and the cost function parameters play a significant role in reporting higher classification performance. The use of kernel functions enables non-linear classification of features. In other words, the use of kernel helps in achieving better classification performance on non-linear data or overlapping features in the higher dimensional space. As such, all the kernels such as linear, radial basis function (RBF), and polynomial functions are used to analyze the accuracy. A summary of the classification accuracy of these different kernel functions is reported in Table 5.2. From Table 5.2, it can be concluded that the RBF kernel reported the highest performance in terms of accuracy among all. It is noted that the training and testing datasets assumed to measure the performance is same as presented in Table 5.2. Therefore, the classification performance of RBF kernel is only reported and studied in detail.

Further, the kernel (γ) and cost function (C) parameters are optimized using PSO technique to enhance the performance of the classifier model from the results reported in Table 5.2. The steps involved in the implementation of the PSO algorithm is summarized in [31]. The PSO technique aims to determine the optimal classifier model by evaluating the fitness of each particle for a specific set of particles at every iteration. Since the current study involves the classification of 16 classes of ECG signals using OAO-SVM model, 16 binary SVM classifiers are optimized with the PSO technique. This study uses the simple SV count technique as a fitness criterion in the PSO optimization network to restrict the error bound condition resulting in the unbiased performance of the recognition model. Using the PSO technique in the training phase of the classifier, the classifier parameters, i.e., C and γ, are gradually optimized by employing the PSO technique. The parameters are selected based on m-fold cross-validation strategy [45] in the training phase. In order to avoid biasing the classifier model, 10-fold cross-validation is

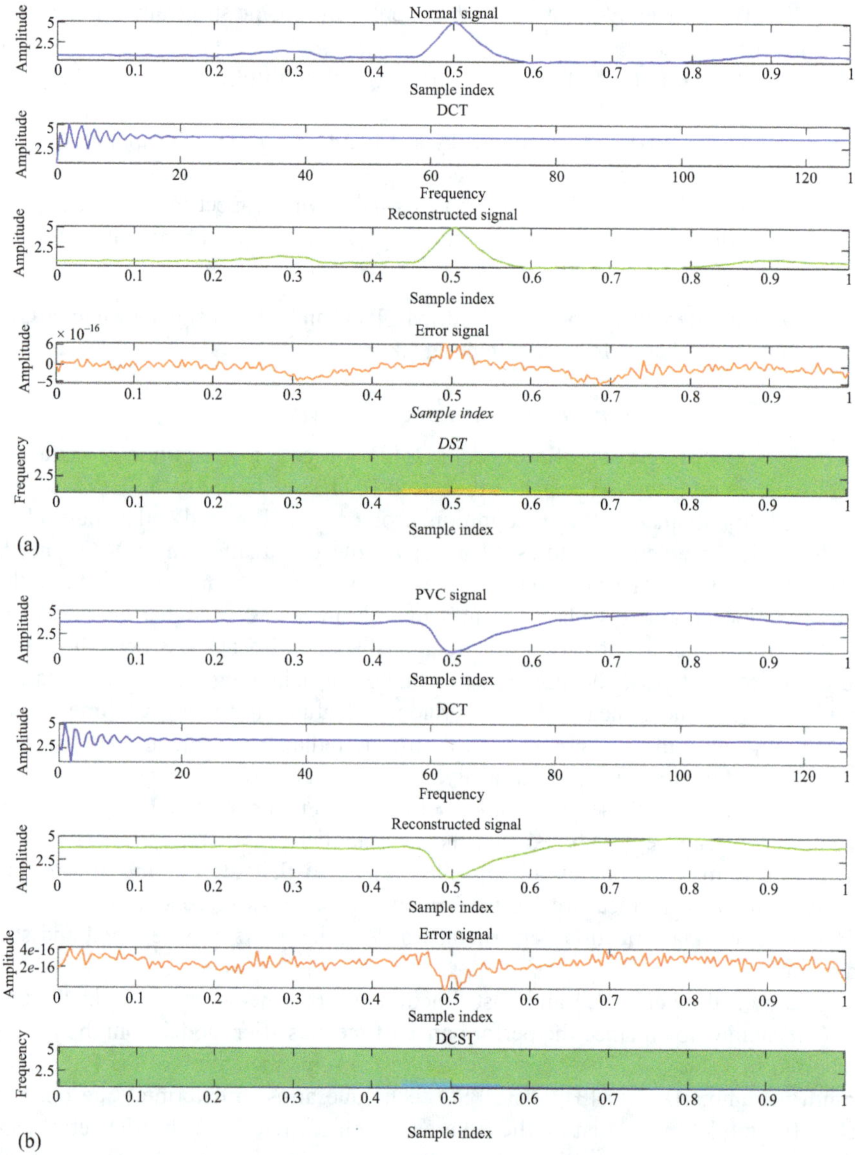

Figure 5.8 CST decomposition of different classes of ECG signals

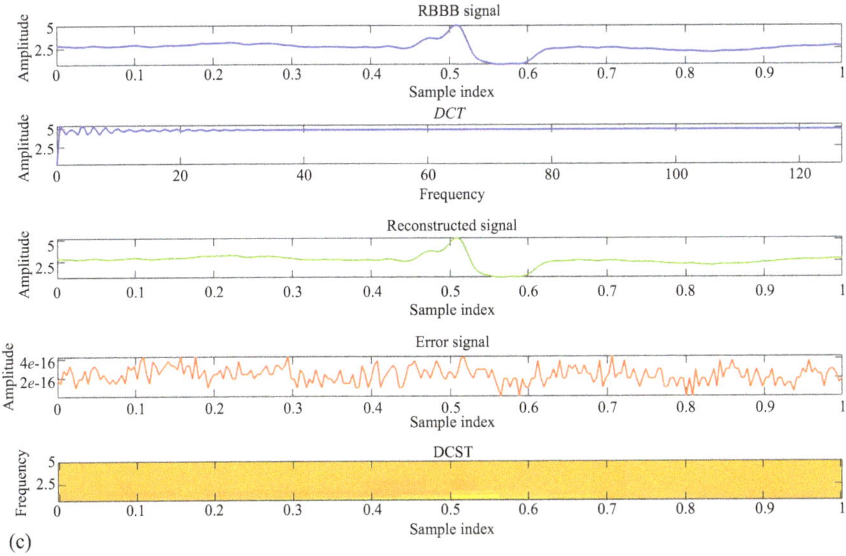

Figure 5.8 (Continued)

Table 5.2 Accuracy obtained for different kernel functions

Kernels	Training accuracy (%)	Testing accuracy (%)
Linear	97.8	90.23
Radial basis function $K(x,x') = \exp\left(-\frac{\lVert x-x'\rVert^2}{2\sigma^2}\right)$	99.7	93.89
Multi-layer perceptron $K(x,x') = \tanh(\rho\langle x,x'\rangle + e)$	99.2	92.91
Polynomial $K(x,x') = \langle x,x'\rangle^d$	99.5	93.47

performed on the entire data set, in order to estimate the best learning parameter values of C and γ which results in best classification performance of the developed model. Figure 5.9 shows the distribution of the normal and LBBB classes of features in the higher dimensional and the support vectors for the developed classifier model.

5.4 Hardware implementation on Wi-Fi integrated embedded platform

The aim of this study is to develop a microcontroller-based hardware platform that must be able to perform the real-time analysis of heartbeats. As such the platform must be capable of signals reception, real-time processing and transfer the

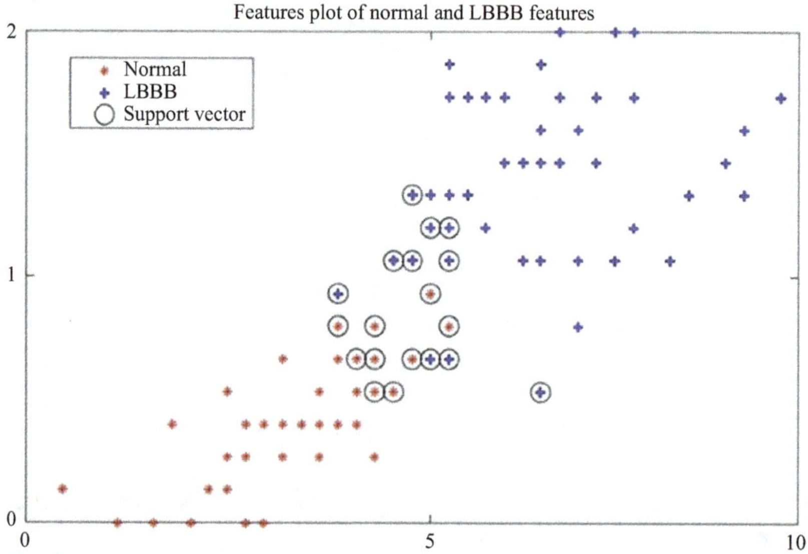

Figure 5.9 Features plot of normal and LBBB signals with support vectors

information to a remote place for telemedicine applications. The feasibility of the idea is demonstrated by developing a hardware prototype comprising 32-bit advanced RISC machine (ARM) microcontroller platform integrated with a wireless technology module.

The hardware setup consists of four significant modules namely the (a) signal generation unit, (b) processing unit, (c) the displaying unit and (d) storage module.

(a) Signal generation unit: This unit generates real-time heartbeats that are used for performing the experiments. An arbitrary function generator (AFG) is used for generating the real-time signals. The heartbeats from the database are generated in text file and transferred to the AFG. It is to note that only testing signals are generated in AFG as the training procedure is performed in off-line mode. The AFG has two channels that can generate the signals up to 200 MHz. In this study, the heartbeats are generated at 1 kHz frequency and the output is taken through the BNC crocodile cable which is sent to processing unit.

(b) Processing unit: This unit processes the input ECG signals to perform real-time recognition of heartbeats using the proposed method as elaborated in the previous section. This unit consists of a 32-bit ARM microcontroller where the proposed methodology is processed. The method is developed using embedded C programming language using KEIL software in the Windows 10 platform. The executable file is transferred to platform to execute the proposed method. The platform is integrated with a Wi-Fi module which sends the class of predicted output by platform 1 to a remote platform, i.e., platform 2 (also interfaced with a Wi-Fi module). The platform 2 is integrated with a display module.

(c) Displaying unit: In this unit, the categories of ECG signals predicted by the developed platform are displayed. This unit consists of a 16×2 liquid crystal display (LCD) module and a digital signal oscilloscope (DSO). The morphology of ECG signals processed is displayed on the MSO while its class LCD.

(d) Storage module: platform 2 is integrated with a storage device (SD-card) 8 GB which stores the class of output predicted by platform 1 as well as the digital data processed. It ensures the data and results to be analyzed further by an experienced cardiologist if required in off-line analysis.

The primary step in implementing the proposed method is to train the hardware platform. The training of the classifier mechanism is performed in off-line mode using the MATLAB® software package (R2018b, version 7.14.0.739) installed on Windows 10 platform. The PSO optimized classifier parameters such as and cost function "C", support vectors (SVs) and kernel "γ" from the trained model are taken and stored on the memory of the platform 1 using the serial communication port. The training procedure makes the platform capable of predicting any input ECG into its subsequent classes. Once the classifier is trained the real-time testing of the proposed methodology is performed to estimate the accuracy of the hardware test platform. The details of the training and testing data are provided in Table 5.1.

The classification performance of the hardware test platform is computed on the ECG signals of a testing dataset. Initially the data is distributed randomly, re-annotated and generated in text file. This text file is transferred to AFG where the analog ECG signals are generated in real time as input. The data available has an amplitude of 10 mV range which is not acceptable by an ADC. Therefore, the data is amplified to 4 V in the AFG to make it acceptable by an ADC. The ECG signals are sent to platform 1 for processing these signals using combination of feature extraction and classification methods. The data is sampled by an ADC on platform 1 (32-bit microcontroller) with a rate such that 256 samples/s is obtained. The resolution of the ADC is 12-bit. The data is encoded with fixed point math by using 32-bit representation. A small pause of time is also introduced between the samples such that the data packets must reach at the same time for the fixed frequency. Once the data reaches ADC, the data is passed through the proposed method for its processing.

The digital ECG signals are initially through the filtering stage where different kinds of noises are eliminated to produce preprocessed signals with improved SNR. The filtering is followed by the R-peak detection stage where a classical Pan-Tompkins technique [35] is applied to locate the R-peaks within the ECG signals. Once the R-peaks are located, a window of length 256 samples is employed across every peak to segment each of heartbeats. The usage of window ensures that the size of signals obtained is of fixed size which is later passed through the feature extraction and recognition stages. The CST method is employed to extract the time-frequency (TF) features for various categories of heartbeats. The TF features extracted bears most of the significant characteristics of the heartbeats and represent them in an efficient manner into a lower d-space. The feature extraction enables platform 1 to distinguish various ECG signals in TF domain. These TF features are given as input to the trained SVM model such that they must be predicted into a particular class. The classification performance of the trained SVM model is estimated at convergence. In the testing phase, a particular class is assigned to the signal as per the voting strategy. The class information of ECG signal is transferred from processing unit (platform 1) to a remote platform (platform 2) using Wi-Fi module integrated with both the platforms to justify the idea of tele-monitoring applications. The platform 2 is integrated with displaying modules where the morphology of the current classified input along with their predicted classes can be seen on DSO and LCD module. These predicted categories of heartbeats are compared with the annotations file provided by ECG database [35] to formulate the confusion matrix. The classified outputs are kept in a text file. These text files are stored in the platform 2 using an SD card. Such kind of storage facilitates the off-line analysis if required by an experienced cardiologist which can help in suggesting medicines to the user.

5.4.1 Performance metrics

After the confusion matrix is estimated, the performance metrics for every category of the heartbeat are computed in terms of five performance metrics, namely, sensitivity (S_E), positive predictivity (P_P), accuracy (A_C), error rate (E_R) and F-score (F_s) [3]. The sensitivity is defined as the ratio of correctly classified instances and total number of instances as $S_E = \mathrm{TP}/(\mathrm{TP} + \mathrm{FN})$ [3]. The P_P is defined as the ratio of correctly classified instances and the total number of detected instances, $P_P = \mathrm{TP}/(\mathrm{TP} + \mathrm{FP})$ [3]. The A_C is defined as fraction of total number of correctly classified instances and the total number of instances classified, $A_C = (\mathrm{TP} + \mathrm{TN})/(\mathrm{TP} + \mathrm{TN} + \mathrm{FP} + \mathrm{FN})$ and F_s is defined as $(2\mathrm{TP}/2\mathrm{TP} + \mathrm{FN} + \mathrm{FP})$ [3]. The aforesaid performance metrics are computed on the benchmark PhysioNet data for the proposed methodology which is analyzed in category-oriented scheme [3].

5.5 Results and discussion

A hardware prototype using the 32-bit ARM-based testing platform (i.e., 400 MHz, Linux environment) is developed implementing the proposed method whose performance is estimated in performing local real-time identification of various classes of heartbeats evaluated under category-oriented assessment scheme. The recognition performance report of the proposed platform is demonstrated by performing the experiment on benchmark MIT-BIH arrhythmia data described in Section 5.1. As such, only testing is conducted in real time on the test data by the trained hardware platform. The performance of the trained platform is presented in terms of a confusion matrix as presented in Table 5.3 for every category of heartbeat in category-oriented assessment scheme. The confusion matrix is formulated by mapping the correctly classified instances and misclassified instances into their

Table 5.3 Confusion matrix under the category scheme

	Correctly classified instances: 81803 Accuracy: 95.80%																
	Misclassified instances: 3582 Error rate: 4.20%																
	Ground truth																
	Class	***N***	***L***	***R***	***A***	***V***	***P***	***a***	**!**	***F***	***x***	***j***	***f***	***E***	***J***	***e***	***Q***	**Σ**
Predicted labels	*N*	61,497	151	0	686	401	0	89	0	95	0	71	27	0	0	0	0	63,017
	L	360	4845	0	9	58	0	0	0	0	0	0	0	0	0	0	0	5272
	R	321	31	4209	81	13	0	0	0	0	0	0	0	0	0	0	0	4655
	A	168	37	0	1391	14	0	0	27	9	0	0	0	0	0	0	0	1646
	V	211	28	0	0	4304	0	0	25	61	0	0	0	0	0	0	0	4629
	P	164	0	77	0	0	4195	0	0	0	0	0	88	0	0	0	0	4524
	a	9	0	0	0	7	0	64	0	0	0	0	0	0	0	0	0	80
	!	16	0	0	0	51	0	0	205	0	0	0	0	0	0	0	0	272
	F	23	0	0	0	18	0	0	0	361	0	0	0	0	0	0	0	402
	x	17	0	0	7	0	0	0	0	0	79	0	0	0	0	0	0	103
	j	19	0	0	9	0	0	0	0	0	0	95	0	0	6	0	0	129
	f	31	13	0	0	0	17	0	0	0	0	0	471	0	0	0	0	532
	E	10	0	0	0	5	0	0	0	0	0	0	0	41	0	0	0	56
	J	8	0	0	0	0	0	0	0	0	0	0	0	0	35	0	0	43
	e	3	0	0	0	1	0	0	0	0	0	0	0	0	0	4	0	8
	Q	4	0	0	0	1	0	2	0	0	0	0	3	0	0	0	7	17
	Σ	62,861	5105	4286	2183	4873	4212	155	257	526	79	166	589	41	41	4	7	85,385

subsequent classes identified by the developed platform implementing the method [3]. The column of the confusion matrix denotes the total number of instances identified by the hardware platform using the proposed method. Whereas the row of confusion matrix denotes the ground truth or annotations used for reference provided in the benchmark database [39]. In total of 85385 testing ECG instances, 81803 instances are correctly identified by the hardware platform reported a higher accuracy of 95.8% along with an error rate of 4.2%. In Table 5.3, it is observed that the accuracy of classes "e" and "q" is quite less when compared to other categories of heartbeats which is due to a smaller number of ECG instances considered for training in these two classes. It is to note that experiments are conducted for all the data available for these two classes in the benchmark PhysioNet data.

After the confusion matrix is computed, the performance metrics such as S_E, P_P and F_s are calculated for every category of heartbeats. Before determining these performance metrics, it is important to calculate the other parameters like true positive (TP), false positive (FP) and false negative (FN) for a particular category of heartbeat and shown in Table 5.4. Under the category-oriented scheme, Table 5.4 presents the overall S_E, P_P, F_s parameters computed for all 16 categories of heartbeats is reported to be 95.8% each respectively. Figure 5.10 depicts the bar plot of the performance metrics obtained in Table 5.4.

The experiments performed under category-oriented assessment scheme may consist of data from the same patient in both the training and testing sets that have assisted in achieving higher accuracy. However, it is suggested to keep the subject data independent, i.e., the testing and training data sets should contain the data from same subject. This may give a more generalized solution to the real time of heartbeats. The performance metrics for the best classifier model for each category

Table 5.4 Performance metrics under category scheme

Class	TP	FN	FP	S_E	P_P	F_S
N	61497	1520	1364	97.58795	97.83013	97.70889
L	4845	427	260	91.90061	94.90695	93.37959
R	4209	446	77	90.4189	98.20345	94.15054
A	1391	255	792	84.5079	63.71965	72.65605
V	4304	325	569	92.97905	88.32341	90.59145
P	4195	329	17	92.72767	99.59639	96.03938
a	64	16	91	80	41.29032	54.46809
!	205	67	52	75.36765	79.76654	77.50473
F	361	41	165	89.801	68.63118	77.80172
x	79	24	0	76.69903	100	86.81319
j	95	34	71	73.64341	57.22892	64.40678
f	471	61	118	88.53383	79.96604	84.03211
E	41	15	0	73.21429	100	84.53608
J	35	8	6	81.39535	85.36585	83.33333
e	4	4	0	50	100	66.66667
Q	7	10	0	41.17647	100	58.33333
Total	81803	3582	3582	95.80488	95.80488	95.80488

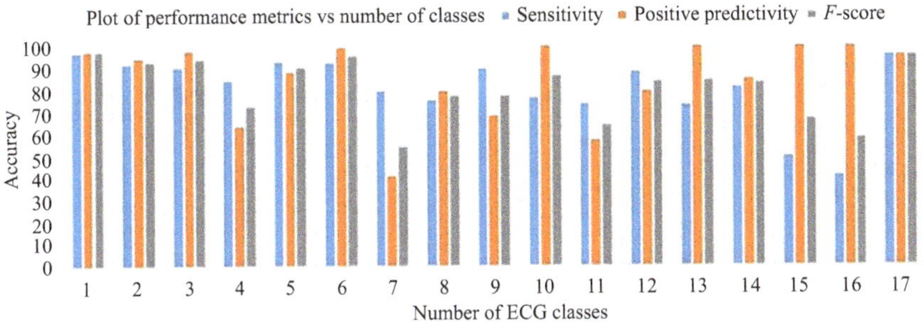

Figure 5.10 Coefficient values in the category-based scheme

of heartbeat are presented in Figure 5.9 under category-oriented assessment scheme.

The categories of heartbeats identified by the hardware platform implementing the proposed method under the category scheme are kept in text file. The report contains the sum of cardiac events recognized by the hardware platform as well as events classified into a particular category. This storage of report and ECG data allows off-line analysis by an experienced cardiologist. When an abnormality or arrhythmia is detected by the prototype, a pop-up message is displayed as "WARNING" on the LCD module as well as an alarm or buzzer is triggered to alert the subject. This enables a patient to not continuously monitor the ECG report summary and facilitates the user by recognizing the abnormality at an earlier stage avoiding any emergency situation.

5.5.1 Comparison with literature

A brief comparison is presented between the results reported by the hardware platform and the existing methods available in the literature under the category-oriented assessment scheme. A fair comparison is quite tedious to make which is due to the fact that different works have been evaluated on a different database and different numbers and classes of heartbeats classified. A few of the works have validated their methods on the data taken from the hospitals or patients. In account of these factors, a fair comparison is presented on the works evaluated on the benchmark MIT-BIH arrhythmia data and reported in Table 5.5.

From Table 5.5, it can be concluded that prototyped embedded platform has achieved higher accuracy under category-oriented assessment scheme when compared with the available methodologies reported in the literature. In comparison with some of the works, the current identifies a number of cardiac events. As such, the number of ECG signals varies greatly among the different categories of heartbeats in the training and testing datasets, the performance metrics parameters reported for a particular class can be considered as more reliable and significant. As the current work achieves a higher accuracy than the existing works, it is implicit to conclude that features extracted in time-frequency space using fast Fourier transform-based discrete wavelet transform (CST) technique are efficient and

Table 5.5 Comparison in class-oriented evaluation scheme with the existing works

Works [ref.]	Feature extraction	Classifier	Classes	Accuracy (%)
Oresko [13]	RR-interval	ANN	5	90
Jeon *et al.* [46]	WT	SVM	3	95.1
Melgani *et al.* [29]	Morphology + PCA	SVM	6	91.67
Cvikl *et al.* [15]	Block processing	OSEA	2	92.36
Nambhash *et al.* [18]	Wavelet	Fuzzy	3	85 (avg.)
Cvikl *et al.* [17]	Geometrical	OSEA	2	92.59
Ince [47]	PCA	ANN + PSO	2	95.58
Martis *et al.* [48]	PCA	LSSVM	5	93.48
Proposed	CST	PSO + TSVM	All MIT	95.80

†WT: wavelet transform; PCA: principal component analysis; ANN: artificial neural networks; LSSVM: least square support vector machines; HOS: higher-order statistics; SVM: support vector machines; TSVM: twin support vector machines.

significant in discriminating between various categories of heartbeats when combined with the PSO optimized SVM for an efficient detection and classification of heartbeats.

The implementation of the proposed method on the embedded platform provides an enriched interface to the consumers or subjects regarding their real-time feedback of the heart. The platform also stores the ECG data along with the summary reports so that a subject may keep the information about the arrhythmias occurring in daily life and investigate their own lifestyle [6]. The developed prototype [42] can be used by subjects in hospitals as well as consumers at their workplace to monitor various categories (i.e., 16 classes in category-oriented assessment scheme) of abnormalities or ECG signals with higher accuracy. Such kind of implementation is made possible by generating real-time signals and processed using IoT-based embedded platform that is best suitable for clinical analysis by consumers in the home environment. This kind of implementation will provide an assistive diagnostic solution to the consumers in leading a healthy life and thereby, improving the healthcare for cardiovascular diseases (CVDs), i.e., smart healthcare.

5.6 Conclusion and future scope

In this chapter, a new method is proposed by combining the CST as a feature extraction technique and artificial bee colony (ABC) optimized SVMs for automated recognition of heartbeats into 16 classes. The proposed method is prototyped on a 32-bit microcontroller test platform for long-term monitoring and analyzing the nonstationary behavior of heartbeats. The validation of the hardware platform is performed on the PhysioNet data while its evaluation is done under two assessment schemes, i.e., subject and category schemes. Improved accuracy of 98.82% and percentage is achieved by the prototype under subject and class-oriented schemes, respectively. The classes of heartbeats detected by the platform are sent to a remote platform using Wi-Fi technology facilitating telemedicine applications. The future scope of this chapter is to include a greater number of arrhythmia signals for analysis, to develop more efficient algorithms and their implementation of mobile platforms. This implementation can be fabricated into a PCB-oriented handheld device as such it can be affordable by common people to lead a healthy lifestyle for cardiovascular diseases.

References

[1] Raj S. 'Development and Hardware Prototype of an Efficient Method for Handheld Arrhythmia Monitoring Device'. *Ph.D. Thesis*. IIT Patna. 2018, pp. 1–181.

[2] Raj S., Ray K. C. and Shankar O. 'Development of robust, fast and efficient QRS complex detector: A methodological review'. *Aust. Phys. Eng. Sci. Med.* 2018, vol. 41(3), pp. 581–600.

[3] Raj S. and Ray K. C. 'A personalized point-of-care platform for real-time ECG monitoring'. *IEEE Trans. Consum. Electron.* 2018, vol. 66(4), pp. 1–9.

[4] Raj S. and Ray K. C. 'A personalized arrhythmia monitoring platform'. *Sci. Rep.* 2018, vol. 8(11395), pp. 1–11.

[5] Raj S., Luthra S. and Ray K. C. 'Development of handheld cardiac event monitoring system'. *IFAC Papers-On-Line.* 2015, vol. 48(4), pp. 71–6.

[6] Raj S., Chand G. S. S. and Ray K. C. 'Arm-based arrhythmia beat monitoring system'. *Microprocess. Microsyst.* 2015, vol. 39(7), pp. 504–11.

[7] Faezipour M., Saeed A., Bulusu S., Nourani M., Minn H. and Tamil L. 'A patient-adaptive profiling scheme for ECG beat classification'. *IEEE Trans. Inf. Technol. Biomed.* 2010, vol. 14(5), pp. 1153–65.

[8] Dey N., Ashour A. S., Shi F., Fong S. J. and Sherratt R. S. 'Developing residential wireless sensor networks for ECG healthcare monitoring'. *IEEE Trans. Consum. Electron.* 2017, vol. 63(4), pp. 442–49.

[9] Chui K. T., Tsang K. F., Chi H. R., Ling B. W. K. and Wu C. K. 'An accurate ECG-based transportation safety drowsiness detection scheme'. *IEEE Trans. Ind. Informat.* 2016, vol. 12(4), pp. 1438–52.

[10] Wang L. H., Chen T. Y., Lin K. H., Fang Q. and Lee S. Y. 'Implementation of a wireless ECG acquisition SoC for IEEE 802.15.4 (ZigBee) applications'. *IEEE J. Biomed. Health Informat.* 2015, vol. 19(1), pp. 247–55.

[11] Gay V. and Leijdekkers P. 'A health monitoring system using smart phones and wearable sensors'. *Int. J. ARM.* 2007, vol. 8(2), pp. 29–36.

[12] Rodriguez J.,Goni A. and Illarramendi A. 'Real-time classification of ECGS on a PDA'. *IEEE Trans. Inf. Technol. Biomed.* 2005, vol. 9(1), pp. 23–34.

[13] Oresko J. J. 'A wearable smartphone-based platform for real-time cardiovascular disease detection via electrocardiogram processing'. *IEEE Trans. Inf. Technol. Biomed.* 2010, vol. 14(3), pp. 734–40.

[14] Garge G. K., Balakrishna C. and Datta S. K. 'Consumer health care: Current trends in consumer health monitoring'. *IEEE Consum. Electron. Mag.* 2018, vol. 7(1), pp. 38–46.

[15] Cvikl M. and Zemva A. 'FPGA-oriented HW/SW implementation of ECG beat detection and classification algorithm'. *Digit. Signal Process.* 2010, vol. 20(1), pp. 238–48.

[16] Özdemir A. T. and Danisman K. 'Fully parallel ANN-based arrhythmia-classifier on a single-chip FPGA'. *Turkish J. Elect. Eng. Comput. Sci.* 2011, vol. 19(4), pp. 667–87.

[17] Cvikl M. and Zemva A. 'FPGA-based system for ECG beat detection and classification'. in *Proc. IFMBE Conf.* 2007, pp. 66–9.

[18] Nambakhsh M. S., Tavakoli V. and Sahba N. 'FPGA-core defibrillator using wavelet-fuzzy ECG arrhythmia classification'. in *Proc. IEEE Eng. Med. Biol. Soc. Conf.* 2008, pp. 2673–6.

[19] Linh T. H., Osowski S. and Stodoloski M. 'On-line heart beat recognition using Hermite polynomials and neuro-fuzzy network'. *IEEE Trans. Instrum. Meas.* 2003, vol. 52(4), pp. 1224–31.

[20] Goh K. W., Lavanya J., Kim Y., Tan E. K. and Soh C. B. 'A PDA based ECG beat detector for home cardiac care'. in *Proc. 27th IEEE EMBC*, Shanghai, China. 2006, pp. 375–8.

[21] Minami K., Nakajima H. and Toyoshima T. 'Real-time discrimination of ventricular tachyarrhythmia with Fourier-transform neural network'. *IEEE Trans. Biomed. Eng.* 1999, vol. 46(2), pp. 179–85.

[22] Fraser G. D., Chan A. D., Green J. R. and Macisaac J. R. 'Automated bio-signal quality analysis for electromyography using a one class support vector machine'. *IEEE Trans. Instrum. Meas.* 2014, vol. 63(12), pp. 2919–30.

[23] Raj S. and Ray K. C. 'Automated recognition of cardiac arrhythmias using sparse decomposition over composite dictionary'. *Comput. Methods Programs Biomed.* 2018, vol. 165, pp. 175–86.

[24] Hu Y. H., Tompkins W. J., Urrusti J. L. and Afonso V. X. 'Applications of artificial neural networks for ECG signal detection and classification'. *J. Electrocardiol.* 1993, vol. 26, pp. 66–73.

[25] Hu Y. H., Palreddy S. and Tompkins W. J. 'A patient-adaptable ECG beat classifier using a mixture of experts approach'. *IEEE Trans. Biomed. Eng.* 1997, vol. 44(9), pp. 891–900.

[26] de Chazal P. and Reilly R. B. 'A patient-adapting heartbeat classifier using ECG morphology and heartbeat interval features'. *IEEE Trans. Biomed. Eng.* 2006, vol. 53(12), pp. 2535–43.

[27] de Chazal P., O'Dwyer M. and Reilly R. B. 'Automatic classification of heartbeats using ECG morphology and heartbeat interval features'. *IEEE Trans. Biomed. Eng.* 2004, vol. 51(7), pp. 1196–206.

[28] Lagerholm M., Peterson C., Braccini C., Edenbrandt L. and Sornmo L. 'Clustering ECG complexes using Hermite functions and self-organizing maps'. *IEEE Trans. Biomed. Eng.* 2000, vol. 47(7), pp. 838–48.

[29] Melgani F. and Bazi Y. 'Classification of electrocardiogram signals with-support vector machines and particle swarm optimization'. *IEEE Trans. Inf. Technol. Biomed.* 2008, vol. 12(5), pp. 667–77.

[30] Raj S., Ray K. C. and Shankar O. 'Cardiac arrhythmia beat classification using DOST and PSO tuned SVM'. *Comput. Methods Programs Biomed.* 2016, vol. 136, pp. 163–77.

[31] Raj S. and Ray K. C. 'ECG signal analysis using DCT-based do stand PSO optimized SVM'. *IEEE Trans. Instrum. Meas*. 2017, vol. 66(3), pp. 470–8.

[32] Sharma P. and Ray K. C. 'Efficient methodology for electrocardiogram beat classification', *IET Signal Process*. 2016, vol. 10(7), pp. 825–32.

[33] Raj S. and Ray K. C. 'A Comparative Study of Multivariate Approach with Neural Networks and Support Vector Machines for Arrhythmia Classification', in *Int. Conf. on Energy, Power and Environment: Towards Sustainable growth*. 2015, pp. 1–6.

[34] Raj S. and Ray K. C. 'Sparse representation of ECG signals for automated recognition of cardiac arrhythmias'. *Expert Syst. Appl.* 2018, vol. 105, pp. 49–64.

[35] Raj S. and Ray K. C. 'Application of variational mode decomposition and ABC optimized DAG-SVM in arrhythmia analysis'. in *Proc. 7th Int. Symp. Embedded Comput. Syst. Design (ISED)*. 2017, pp. 1–5.

[36] Andreao R. V., Dorizzi B. and Boudy J. 'ECG signal analysis through hidden Markov models'. *IEEE Trans. Biomed. Eng.* 2006, vol. 53(8), pp. 1541–9.

[37] Pyakillya B., Kazachenko N. and Mikhailovsky N. 'Deep Learning for ECG classification'. *J. Phys.: Conference Series*. 2017, vol. 913, pp. 1–5.

[38] Pourbabaee B., Roshtkhari M. J. and Khorasani K. 'Deep Convolutional Neural Networks and Learning ECG Features for Screening Paroxysmal Atrial Fibrillation Patients'. *IEEE Trans. Syst. Man Cybern*. 2018, vol. 48 (12), pp. 2095–104.

[39] Moody G. B. and Mark R. G. 'The impact of the MIT-BIH arrhythmia database'. *IEEE Eng. Med. Biol. Mag.* 2001, vol. 20(3), pp. 45–50.

[40] Stockwell R. G. 'A basis for efficient representation of the S-transform'. *Digit. Signal Process.* 2007, vol. 17(1), pp. 371–93.

[41] Tomar D. and Agarwal S. 'A comparison on multi-class classification methods based on least squares twin support vector machine'. *Knowledge Based Systems* 2015, vol. 81, pp. 131–47.

[42] Hsu C. W. and Lin C.-J. 'A comparison of methods for multiclass support vector machines'. *IEEE Trans. Neural Netw*. 2002, vol. 13(2), pp. 415–25.

[43] Chakraborty C. 'Chronic wound image analysis by particle swarm optimization technique for tele-wound network'. *Springer: Int. J. Wireless Pers. Commun*. 2017, vol. 96(3), pp. 3655–71.

[44] Pan J. and Tompkins W. J. 'A real-time QRS detection algorithm'. *IEEE Trans. Biomed. Eng.* 1985, vol. 32(3), pp. 230–6.

[45] Stone M. 'Cross-validatory choice and assessment of statistical predictions'. *J. Roy. Stat. Soc. B (Methodol.)*. 1974, vol. 36(2), pp. 111–47.

[46] Jeon T., Kim B., Jeon M. and Lee B. 'Implementation of a portable device for real-time ECG signal analysis'. *BioMedical Engineering-On-Line*. 2014, vol. 13, pp. 160.

[47] Ince T., Kiranyaz S. and Gabbouj M. 'A generic and robust system for automated patient-specific classification of ECG signals'. *IEEE Trans. Biomed. Eng.* 2009, vol. 56(5), pp. 1415–26.
[48] Martis R., Acharya U., Mandana K., Ray A. and Chakraborty C. 'Cardiac decision making using high order spectra'. *Biomed. Signal Process Control.* 2013, vol. 8(2), pp. 193–203.

Chapter 6

Data mining in telemedicine

Md Fashiar Rahman[1], Yuxin Wen[2], Honglun Xu[1], Tzu-Liang (Bill) Tseng[3] and Satya Akundi[4]

To date, the field of telemedicine is at a critical standpoint and faces a wide variety of challenges. Voluminous data are generated through the interaction among the telemedicine stakeholders, which are ever increasing. It is well conjectured that the successful implementation of telemedicine largely depends on the effective and efficient knowledge extraction from this available data cloud. However, due to lack of proper integration of the data mining techniques, the stakeholders are not getting the full-fledged benefit from this promising platform. Considering the aforementioned fact, this book chapter provides a contrivance to integrate data mining techniques into telemedicine connecting all the stakeholders into a single podium using data engine. It illustrates the prospects of different data mining techniques and their integration for telemedicine. These techniques combine all the basic classification and clustering method including the state-of-the-art artificial neural network (ANN) and deep learning procedure for disease prediction. Two case studies, heart diseases, and breast cancer prediction have been demonstrated applications of the integrated data mining engine.

6.1 Introduction to data mining

Data mining, an interdisciplinary subfield of statistics and computer science, enables us to extract information by different intellectual methods from large unstructured datasets and converts them into a comprehensible structure for further application. Data mining is the process of discovering patterns involving methods at the intersection of statistics, machine learning, and database systems in large datasets. Over the past decade, data mining has become more and more useful in many areas, especially in knowledge extraction. Knowledge could be at various levels, such as a complicated chemical formula describing the relationship between

[1]Computational Science Program, University of Texas, El Paso, USA
[2]Department of Electrical and Computer Engineering, University of Texas, El Paso, USA
[3]Department of Industrial, Manufacturing and System Engineering, University of Texas, El Paso, USA
[4]Department of Manufacturing & Industrial Engineering, University of Texas, Rio Grande Valley, USA

different materials or knowing the number of doctors or nurses working on a day. Although some kinds of knowledge are known and widely used, there is most likely a lot of unknown knowledge stored in in-house databases that need to be investigated further. Knowledge extraction is the creation of knowledge from unstructured sources of information (such as text, documents, and images) and structured sources of information (like relational databases and XML). The elaborate knowledge needs to be in a machine-readable and machine-interpretable format and must represent knowledge in a way that makes inferencing easier. Even though it is methodically similar to data extraction, the key criteria are that the result of extraction goes beyond generating structured information or transforming it into a relational scheme.

Over the past few years, several methods of data mining have been developed for knowledge extraction. These can be summarized into three categories: (1) Clustering methods, which involve dividing a data set into sub-sets of items so as to items in each cluster are more similar than items in the same cluster. The similarity is usually defined as a metric to be constructed in order to be relevant to the clustering [1]. In knowledge extraction, clustering is used as a classification tool. Clustering research emphases on the challenge of developing appropriate metrics and/or clustering methods designed to build clusters that meet certain specific conditions of optimality. (2) Rule induction methods, which focus on the prediction of one class unlike tree induction techniques based on many classes. It applies heuristics and does not require to balance the data sets [2]. Recently, research on rule induction has focused on objective methods based on multi-criteria. (3) Knowledge discovery in database (KDD) method, which is an interdisciplinary area that focuses on methodologies to extract useful data knowledge. This method is also a non-trivial process in which valid, new, potentially useful and ultimately understandable patterns from large data collections are identified. Due to the Internet and the widespread use of databases, the ongoing rapid growth of online data has created an immense need for KDD methodologies [3]. KDD refers to the general process and discipline of extracting useful knowledge from databases, including data storage, data cleaning, and data manipulation tasks to interpret and exploit results. Data Mining now refers to one stage to extract useful rules and patterns from the data within the KDD process. The key research within the Knowledge Extraction Group is the development of algorithms to perform the various stages of the KDD process. This refers not only to the actual stage of data mining but also to sampling, cleaning, and pre-processing of data.

6.2 Data mining in telemedicine

Telemedicine started with the idea to serve patients in remote areas for easy access to health facilities or in areas where medical professionals are not available. Today, the application of telemedicine is expanding besides serving its intended purpose. It is becoming a platform for easy and accessible medical care. Patients are starting to expect more convenient options and have access to more information about their health. They want to get immediate care for minor or urgent health conditions without wasting their time in the waiting room of the doctor. The expectation of getting easy and accessible care has been changed the trajectory of telemedicine. With the help of technology, telemedicine brings medical professionals and patients on the same virtual platform by removing the geographical and physical barriers. Now, telemedicine is the most affordable, accessible, and universal tool from the patients' viewpoint. For example, there are several online platforms like Skype, Zoom, and FaceTime, which are providing the benefit of audio-video conversation. People can easily use these platforms to reach medical professionals to discuss their problems and get an informed diagnosis in the case of urgent need. Furthermore, simple home-use medical devices or applications can play a vital role here. These devices can be used to diagnose preliminary infections, monitor glucose levels or measure blood pressure and gather them into the data warehouse for doctor's diagnosis, without the face-to-face doctor-patient interaction.

6.2.1 Role of data mining in telemedicine

The landscape of telemedicine is changing faster than ever before and so as the complexity of the whole system. Telemedicine is a multidisciplinary and cross-functional platform, which involves service providers, insurers, pharmaceuticals, practitioners, and patients. The successful implementation of telemedicine concept requires concurrent response and information sharing among all these parties. Obviously, this entire process generates voluminous structured or unstructured data, which needs to be used effectively to discover the required knowledge. In addition, the practice of telemedicine is no longer limited to simple telecommunication technology, like telephones and radio. Today, this service involves a very friendly and informal way by connecting through any possible media or devices. Hence, telemedicine platforms need to give physicians an organized, secure system for practicing medicine remotely, tracking patient health data, sharing medical records with consulting physicians, documenting all remote patient visits, charging patients and getting reimbursed from third-party payers, and so much more. Obviously, both telemedicine and analytics are major areas of interest in this platform. These two areas go hand in hand, as big data analytics are helping to advance telemedicine and empower both physicians and patients. Here are eight ways big data is playing a role in telehealth.

6.2.1.1 Patient health tracking and predictive analytics

The first and foremost advantage of the application of data mining in telemedicine is the early identification of health problems to protect the patient from severe health conditions. The use of various smart devices like wearable fitness trackers and the Internet of Medical things (IOMT) make this possible by collecting patient data on a real-time basis. Application of data mining techniques to this data ensures that patients' vitals and statistics are constantly monitored such as blood pressure and heart rate. This system of monitoring can help keep high-risk individuals out of the hospital, and allow doctors, patients, and caregivers to track the patient's overall health. This not only helps to predict life-threatening events and keeps more patients out of the hospital; but also, it cuts down on costs and allows patients to live healthier, more comfortable lives. Real-time data can even help doctors administer the correct medication dosages, improving care. Besides, the data collected and stored in the cloud facilitates the predictive analytics of possible future outcomes. Doctors can create risk scores based on data gathered from various sources, which is important for the identification of individuals at elevated risks of developing chronic ailments at the early stage of disease progression.

6.2.1.2 Post-discharge observation

Following any critical hospitalization, post-discharge monitoring is necessary to ensure patients' health recovery conditions. Usually, patients need to set up several appointments with physicians, which is cumbersome, especially for elderly and debilitated patients who cannot make frequent trips to the hospital. Telemedicine with the integration of data mining techniques can alleviate these unnecessary visits of patients to the doctor's clinic while maintaining effective and efficient follow-up. Vital patient stats like blood pressure and heart rate are collected by the use of health devices, which have advanced sensors attached to them. The data collected is processed using analytics techniques to leverage regular checkups. The clinicians are able to make use of numerous healthcare-based apps to remotely monitor the patient's condition and be on the lookout for signs of disease progression. This helps to keep the patients out of the hospitals and keeps the cost relatively low by avoiding unnecessary hospitalization.

6.2.1.3 Convenient and accurate diagnosis

In telemedicine, diagnosis can be difficult as the doctor cannot get the physical touch or listen to the patient's heart or stomach. Sometimes the doctor relies solely on patient's description of symptoms and the signs of diseases. Now instead of subjective symptoms narrated by the patient, the doctors can base their diagnosis on the patient data collected regularly by wearable devices. Using a patient's electronic health records (EHRs), combined with the doctor's observations, can help identify high-risk patients and diagnose patients more effectively.

6.2.1.4 Precise medication and observation

Application of data analytics in telemedicine shifts the traditional generic medicine into the domain of precision medicine. Precision medicine is influenced by several factors such as lifestyle, environmental conditions for each individual. Patients' EHRs and genomics data can be collected using different wearable devices and healthcare-based apps. Data analytics make it possible to compute the relevant data collected from the various sources and tapped into for developing a medication that caters to patients individually. Besides, healthcare professionals can keep eye continuously on patients' recovery progression and take appropriate action on individual's treat plan.

6.2.1.5 Specialist outreach

The telemedicine platform generates tons of data including patients' EHRs and electronic medical records (EMRs) and stores them on the data warehouse or data cloud. One of the great advantages of telemedicine is that it can access the patient data at any time from any location. Thus, treatment can be prescribed irrespective of the geographical location of the patient and the healthcare provider. Therefore, if a patient is referred to the specialist who is at different location than the patient, telemedicine gives the opportunity to reach that specialist easily. Secure access to the cloud ensures that physical location is no longer a variable in availing the best treatment possible. Besides, it allows the healthcare provider to use the doctor's time through flexible scheduling, as well as increasing the effectiveness of care.

6.2.1.6 Observing infection trends and timely intervention

Disease outbreaks are a serious concern in healthcare industry. When infectious diseases start to spread in an area or community, it becomes hard for the healthcare provider to manage and provide proper treatment to infected population; sometimes the situation goes beyond control. However, application of data analytics can leverage the prediction of such types of diseases and studying the patterns and trends of infection outbreaks. Big data in the form of Internet search queries are also being utilized for understanding disease trends, predicting the spread of infectious diseases. Once the regions affected by the infection are identified, the benefits of telemedicine become known. A physician can interact with the affected populations using healthcare apps, teleconferencing or different web-based media and intervene with the appropriate treatments to prevent the further spread of infection.

6.2.1.7 Tackling disaster emergency

Telemedicine can play an important part in tackling emergency situations. In an event of a disaster, people find themselves in the middle of incomprehensible situations. Sometimes, emergency management agencies and associated help cannot reach the affected people in time. As a result, people get sick and infection spreads. Data integrated telemedicine platforms can handle this situation by deploying proper treatment in right time. Unmanned aerial vehicles, commonly known as drones, already proved its successful implementation in disaster relief [4]. Drones collect data and use them to navigate and perform reconnaissance after a disaster. They can be deployed into an area hit by a natural disaster and show healthcare and disaster relief officials what is really going on at the ground level. Then, drones can be deployed to deliver supplies, including medical equipment, to areas where they are needed the most.

6.2.1.8 Detection of fraud and abuse

Due to the convenient service of telemedicine, it is becoming popular among the patients and medical professionals as well. Voluminous data including patients' personal data and financial terms and conditions are cross-related in the telemedicine platform. It should not neglect the possibility to arise the fraudulent issues. Application of data mining successfully integrated into the commercial sector for fraud detection, for example, in the detection of fraudulent credit card transactions. Similarly, data mining can be integrated into telemedicine platform to detect healthcare insurer fraud and to protect patients' privacy and security. Detection of fraud and abuse for healthcare insurers can enable them to reduce their losses and track offenders.

6.2.2 Big data sources and characterization

The service in telemedicine depends on successful interaction between the patient and healthcare provider. Technology plays a critical role here. Smartphone applications, home monitoring equipment, genomic sequencing, and social determinants of health are adding significantly to the scope of healthcare data. Healthcare providers and insurers also feed their information to the cloud for easy access to the patient. The information flow could be two directional from patient to doctor or cross-linked among all parties. The voluminous data and their flow of direction create new challenges for health systems in data management and storage. Data collection can be both structured and unstructured. However, to make the data retrieval process successful and efficient, medical data should be stored in the warehouse based on the characteristics of data. Definitely, different types of data contain a different type of information, which can help all the telemedicine stakeholders to retrieve variety of knowledge when they needed. Medical data can be characterized in three broad categories, namely qualitative, quantitative, and multimedia data.

6.2.2.1 Qualitative data

Qualitative data deals with numbers and things that can be measured objectively. When a patient visits a doctor's office, his/her health information (data) is collected and stored to the data warehouse for further processing, analyzing, and dissemination. This copious data may involve measurable information related to heart or stomach, such as patient's heart rate during a particular visit. However, there is potentially more to it than that. Broadly speaking, this type of data refers to health-related information that is associated with regular patient care or as part of a clinical trial program. General numeric information includes pulse rate, repository rate, temperature, and other diagnostic-related information like laboratory test results from blood tests, genetic tests, and culture results and so on.

6.2.2.2 Quantitative data

Quantitative data deals with characteristics and descriptors that cannot be easily measured but can be observed subjectively.

1. Patient/disease registries are systems to collect patients details information including his/her diseases history, various types of symptoms, medication history, and geographic and demographic information.
2. Treatment information includes the treatment history provided to a patient. For instance, is the person receiving any medication? If so, how much (what dose) and how often or the start date of medication?

3. Health surveys, which can help evaluate or tally statistics like the most common chronic illnesses a nation faces.
4. Administrative data, non-clinical data focused on record-keeping surrounding a service, such as a hospital admission and discharge information. This can be part of an EHR as well.
5. Claims data, which is information regarding insurance claims.

6.2.2.3 Multimedia data

Multimedia data becomes very effective in the field of telemedicine. This type of data includes all types of medical imaging like CT scans, MRI scans, X-ray, mammography, ultrasonography, etc. Recently, video repository, showing the different disease symptoms, is also being effectively used in decision-making.

Organizations must come up with secure, scalable, elastic, and analytically agile data warehousing solutions that leverage data analytics to enhance the telemedicine service. This requires to understand about the data sources, data type, applications of data analytics, and their underlying analytical techniques. Table 6.1 articulates all these concepts briefly.

6.3 Integration of data mining techniques into telemedicine

6.3.1 Data mining framework

Telemedicine requires the integration of EMRs and EHRs among the cross-linked stakeholders. The previous section has mentioned about the data collection from various sources and their types. Different healthcare apps and electronic devices are collecting these data from the sources and feeding them into the data warehouse or cloud. It creates a comprehensive healthcare information system containing large volume of information including patients' demographic and medical history such as medication, lab test results, radiology information, procedures, and many others. Definitely, this information system is constantly growing. The imminent growth of the voluminous and heterogeneous data leads to the necessity of data management and data mining techniques in order to extract and explore the significant knowledge from the data. In the last two decades the data mining algorithms have been enriched significantly and intervened successfully in the different areas of applications ranging from business intelligence to health informatics [5]. Data mining methods are applied to the large sets of data stored in the data cloud or data warehouse to discover the significant patterns, trends, rules, relations, and correlations contained within the data. The extraction of information and knowledge would be very difficult without data mining techniques. The process of applying data mining techniques to telemedicine is represented in Figure 6.1.

The main purpose of the data mining framework includes diagnosis, treatment, monitoring, and education of patients that allow ready access to expert advice and patient information. This framework connects all the stakeholders in a single telemedicine platform, which consists of four major stages. In the first stage, data are

Table 6.1 *Big data profile of the telemedicine system*

Sources of big data	Types of data and examples	Application of analytics	Backend analytics techniques
Patients	– Genomic database – Demographic database – The device generated data i.e. blood pressure, blood sugar, pulse rate, and follow-up information	– Classification of patient communities – Providing warning on patients' current health conditions	– Clustering and classification algorithms i.e. partitioned clustering, density-based clustering, *k*-NN, etc. – Time series analysis
Medical practitioners	– Patients' medical history – Diseases symptoms database – Medication records	– Understanding patients' health status – Teal-time and remote health monitoring – Providing preliminary treatment	– Support vector machine (SVM), decision tree, Bayesian network algorithm – Association rule mining
Clinical system	– Admission and discharge information – Treatment plan – Patients' health survey – Resource utilization log – Doctor's and nurse's schedule – Service cost information	– Post-discharge observation – On-demand patients' health statistics – Flexible and convenient manpower scheduling – Resource optimization	– Adaptive fuzzy cognitive maps – Operation research techniques like linear and complex system optimization, scheduling techniques, etc. – Text mining
Pathology	– Details information about diseases symptoms – Medical imaging like X-ray, MRI, CT-scan, mammography, etc. – Diseases consequence	– Identification of diseases symptoms – Prediction of diseases – Consequence analysis	– Machine leaning algorithms like an ANN, convolutional neural network, and image data mining, fuzzy *c*-means clustering
Pharmaceuticals	– Medicine genre – Medicine dosage records – Drug sales reports	– Precision medicine – Observation of usage and purchase patterns of drugs	– Statistical modeling techniques, association rule mining, deep learning techniques, time series analysis
Healthcare insurers	– Claims data – Cost sharing information – Details health coverage	– Detection of fraud and abuse – Reliable analysis of claims	– Outlier analysis, nearest neighbor approaches, data query techniques
Clinical researchers	– Current scenarios of particular diseases – A recent update in the medical area and medication invention	– Diseases outbreaks prediction – Keep the telemedicine up to date	– Machine learning, deep learning algorithms, diagnostics and prognostics analysis, etc.

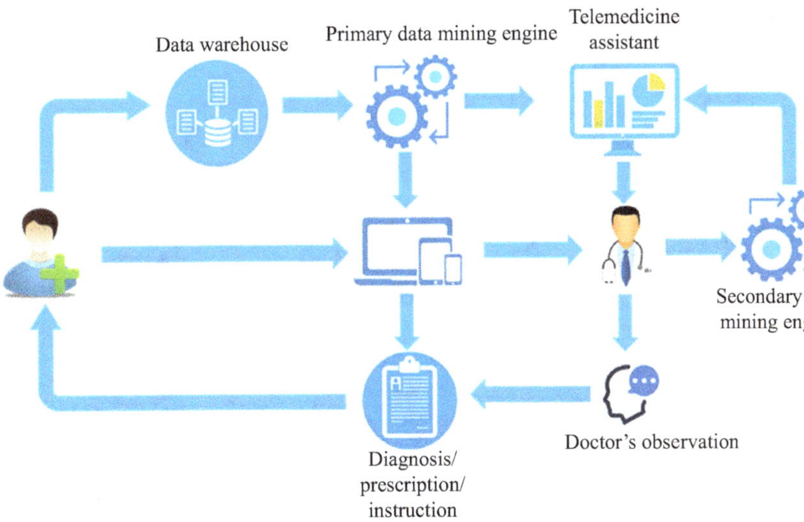

Figure 6.1 Data mining framework for telemedicine

collected from all the stakeholders such as patients, healthcare providers, insurance providers, pharmaceuticals, and other related agencies. These data are preprocessed through data cleaning and converting into a structured format and then store them in the data warehouse or cloud. In the second stage, all the data are fed into the data mining engine to extract knowledge. The data mining engine is developed using various data analysis techniques and tools that can process the data upon the request from the doctor, patient or any other stakeholder's terminal. This phase of data mining is able to process data continuously to monitor or track some basic health issues and send warning to the patients or doctors through the devices connected to it. The final outcome of this data mining engine is to generate a ready access dashboard (here named as telemedicine assistant) containing all the preliminary and historic information for any particular entities, as shown in Figure 6.2. For example, if a doctor wants to know the disease history for a particular patient, he/she will be able to get a ready access report from this data mining engine upon request. In later stage, doctor can input some further symptoms or information to update the report in real time using the secondary data mining engine. In the last stage, after getting the report from the data engine, the doctors can interpret the report to obtain useful information and disseminate some prompt action or provide useful treatment to the patient.

6.3.2 Data mining techniques

The data mining engine is the core part of the framework, which applies a variety of advanced data mining techniques for extracting important knowledge from raw data. All these techniques are developed based on very highly sophisticated algorithm from statistics, artificial intelligence, machine learning, and a database

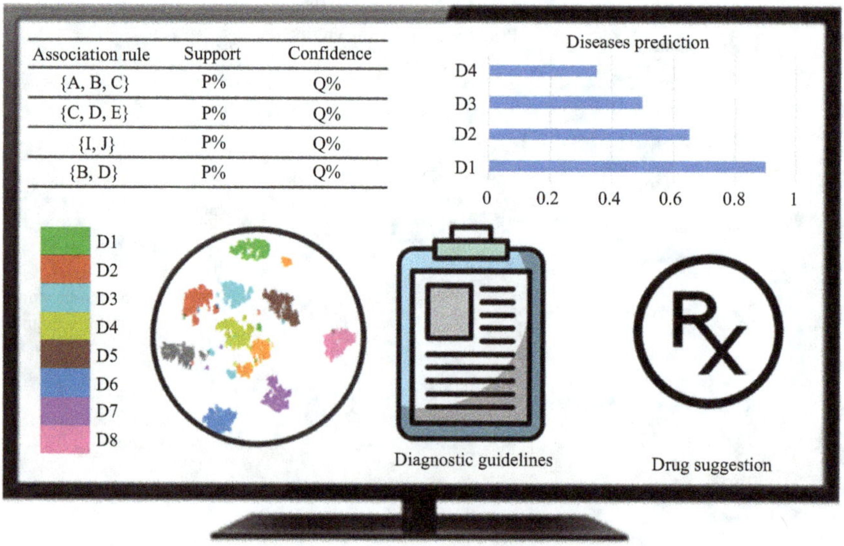

Figure 6.2 Ready access dashboard to help in decision-making

system. Some main data mining procedures are referred below to leverage the data mining engine.

6.3.2.1 Association rules mining

In medical science, there is a strong assumption that the occurrence of one disease can result in other associated diseases. For example, hypertension can lead to the occurrence of heart-block, which can eventually end up with another massive problem like cardiac arrest. Hence, it is very important to understand the consequences of different diseases. Healthcare sectors are accumulating large quantities of information about patients and their medical conditions every day. It is high time for the telemedicine institutes to take advantage of this big data and make it useful by carrying out relational analysis of various diseases. Data mining-based techniques, such as association rule mining [6] is a very effective and popular algorithm to gain a clearer understanding and relation of different physical and scientific phenomenon in large databases. Hence, the association rules mining algorithm can be applied to extract knowledge from clinical data for predicting correlation of diseases carried by a patient. Usually, a patient contacts the doctor for his primary diseases. Given a database for the patient's previous record or secondary diseases, it is very quick and efficient to analyze the correlation with different cases and come up with a good prescription.

Association rules provide information in the form of if-then statements. These rules are computed from the data and, unlike the if-then rules of logic, association rules are probabilistic in nature. In addition to the antecedent (if) and the consequent (then) item sets, an association rule has two numbers, support, and confidence as shown in Table 6.2, that express the degree of uncertainty about the rule.

Table 6.2 Example of some association rules

Item sets	Support (%)	Confidence (%)
$\{A, B\} \Rightarrow \{C\}$	0.8	40
$\{X\} \Rightarrow \{Y\}$	0.9	60
$\{P, Q\} \Rightarrow \{R\}$	0.7	55

The support is simply the frequency that includes all diseases in the antecedent and consequent parts of the rule. The support is sometimes expressed as a percentage of the total number of records in the database. Confidence explains how likely a disease A may occur when B occurs. The support and confidence are defined using (6.1) and (6.2).

$$\text{Support} = \frac{\sigma(XUY)}{N} \tag{6.1}$$

$$\text{Confidence} = \frac{\sigma(XUY)}{\sigma(X)} \tag{6.2}$$

where σ is the support or frequency of diseases.

For example, a medical database has 100,000 diseases record listed with primary and secondary diseases, out of which 2,000 include both diseases A and B, and 800 of these include C. The association rule $\{A, B\} \Rightarrow \{C\}$ means that "If diseases A and B occur, then disease C also occurred to the same patient". This rule has the support of 800 frequency of C (alternatively 0.8% = 800/100,000), and a confidence of 40% (= 800/2,000). One way to think of support is that it is the probability that a randomly selected patient in the database will have all diseases in the antecedent and the consequent, whereas the confidence is the conditional probability that a randomly selected patient will include all the diseases in the consequent, given that the patient includes all the diseases in the antecedent.

6.3.2.2 Artificial neural network

In telemedicine, disease prediction is very crucial to protect patients from severe health conditions. Machine learning and artificial intelligence have already been developed to tackle this type of medical care problem. Recently, ANN becomes a powerful tool to enhance the current medical techniques including to assist in medical diagnosis [7]. Given the preliminary knowledge, ANN can significantly improve the generalization ability to learn systems through training a finite number of hidden layers. The technique has an advantage over conventional solutions as it can mimic computational principle of neural networks of an animal. In ANNs, units correspond to neurons in biological neural networks, inputs to dendrites, connection weights to electrical impulse strengths, and outputs to axons. An analogy between biological neuron and ANN is shown in Figure 6.3.

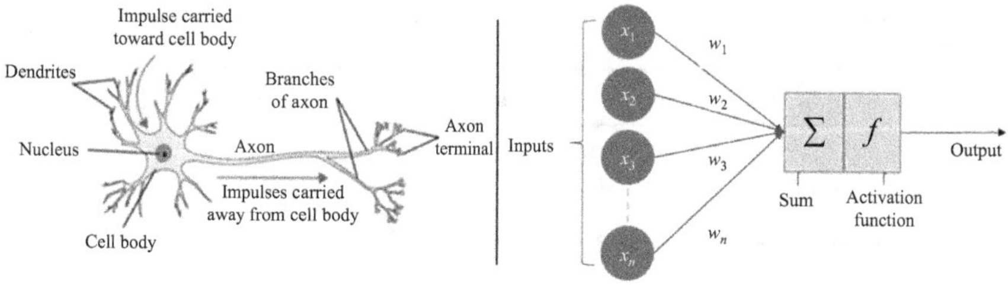

Figure 6.3 Biological neuron versus ANN

With technologies becoming more advanced, it is very possible to integrate artificial intelligence techniques into the telemedicine filed. Smart devices, nowadays, turn into an individual's digital twin, as they can sense and record all the necessary health conditions including blood pressure, pulse rate, calorie level, various genetic information, etc. All these information or entities can be considered as the input features of the neural network and feed into a pre-trained model to predict the diseases in real time. For example, ANN can assess the risk factors of osteoporosis. Osteoporosis is one of the very common diseases, which makes the bone so fragile that can lead to bone break with minor activity, even coughing. Luckily, the disease is preventable and treatable. The drastic effects of these diseases can be effectively decreased by revealing those people at risk, alerting and encouraging them to take preventive measures. Evaluating risk of osteoporosis can be viewed as a predictive problem, which can be resolved with an ANN.

6.3.2.3 Deep learning

The medical images are usually interpreted by a human specialist, which is limited due to its subjectivity, complexity of the image, variation of opinion across different interpreters, and fatigue. In the last decade, many researchers came up with the deep learning concepts with different algorithm namely convolution neural network (CNN), deep neural network, deep belief network, deep autoencoder, deep Boltzmann machine, and so forth. After the successful implementation of deep learning in other real world applications, it is also providing exciting solutions with good accuracy for medical imaging and is seen as a key method for future applications in health sector [8].

It is estimated that in future the accuracy of deep learning will suppress human capability and most of the diagnosis will be performed by intelligent machines to predict disease, prescribe medicine, and guide in treatment. This will revolutionize the various medical field like ophthalmology, pathology, cancer detection, radiology or prediction, and personalized medicine. Several recent researches showed that CNN is very successful in detection of breast cancer and lung cancer [9,10]. Surely, these are the blessing for healthcare industry, especially for telemedicine. For instance, dermatology is one of the key areas where telemedicine is offering its service. Definitely, dermatologist would like to rely on skin image rather than the patient's relaying of symptoms. Deep learning, more

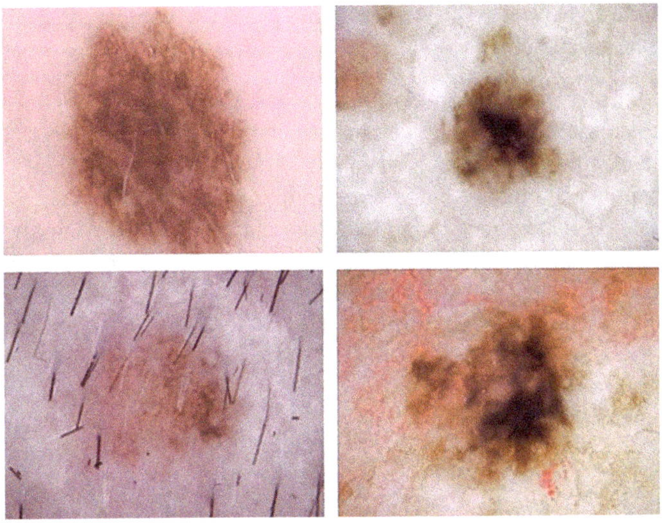

Figure 6.4 Skin cancer images: benign type (left column) and malignant type (right column) (Source: International Skin Imaging Collaboration Dataset)

specifically, the CNN can play a critical role here. CNN is well capable of segmenting, detecting, and localizing the disease symptoms in both 2-dimensional and 3-dimensional images. Patient can send the image of infected area through the healthcare apps and doctor can screen the image using a ready access CNN architecture to get deep understanding. Later doctor can prescribe the necessary action plan by blending discovered knowledge with his expertise. Figure 6.4 demonstrates two types of skin cancer images, benign and malignant. Thus, the application of deep learning in the telemedicine can leverage to fulfill the need of medical expertise in a particular domain.

6.3.2.4 Clustering algorithms

The clustering algorithm, which is the most important unsupervised learning technique, is the task of grouping a given data set into homogeneous clusters based on their similarities. In healthcare applications, it is an important method for efficiently detecting unknown and valuable information from huge heterogeneous health data. The main advantage of clustering is that less or no information is needed when analyzing the data [11]. In recent decades, clustering algorithms have been widely used in healthcare and telemedicine domain. For example, medical images have great potential to enhance the disease diagnosis, help predict the disease progression in telemedicine. Image clustering can provide great help to disease identification. A wide variety of methodologies have been presented for imaging clustering. Another application is clustering-based compression approaches which can help improve information transfer rate and storage capacity when connecting to cloud databases when related to telemedicine [12]. The commonly used clustering algorithms are discussed below:

(a) Partitioned clustering algorithm

In partitioned clustering method, the aim is to partition n objects into k clusters and improve the clustering quality based on an objective function. There is a need to define the number of clusters before partitioning the datasets into groups. k-means clustering is one of the most commonly used partitioned clustering algorithms. It classifies objects in multiple groups by similarity measures, such that objects within the same cluster are as similar as possible, whereas objects from different clusters are as dissimilar as possible [13]. The object function for minimization is defined as (6.3).

$$J = \sum_{j=1}^{k}\sum_{i=1}^{n} \left\|x_i^{(j)} - c_j\right\|^2 \tag{6.3}$$

where c_j represents centroids. A centroid is a location representing the center of the cluster. Sanchez-Morillo *et al.* [14] provided a pilot study aimed at early detecting acute exacerbation of respiratory symptoms using the k-means clustering algorithm. In [15], a hybrid hierarchical k-means clustering algorithm is used for detecting implausible EHRs vital signs and laboratory tests.

(b) Hierarchical clustering algorithm

The hierarchical clustering algorithm is mainly based on generating a cluster hierarchy by using heuristic splitting or merging techniques, which can be divided into two categories: agglomerative (bottom-up) or divisive (top-down) [16]. Agglomerative hierarchical (bottom-up) algorithms merge the objects that are close to each other then go to the next level, where it merges together clusters that are similar to each other. It operates this way until one cluster is formed. Divisive hierarchical clustering (top-down) starts with all data assigned to one cluster and then split them into disjoint clusters until each individual is reached. Belciug [17] used the hierarchical clustering approach for grouping the patients according to their length of stay in the hospital which can enhance the capability of hospital resource management.

(c) Density-based clustering algorithm

Density-based clustering works by identifying "dense" clusters of points, allowing it to learn clusters of arbitrary shapes and identify outliers in the data. Due to the ability to discover arbitrary-shaped clusters while preserving spatial proximity of data points, density-based clustering algorithm is a better choice for segmentation of structures such as skin lesions, tumors of breast, bone, and brain of medical images. Celebi *et al.* [18] presented a segmentation of pigmented skin lesion images based on density-based spatial clustering of applications with noise (DBSCAN) algorithm. Bandyopadhyay segmented brain tumor from Magnetic Resonance images (MRI) of human brain using k-means and DBSCAN clustering algorithm. It was proved that DBSCAN is efficient to handle noise points over k-means clustering [19].

(d) The fuzzy c-means clustering algorithm

Fuzzy *c*-means is a method of clustering which allows one piece of data to belong to two or more clusters with varying degrees of membership. In particular, a certain data-point that lies close to the center of a cluster will have a high degree of membership to that cluster and another data-point that lies far away from the center of a cluster will have a low degree of membership to that cluster [20]. A novel neighborhood intuitionistic fuzzy *c*-means clustering algorithm with a genetic algorithm (NIFCMGA) is proposed in [21]. It has been successfully applied to the clustering of different regions of magnetic resonance imaging and computerized tomography scanning. In a comparison of other clustering methods, the NIFCMGA clustering technology can also clearly index the tumor and reduce noise effects.

(e) Other clustering algorithms

More advanced or hybrid algorithms for clustering algorithms can be found in the literature. Hancer *et al.* [22] presented an artificial-bee-colony-based image clustering approach to finding the clusters of images, Lin *et al.* [21] presented functional principal component analysis and a randomized sparse clustering algorithm. Hsu [12] proposed a three dimensional histogram competitive Hopfield neural network clustering algorithm, which can greatly assist the doctors in real-time diagnosis.

It should be noted that most clustering algorithms above only allow objects to belong to one cluster. However, most real-world medical datasets have inherently overlapping information, which cannot be fully explained using one or exclusive clustering. In this case, overlapping clustering methods should be applied to help doctors to get a better diagnosis. One of the most common overlapping clustering algorithms is partition-based methods because of their simplicity and effectiveness. Examples include overlapping *k*-means, weighted overlapping *k*-means, and so forth [23].

6.3.2.5 Classification algorithms

Classification is a supervised learning technique. In classification, the idea is to predict the target class by analyzing the training dataset and finding proper boundaries for each target class. Different from the clustering, the class categories are known in classification. For example, a patient can be classified as "low risk" or "high risk" depending on the basis of the patient disease symptoms. Various classification algorithms used in healthcare and telemedicine applications are provided here.

(a) Support vector machines (SVM)

The objective of SVM is to find a hyperplane in an *N*-dimensional space that distinctly classifies the data points. The optimal hyperplane is that it has the largest distance to the nearest training-data point of any class (so-called functional margin). SVM is one of the most popular approaches that are used by researcher in healthcare field for classification. Barakat *et al.* [24] employed SVMs for the diagnosis and prediction of diabetes. Wannous *et al.* [25] designed a complete color processing chain. The developed tool can ensure stability independent of the image capture conditions or expert variability, which is a requirement in telemedicine environment, to achieve accurate and robust classification of skin tissues.

(b) K-nearest neighbor (K-NN)
K-NN classifier is one of the simplest classifiers, which is a type of instance-based learning, or lazy learning that categorizes an input by using its *k* nearest neighbors. K-NN is non-parametric method, which means that it does not make any assumptions about the probability distribution of the input. Jen *et al.* [26] used K-NN to analyze the relationship between cardiovascular disease and hypertension and the risk factors of various chronic diseases in order to build an early warning system to reduce the complication occurrence of these diseases.

(c) Decision trees (DT)
DT is a simple yet effective classification algorithm that uses a tree-like model of decisions and their possible consequences. Khan *et al.* [27] used DT for predicting the survivability of breast cancer patient and Chien *et al.* [28] proposed a universal hybrid DT classifier for classifying the activity of patients having chronic disease. They further improved the existing decision tree model to classify different activities of patients in more accurate manner [29].

(d) Other classification algorithms
Other research domains have led to a wide variety of other algorithms. Seera and Lim [30] proposed a hybrid intelligent system that consists of the Fuzzy Min–Max neural network, the Classification and Regression Tree, and the Random Forest model for medical data classification. A series of empirical studies using three benchmark medical data has been conducted to evaluate the efficacy of the hybrid model, which demonstrates its usefulness as a decision support system in practical environments. A telemedicine-based wound tissue prediction model was proposed for chronic wound image characterization in telemedicine environment [31]. The image with demographic information was captured by tele-medical agents using smartphone and send it to a tele-medical hub to classify the wound tissue type using linear discriminant analysis.

6.3.2.6 Bayesian network algorithm

Bayesian networks (BNs), also known as belief networks, is a probabilistic graphical model that represents model random variables and their influences between them via a directed acyclic graph (DAG). In DAG, each edge corresponds to a conditional dependency, and each node corresponds to a unique random variable. Bayesian networks have been a powerful tool in medical diagnostics. For example, a Bayesian network could represent the probabilistic relationships between diseases and symptoms. Given symptoms, the network can be used to compute the probabilities of the presence of various diseases.

Give respiratory diseases diagnosis as an example, let's assume that 20% of the individual in the population smoke, denoted as $P(S = yes) = 0.2$. It is also assumed that 3% of smokers get lung cancer, denoted as $P(L = yes|S = yes) = 0.3$. Figure 6.5 shows an initialized Bayesian network of respiratory diseases based on our

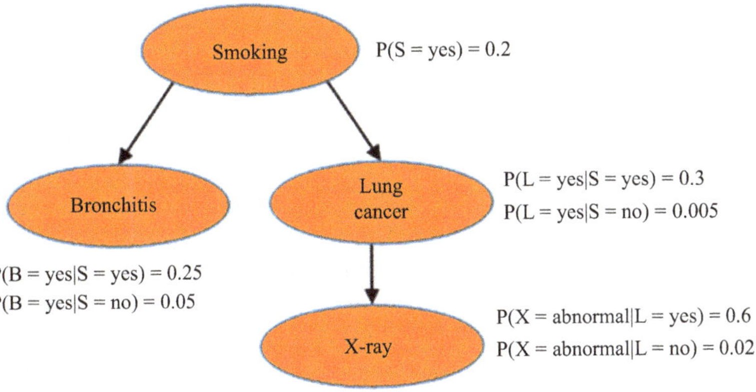

Figure 6.5 Initialized Bayesian network

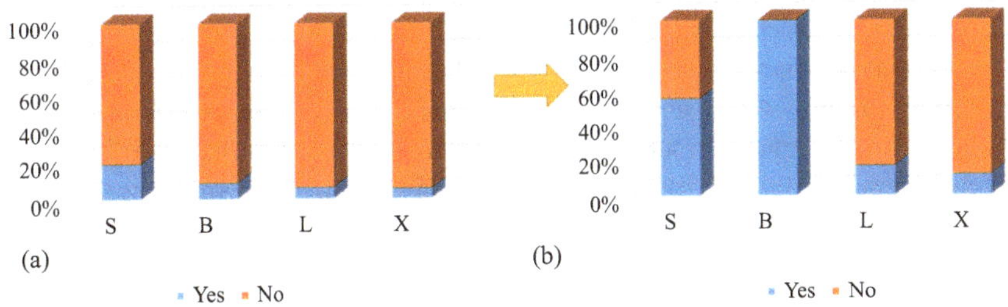

Figure 6.6 Bayesian network updating (a) initial probabilities and (b) updated probabilities

assumption. Without any observations, it achieved the probability of getting lung cancer is 0.064, namely P(L = yes) = 0.064 as shown in Figure 6.6. Suppose a patient visits with bronchitis, it instantiates with P(B = yes) = 1, then update the network. From the updated results in Figure 6.6(b), it is observed that the probability of lung cancer increases from 0.064 to 0.168 and so does the probability of other nodes. It is noticed that the probability of smoking increased significantly because smoking is one leading cause of bronchitis.

Bellot *et al.* [32] designed a smart agent-based telemedicine system using dynamic Bayesian networks aimed at giving a daily diagnosis on the hydration state of kidney disease people. In [33], Bayesian networks were used for risk prediction in the era of precision medicine. Lin *et al.* [34] proposed smooth Bayesian network model for early identification of high-cost patients with chronic obstructive pulmonary disease to decrease hospitalization rates and healthcare spending.

6.3.2.7 Adaptive fuzzy cognitive maps

Fuzzy cognitive map (FCM) is a relational representation among the various interactive elements like concepts, events, project resources, etc., to demonstrate the strength of impact of these elements. This technique is used for causal knowledge acquisition and representation. It also supports causal knowledge reasoning process in solving the decision-making problems, modeling and simulating complex systems. The strength of impact is determined through the FCMs weights which generate through a learning algorithm similar to the ANNs, genetic algorithms, swarm intelligence, and evolutionary computation, etc. [35]. The adaptation and learning algorithms are used to adapt the FCM model and adjust its weights. Due to the ability in representing structured knowledge, FCM has gained considerable interest in the various fields including business, economics, project planning, and reliability engineering. Recently, many efforts have been made to use FCM in medical applications to model systems, provide diagnosis, develop decision support systems, and medical assessment [36,37]. For example, FCM can be used to investigate the temporal dependencies between medical interventions (such as prescribing drugs) and health effects expressed by changes in patients' conditions. Discovering this type of temporal dependencies is very important in the field of telemedicine, especially for the post-discharge patient observation or remote health monitoring.

In research conducted by Wojciech and Alicja [38] showed the temporal dependencies for diabetes patients who are insulin deficient. The effect of the insulin dose varies with time and can be approximately estimated by doctors. The frequency of injections and blood glucose measurements are very important in this case. Here, the medical concept is developed based on the insulin dose and the blood glucose measurements using notation and code. Three levels of insulin dose are used which are represented using three codes i.e. 33, 34, and 35 for regular, NPH and ultralente, respectively*. The measurements are symbolized with the set of numbers as shown in Table 6.3.

The concepts that refer to the glucose measurements are assigned to separate labels for different parts of the day. However, the concepts of the insulin doses are not divided this way. To resolve this issue, the day scale of 0-24 hours was divided into four time slots denoted by 1 (0–9), 2 (9–13), 3 (13–19), and 4 (19–24). Every time slot was defined by its "begin" and "end" times, given units of hours. Thus, the concept 343 means that the insulin NPH is injected at the third slot of a day or in evening. After the setup of the medical intervention and measurement concepts, FCM can be deployed to obverse their interdependencies for the individual or entire

Table 6.3 Representation of measurements

Code	Measurement
58	Pre-breakfast blood glucose
59	Post-breakfast blood glucose
60	Pre-lunch blood glucose
61	Post-lunch blood glucose
62	Pre-supper blood glucose
63	Post-supper blood glucose

*The details names and abbreviation of the insulin types are not provided in the original resource

patients. Usually, the interdependency is expressed with the weights of FCM edges, which ranges from −0.01 to 0.1. The generalization of FCMs over the entire population is very complex. Due to the complexity, an exemplary FCMs with the values of weights greater than 0.01 and less than −0.01 are shown in Figure 6.7.

The arcs can be interpreted as the interaction between concepts and their possible effects. For example, in the FCMs showed in Figure 6.8, the highest negative value of the weight, i.e., −0.060399, is achieved for the arc 342 → 582. This signifies that the NPH (code 34) insulin dose lowers the level of pre-breakfast

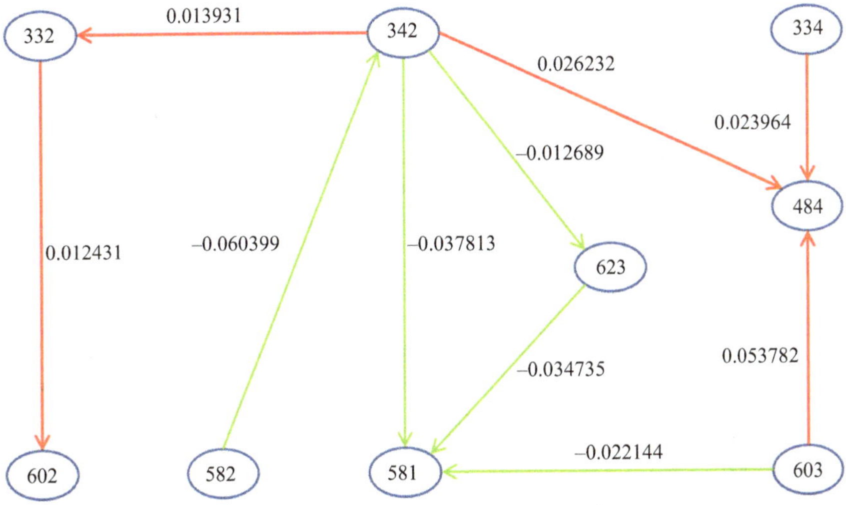

Figure 6.7 Fuzzy cognitive map

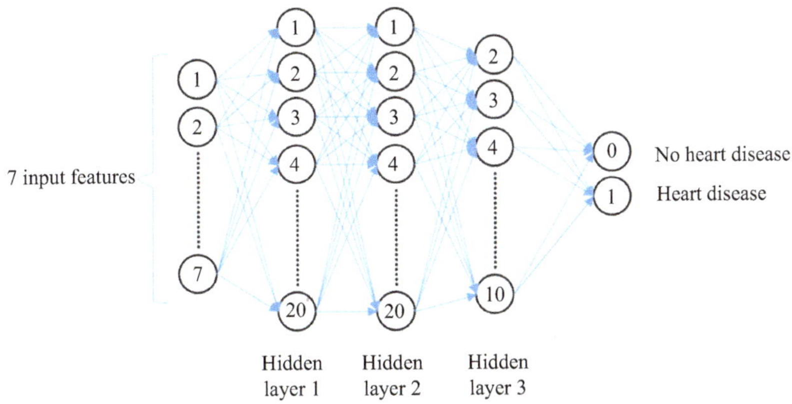

Figure 6.8 Architecture of the MLP classifier

blood glucose (code 58) label when it is injected in the second slot (as third digit of the concept is 2) of a day. On the other hand, some positive values greater than 0.01 can be achieved like the arc 603 → 484 i.e. 0.022144. However, this large value is not surprising if the wrong time slot is assigned to the concept. In conclusion, analysis of this type of interdependency can facilities many aspects of medical concepts from the perspective of telemedicine.

6.3.2.8 Text mining

Text mining, commonly known as text data mining, is the process of discovering knowledge from voluminous text. It usually involves the procedure of structuring input text, finding out the patterns of the structured data and finally evaluation and interpretation the output. Some common text mining tasks include text categorization, text clustering, concept/entity extraction, sentiment analysis, document summarization, and entity relation modeling. The supreme goal is to fit text into data for analysis using natural language processing and analytical methods. Recently, the application of text mining has been deployed successfully in a variety of fields starting from government to business. All these fields use text mining for records analysis and searching documents relevant to their daily activities. For example, legal professionals may use text mining for e-discovery, while government and security agencies may use for national security and intelligent purpose.

Recently, text mining leaps into the biomedical field to assist studies in protein docking, protein interaction, and protein-diseases associations [39,40]. The overarching idea of text mining fits well into the field of telemedicine. The telemedicine stakeholders continue to generate a large amount of data including patients' textual datasets, demographic information, and adverse reports. Text mining can facilitate the stratification and indexing of specific patient record i.e. textual dataset of symptoms, side effects, diagnostic tests, and other EHRs, which enables the medical practitioners to extract knowledge from unstructured documents in the telemedicine domain. In addition, security in telemedicine is a very sensitive matter as it deals with the patients' confidential information. This derives the service providers and insurers to be responsible to ensure patients' safety and privacy. Here, text mining can play a role of detecting attempts of gaining unauthorized access to a telemedicine web application [41].

6.4 Case study

This section demonstrates two health care-related case studies. The objective of this demonstration is to explain how the data mining tools can be used in telemedicine platform and how efficient it is. The dataset used in these two case studies are related to heart diseases and breast cancer diagnosis[†]. ANN is used in both cases to predict the presence of heart diseases and breast cancer for a particular patient.

[†]The dataset are collected from the UC Irvine machine learning repository

6.4.1 Heart diseases prediction

The original dataset contains 14 attributes, but to make the case simple, it refers to using a subset of 8 of them. The dataset has 297 entities with 8 fields, namely age, sex, chest pain type (cp), resting blood pressure (trestbps), serum cholesterol label (col), fasting blood sugar (fbs), resting electrocardiographic results (restecg), and maximum obtained heart rate (thalach). The last field refers to the presence of heart diseases in the patient. It is integer valued 0 (no presence) and 1 (presence of heart diseases). The chest pain type (cp) is the categorical variable containing four integer values with 1, 2, 3, and 4 representing typical angina, atypical angina, non-anginal pain, and asymptomatic, respectively. The resting blood pressures are in mmHg and the serum cholesterol is in mg/dl. The Fasting blood sugar (fbs) is presented with two integer values, 1 if fbs is greater than 120 and 0 otherwise. Table 6.4 shows some exemplary entities from the dataset.

A feed forward ANN, Multilayer perceptron (MLP)[‡], is used to train the dataset and build the heart diseases, predictive model. In this training process, the MLP classifier uses 3 hidden layers containing 20, 20, and 10 nodes, respectively. Figure 6.8 demonstrates the architecture of the MLP classifier. The training starts with the initial learning rate 0.001 and iterates 2,000 times until it convergences. All other parameters were set defaults as the scikit-learn MLP classifier suggests. For example, the activation function for hidden layer was "relu" and weight optimization technique was "adam". The dataset was divided into training and testing sets. Among the 297 entities, 250 entities were used for training purposes and rest of the entities were used for testing purposes. Notice that, the chest pain type is a categorical variable with integer-valued from 1 to 4. It needs to be prepossessed before it is fed into the training model. Hence, the categories column (except the binary category) is converted into one-hot encoding[§] and rest of the columns

Table 6.4 Heart diseases data (five entities)

	Age	Sex	cp	trestbps	chol	fbs	thalach	label
1	63	1	1	145	233	1	150	0
2	67	1	4	160	286	0	108	1
3	67	1	4	120	229	0	129	1
4	37	1	3	130	250	0	187	0
5	41	0	2	130	204	0	172	0

[‡]MLP is a class of feedforward artificial neural network. It consists of at least three layers of nodes: an input layer, a hidden layer and an output layer. Except for the input nodes, each node is a neuron that uses a nonlinear activation function.

[§]One hot encoding is a process by which categorical variables are converted into a form that could be provided to ML algorithms to do a better job in prediction.

are normalised. After finishing the training process, about 99% accuracy on the training datasets and 92% accuracy on testing datasets are achieved.

$$model = MLPClassifier(hidden\_layer\_sizes = (20, 20, 10), lr = 0.001,$$

$$max\_iter = 2000)model.fit(Xtrain, Ytrain)testResult = model.predict(testdata)$$

Some testing results are shown in Table 6.5. Notice that, the model did not see these testing data before.

After building the predictive model, now it can be used to predict the presence of heart diseases in particular patients. In real time when a doctor interacts with the patients, he/she can obtain the required patient's information like age, sex, type of chest pain in the category of 1, 2, 3, or 4, etc. With the help of telemedicine smart technology or from the data warehouse, the doctor can access the patient's resting blood pressure, serum cholesterol label, fasting blood sugar, maximum heart rate or other information. Based on this observation, the doctor can input the data into the system to predict whether a patient prone to heart disease or not. For example, if a doctor has the information as 57, 0, 2, 130, 236, 0, and 174 for age, sex, chest pain type, resting blood pressure, serum cholesterol, fasting blood sugar, and maximum heart rate, respectively. He feeds these parameters into the model and noticed that the patient is likely to have heart diseases as shown in Figure 6.9.

Table 6.5 Test on heart diseases dataset

	Age	**Sex**	**cp**	**trestbps**	**chol**	**fbs**	**thalach**	**Prediction**	**Actual**
1	57	1	2	124	261	0	141	1	1
2	60	0	1	150	240	0	171	0	0
3	43	1	4	115	303	0	181	***1***	***0***
4	40	1	4	152	223	0	181	1	1
5	56	1	2	130	221	0	163	0	0

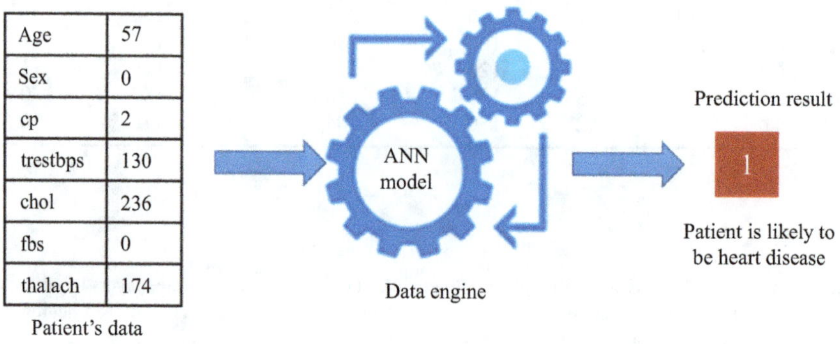

Figure 6.9 Model integration into the data engine

6.4.2 Breast cancer prediction

Breast cancer is one of the very common diseases for women. It is estimated that one out of eight women will develop breast cancer in their lifetime. However, proper diagnosis and treatment can increase the number of survivals. Patients can save themselves from this cancer through regular follow-up and consultation with their physicians. However, most of the women develop breast cancer due to their unawareness of this disease, even though the condition a woman's breast can be easily diagnosed and possible to predict the presence of cancer through the analysis of diagnostic data coming from mammography. Once the status is identified, the patient can follow-up with the doctor remotely using telemedicine platform to get effective suggestions and treatment.

The data used in this case study has a total of 569 patients' breast diagnosis information. The data has 10 parameters, which are explained below:

1. radius_mean: mean of distances from the center to points on the perimeter
2. texture_mean: standard deviation of gray-scale values
3. perimeter_mean: mean size of the core tumor
4. area_mean
5. smoothness_mean: mean of local variation in radius lengths
6. compactness_mean: mean of perimeter^2/area – 1.0
7. concavity_mean: mean of the severity of concave portions of the contour
8. concave_points_mean: mean for the number of concave portions of the contour
9. symmetry_mean
10. fractal_dimension_mean: mean for "coastline approximation."

A sample dataset of 5 patients is shown in Table 6.6. The first column is the patients' ID and the second column indicates their corresponding diagnosis result, where M for malignant type breast cancer and B for benign type of cancer. The rest of the columns contain the numeric values for the parameter listed above.

To train this data, the ANN architecture as shown in Figure 6.10 is used. The training starts with the initial learning rate of 0.001 and iterates 2,000 times until it convergences. All other parameters were set to defaults according to the scikit-learn MLP classifier documentation. The dataset was divided into training and testing sets. The entire dataset was shuffled and kept the last 100 entities for the

Table 6.6 Breast cancer data

ID	L	rad	tex	peri	area	smth	cpt	cvt	cnv	smt	frac
844959	M	17.99	10.38	122.8	1,001	0.1184	0.2776	0.3001	0.1471	0.2419	0.0787
842517	M	20.57	17.77	132.9	1,326	0.0847	0.0786	0.0869	0.0701	0.1812	0.0566
843009	M	19.69	21.25	130	1,203	0.1096	0.1599	0.1974	0.1279	0.2069	0.0599
851042	B	13.54	14.36	87.46	566.3	0.0978	0.0813	0.0666	0.0478	0.1885	0.0577
851065	B	13.08	15.71	85.63	520	0.1075	0.127	0.0457	0.0311	0.1967	0.0681

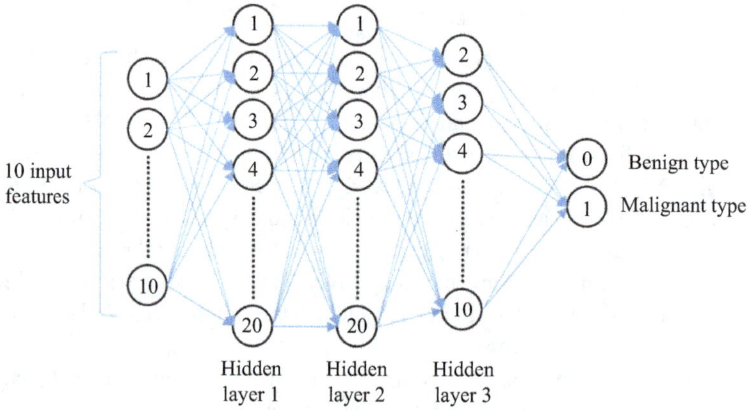

Figure 6.10 Architecture of MLP classifier for breast cancer diagnosis

Table 6.7 Testing result on breast cancer dataset

	rad	tex	peri	area	smth	cpt	cvt	cnv	smt	frac	P	A
1	19.44	18.82	128.1	1,167	0.1089	0.145	0.2256	0.119	0.182	0.061	M	M
2	11.74	14.69	76.31	426	0.0809	0.097	0.0673	0.026	0.149	0.068	B	B
3	12.83	15.73	82.89	506.9	0.0904	0.0827	0.0583	0.0308	0.171	0.0591	B	B
4	15.46	23.95	103.8	731.3	0.1183	0.187	0.203	0.0852	0.181	0.0708	M	M
5	13.16	20.54	84.06	538.7	0.0734	0.0528	0.0180	0.0126	0.171	0.0589	B	B

testing purpose. The rest of the entities were used for training purposes. There are no categorical variables, hence all the columns were normalized before training the model. The original diagnosis result (label) of the dataset was converted to the binary variable i.e. 1 for M (malignant type) and 0 for B (benign type). After finishing the training process, more than 99% accuracy on the training datasets and 93% accuracy on testing datasets is obtained. Some testing results are shown in Table 6.7. Here, the second last column (P) indicates the prediction of breast cancer type while the last column (A) shows the actual label.

These types of predictions can help the medical professionals in providing quick responses regarding patient health. Based on this prediction, doctors can do further investigation or can give some prescription or suggestion to the patient.

6.5 Challenges of deploying data mining techniques into telemedicine

With the emergence of EMRs and EHRs, the volume of medical data is growing exponentially. The abundance of medical data can lead to a number of benefits for healthcare providers, including more cost-effective ways to store information, greater accuracy of diagnosis and improved workflow. However, the datasets usually are very large, complex, heterogeneous, and hierarchical and vary in quality. The application of data mining, knowledge discovery techniques to the explosion of datasets is presenting significant challenges for healthcare IT organizations. The first challenge is data preprocessing. Due to complexity of clinical data such as clinical notes, images, videos, pathology, reports, biospecimen data, data preprocessing, and transformation are required before data mining techniques can be applied. How to link data from multiple sources is challenging. In the past decade, a great effort has been made to develop data standards, such as systematized nomenclature of medicine-clinical terms (SNOMED CT), medical subject headings (MeSH), Clinical Data Interchange Standards Consortium (CDISC), controlled vocabularies and ontologies for structural or semantic representations of data and metadata. However, among the standards themselves, the heterogeneity still exists. In the telemedicine context, the increasing adoption of wearable devices has great potential to help diagnosis for patients. Those devices generate large amounts of data providing richer picture of the patient's condition, which can support patients and physicians in disease management and treatment. However, given the relative simplicity of most past tele-monitoring trials, the knowledge on how to interpret data from wearable devices is underdeveloped [42]. The second challenge is big data storage. For example, a wide variety of digital imaging technologies may simultaneously produce a large amount of data or images for each patient. Hence, the process and storage of them are considered as a big problem. The third challenge is real-time mining. In healthcare and telemedicine scenarios, there are situations that require not only access to data, but also processing it in real-time manner and on an integrated view of the patient's medical history and the hospital information system. With the explosion of big data, there is a growing gap between more powerful storage and retrieval systems and the clinicians' ability to effectively analyze and act on the information they contain. The fourth challenge is medical data visualization. The medical features representation by using the data visualization can provide better data analytical performance. For example, it can help to identify dangerous situations for patients thus communicate with patients efficiently, which could guarantee quality control of patients' treatments, and reduce health-care costs. Unfortunately, interpreting big data and efficiently showing information for good understanding are difficult tasks due to the complexity of medical data format [43]. The last but not the least challenge is medical data security and privacy during data mining. Medical data are primarily generated through the delivery of patient care. Therefore, mining of medical data inevitably is involved with privacy and legal issues. The patient's records must be seen only by the authorized personnel and the medical record's integrity should be maintained between the doctors and the patients and vice-versa. However, digitized medical data could potentially be misused, damage caused cannot be reversed [44]. The fear of inadequate data protection negatively influences the positive assessment of health technology among doctors and patients.

6.6 Conclusion

In the last decade, data mining draws great attention in the field of telemedicine. It provides a comprehensive way to enable thorough understanding of needs for the healthcare organization. As illustrated in this chapter, data mining is very efficient in knowledge discovery, which can be used to make trustworthy decision that brings success to the telemedicine. In return, all the stakeholders of the telemedicine platform are getting benefits, especially the patients. It is observed that patients are more likely to depend on remote health monitoring and observation. Data mining requires appropriate technologies and analytical techniques for its successful implementation. Obviously, technologies are more sophisticated than before. Many tech giant companies are focusing on the development of technology for the telehealth industry. In parallel, different analytical techniques become enriched in both theory and application. Now, data mining requires a system to integrate all the components for reporting and tracking the data generated in the telehealth organization. Once the system is ready, data mining can continue to discover knowledge and provide feedback to the telemedicine stakeholders, which can be one of the key components to create a good business strategy. Today, there have been many efforts with the goal of successful integration and application of data mining in the telehealth industry. Primarily, these efforts include the possibility of finding out the different phenomenon and hidden patterns in data sets in the healthcare domain. Recently, many researchers have showed their effort in machine learning techniques to enhance the disease predictive power based on the available medical data and patients' health-related information. All these efforts make the clinical diagnosis and disease prediction easy and trustworthy. However, the medical data are copious in nature, sometimes unstructured, different and widely distributed. The data must be collected and stored in a cloud in structured and organized forms to feed them into the data mining engine. The data mining engine, which is already enabled with data analytics techniques to process structured data and to discover knowledge. The knowledge that can help in providing medical and other services to the patients. The telemedicine industry that uses data mining applications has the possibility to predict future requests, needs, desires, and conditions of the patients and to make adequate and optimal decisions about their treatments. With the future development of information communication technologies, data mining will achieve its full potential in the discovery of knowledge hidden in the medical data. Thus, the integration of data mining techniques into the telemedicine platform will bring two-way privilege for both the healthcare professionals and patients.

References

[1] Rokach L, and Maimon O. Clustering methods. In Data Mining and Knowledge Discovery Handbook. 2005 (pp. 321–52). Springer, Boston, MA.

[2] Apté C, and Weiss S. Data mining with decision trees and decision rules. Future Generation Computer Systems. 1997;13(2–3):197–210.

[3] Fayyad U, Piatetsky-Shapiro G, and Smyth P. From data mining to knowledge discovery in databases. AI Magazine. 1996;17(3):37.

[4] Rosser JJ, Parker BC, and Vignesh V. Medical Applications of Drones for Disaster Relief: A Review of the Literature. Surgical technology international. 2018 Nov;33.

[5] Han J, Kamber M, and Pei J. Data mining concepts and techniques, third edition. The Morgan Kaufmann Series in Data Management Systems. 2011 (pp. 83–124). Elsevier, Waltham, MA.

[6] Kotsiantis S, and Kanellopoulos D. Association rules mining: A recent overview. GESTS International Transactions on Computer Science and Engineering. 2006;32(1):71–82.

[7] Amato F, López A, Peña-Méndez EM, Vaňhara P, Hampl A, and Havel J. Artificial neural networks in medical diagnosis. Journal of Applied Biomedicine. 2013;11(2):47–58.

[8] Razzak MI, Naz S, and Zaib A. Deep learning for medical image processing: Overview, challenges and the future. In Classification in BioApps. 2018 (pp. 323–50). Springer, Cham.

[9] Sun W, Tseng TL, Zhang J, and Qian W. Enhancing deep convolutional neural network scheme for breast cancer diagnosis with unlabeled data. Computerized Medical Imaging and Graphics. 2017;57:4–9.

[10] Zhang J, Xia Y, Cui H, and Zhang Y. Pulmonary nodule detection in medical images: a survey. Biomedical Signal Processing and Control. 2018;43:138–47.

[11] Haraty RA, Dimishkieh M, and Masud M. An enhanced k-means clustering algorithm for pattern discovery in healthcare data. International Journal of Distributed Sensor Networks. 2015;11(6):615740.

[12] Chakraborty C. Performance analysis of compression techniques for chronic wound image transmission under smartphone-enabled tele-wound network, Int. Journal of E-Health and Medical Communications (IJEHMC). 2019; 10(2):1–15.

[13] Hartigan JA, and Wong MA. Algorithm AS 136: A k-means clustering algorithm. Journal of the Royal Statistical Society. Series C (Applied Statistics). 1979;28(1):100–8.

[14] Sanchez-Morillo D, Fernandez-Granero MA, and Jiménez AL. Detecting COPD exacerbations early using daily telemonitoring of symptoms and k-means clustering: a pilot study. Medical & Biological Engineering & Computing. 2015;53(5):441–51.

[15] Estiri H, Klann JG, and Murphy SN. A clustering approach for detecting implausible observation values in electronic health records data. BMC Medical Informatics and Decision Making. 2019;19(1):142.

[16] Bansal JC, Sharma H, and Jadon SS. Artificial bee colony algorithm: a survey. International Journal of Advanced Intelligence Paradigms. 2013;5 (1–2):123–59.

[17] El-Darzi E, Abbi R, Vasilakis C, Gorunescu F, Gorunescu M, and Millard P. Length of stay-based clustering methods for patient grouping. In Intelligent Patient Management. 2009 (pp. 39–56). Springer, Berlin, Heidelberg.

[18] Celebi ME, Aslandogan YA, and Bergstresser PR. Mining biomedical images with density-based clustering. In International Conference on Information Technology: Coding and Computing (ITCC'05)-volume II. 2005 Apr 4 (Vol. 1, pp. 163–8). IEEE.

[19] Bandyopadhyay SK, and Paul TU. Segmentation of brain tumour from MRI image analysis of k-means and DBSCAN clustering. International Journal of Research in Engineering and Science. 2013;1(1):48–57.

[20] Bezdek JC, Ehrlich R, and Full W. FCM: The fuzzy c-means clustering algorithm. Computers & Geosciences. 1984;10(2–3):191–203.

[21] Huang CW, Lin KP, Wu MC, Hung KC, Liu GS, and Jen CH. Intuitionistic fuzzy *c*-means clustering algorithm with neighborhood attraction in segmenting medical image. Soft Computing. 2015;19(2):459–70.

[22] Hancer E, Ozturk C, and Karaboga D. Artificial bee colony based image clustering method. In 2012 IEEE Congress on Evolutionary Computation. 2012 June 10 (pp. 1–5). IEEE.

[23] Khanmohammadi S, Adibeig N, and Shanehbandy S. An improved overlapping k-means clustering method for medical applications. Expert Systems with Applications. 2017;67:12–18.

[24] Barakat N, Bradley AP, and Barakat MN. Intelligible support vector machines for diagnosis of diabetes mellitus. IEEE Transactions on Information Technology in Biomedicine. 2010;14(4):1114–20.

[25] Wannous H, Treuillet S, and Lucas Y. Robust tissue classification for reproducible wound assessment in telemedicine environments. Journal of Electronic Imaging. 2010;19(2):023002.

[26] Jen CH, Wang CC, Jiang BC, Chu YH, and Chen MS. Application of classification techniques on development an early-warning system for chronic illnesses. Expert Systems with Applications. 2012;39(10):8852–8.

[27] Khan MU, Choi JP, Shin II, and Kim M. Predicting breast cancer survivability using fuzzy decision trees for personalized healthcare. In 2008 30th Annual International Conference of the IEEE Engineering in Medicine and Biology Society. 2008 August 20 (pp. 5148–51). IEEE.

[28] Chien C, and Pottie GJ. A universal hybrid decision tree classifier design for human activity classification. In 2012 Annual International Conference of the IEEE Engineering in Medicine and Biology Society. 2012 August 28 (pp. 1065–8). IEEE.

[29] Chakraborty C, Gupta B, Ghosh SK, Das D, and Chakraborty C. Telemedicine Supported Chronic Wound Tissue Prediction Using Different Classification Approach. Journal of Medical Systems. 2016;40(3):1–12.

[30] Seera M, and Lim CP. A hybrid intelligent system for medical data classification. Expert Systems with Applications. 2014;41(5):2239–49.

[31] Chakraborty C, Gupta B, Ghosh SK, Das DK, and Chakraborty C. Telemedicine supported chronic wound tissue prediction using classification approaches. Journal of Medical Systems. 2016;40(3):68.

[32] Bellot D, Boyer A, and Charpillet F. Designing smart agent based telemedicine systems using dynamic Bayesian networks: an application to kidney disease people. 4th International Workshop on Enterprise Networking

and Computing in Health Care Industry – HEALTHCOM 2002, Nancy, France, p. 8.

[33] Arora P, Boyne D, Slater JJ, Gupta A, Brenner DR, and Druzdzel MJ. Bayesian networks for risk prediction using real-world data: a tool for precision medicine. Value in Health. 2019;22(4):439–45.

[34] Lin S, Zhang Q, Chen F, Luo L, Chen L, and Zhang W. Smooth Bayesian network model for the prediction of future high-cost patients with COPD. International Journal of Medical Informatics. 2019;126:147–55.

[35] Salmeron JL, and Froelich W. Dynamic optimization of fuzzy cognitive maps for time series forecasting. Knowledge-Based Systems. 2016;105:29–37.

[36] Papageorgiou EI, Stylios CD, and Groumpos PP. An integrated two-level hierarchical system for decision making in radiation therapy based on fuzzy cognitive maps. IEEE Transactions on Biomedical Engineering. 2003;50(12): 1326–39.

[37] Georgopoulos VC, and Stylios CD. Supervisory fuzzy cognitive map structure for triage assessment and decision support in the emergency department. In Simulation and Modeling Methodologies, Technologies and Applications. 2015 (pp. 255–69). Springer, Cham.

[38] Froelich W, and Wakulicz-Deja A. Mining temporal medical data using adaptive fuzzy cognitive maps. In 2009 2nd Conference on Human System Interactions 2009. May 21 (pp. 16–23). IEEE.

[39] Papanikolaou N, Pavlopoulos GA, Theodosiou T, and Iliopoulos I. Protein–protein interaction predictions using text mining methods. Methods. 2015;74:47–53.

[40] Liem DA, Murali S, and Sigdel D *et al.* Phrase mining of textual data to analyze extracellular matrix protein patterns across cardiovascular disease. American Journal of Physiology-Heart and Circulatory Physiology. 2018;315(4):H910–24.

[41] Adeva JG, Pikatza JM, Florez S, and Sobrado FJ. Intrusion detection using text mining in a web-based telemedicine system. In Australasian Joint Conference on Artificial Intelligence. 2005 (pp. 1009–14). Springer, Berlin, Heidelberg.

[42] Mlakar M, Puddu PE, Somrak M, Bonfiglio S, and Luštrek M. Chiron and HeartMan research projects. Mining telemonitored physiological data and patient-reported outcomes of congestive heart failure patients. PloS One. 2018;13(3):e0190323.

[43] Galletta A, Carnevale L, Bramanti A, and Fazio M. An innovative methodology for big data visualization for telemedicine. IEEE Transactions on Industrial Informatics. 2018;15(1):490–7.

[44] Simon S, Evans JS, Benjamin A, Delano D, and Bates D. Patients' attitudes toward electronic health information exchange: qualitative study. Journal of Medical Internet Research. 2009;11(3):e30.

Chapter 7

Social work and tele-mental health services for rural and remote communities

Lia Bryant[1], Bridget Garnham[1], Deirdre Tedmanson[2] and Sophie Diamandi[1]

Rural and remote communities often have complex and diverse mental health needs and inadequate mental health services and infrastructure. Information and communication technologies provide an array of means for connecting rural and remote communities to specialist mental health practitioners as used in psychiatry and psychology. Social work practitioners have additional skills to bring to tele-mental health and in particular, the socio-cultural dimensions that impact on mental health and therefore the ability to recognize and explore these with participants, as well as, refer participant to resources and services outside of or in addition to psychology or medical fields. However, despite this potential, a review of international literature reveals that information and communication technologies (ICTs) have not attained widespread uptake in social work practice in rural communities. This chapter reviews the social work literature on ICTs, the tele-psychology and psychiatry literature and provides suggestions on how to enhance engagement with ICT by social workers to implement and provide social work services tailored to rural and remote community needs, values and preferences.

7.1 Introduction

A deficiency of mental health services combined with a substantial unmet need for mental health support is an on-going issue across rural communities that contributes to significant mental health disparities between urban and rural Australia. Australia is a vast landmass with 'six million people dispersed across the 7.5 million square kilometres' [1, p. 1]. However, 70% of the population resides in major cities with 18% occupying inner regional, 9% outer regional and 2% remote and very remote areas [2]. This often translates into rural and remote communities being geographically and socially isolated, inadequately resourced by Government

[1]School of Psychology, Social Work and Social Policy, University of South Australia, Magill, Adelaide, Australia
[2]University of South Australia College, Adelaide, South Australia, Australia

social service infrastructure and unable to attract and retain professional and specialist mental health practitioners. Whilst prevalence of mental illness is similar across the nation, the proportion of psychiatrists and psychologists in rural areas are 36% and 57% of those in major cities respectively [3].

Given the apparently insurmountable challenges of resourcing rural and remote communities in place, ICTs with applications for connecting rural communities to specialist mental health practitioners, self-help information and services and supports irrespective of physical location are increasing being developed. However, despite the potential offered by ICT to address service gaps and improve access, deliver cost-effective and innovative services and improve mental health for rural residents, a review of Australian and international literature reveals that ICT has not attained widespread uptake into social work practice or implementation in rural communities. Indeed, a theme focused on this paradox courses its way through the literature and provides some insights into the reluctance of the social work profession to engage ICT in practice. This chapter reviews the social work literature on ICT and draws on research on the efficacy of tele-psychology to address some of the concerns voiced by the profession concerning the nature of the therapeutic alliance and interpersonal communication via videoconferencing. Finally, the chapter provides suggestions for how to enhance engagement with ICT by social workers to implement and provide mental health services and supports tailored to community values, needs and preferences that are commensurate with the values of the social work profession.

7.2 Rural heterogeneity and complexity challenge mental health service provision

The lack of health and welfare services in rural areas and their decreasing availability over time is an issue that has been well documented [e.g. 4–8]. It is now an expectation that living in rural places is commensurate within adequate healthcare and service provision. Whilst distance and spatial dispersion are challenges, equally challenging are how to deliver services to the complex constitution of rural Australia made up of multiple subjectivities, experiences, histories and practices [9]. The understanding of rurality as a unifying concept has had dire implications for service delivery with people who are constituted outside the dominant understandings of 'rural subject' rendered invisible. For example, Cloke *et al.* [10] have argued that rurality and homelessness are discursively non-coupled and Hughes [11] has shown that despite the growth of single parents in rural areas, the rural is overwhelmingly perceived of as sustained by the traditional heterosexual family [9]. A range of specific health and welfare needs in relation to diversity and difference requires addressing in rural areas in ways that enable a more appropriate matching of services and needs.

In relation to service gaps and multiplicity of need, mental health services are one of the most complex and inaccessible in rural Australia. Rural areas tend to experience higher rates of psychological distress [12,13] linked to adverse social conditions in rural communities including higher rates of poverty and unemployment, poorer standards of education, housing and health and other facets of social disadvantage and marginalization that impact upon the well-being and mental health of rural people [14,15]. In addition, there are precipitating contexts for poor mental health that are particularly part of rural experiences such as environmental degradation [16], drought and reduced water allocation for farmers [17] and bushfire and flood disasters [18].

Very often rural communities do not have mental health units or specialist services and so people seeking help for mental health issues need to present to emergency departments or GPs and may be transferred to mental health services outside the community and away from family [12,19]. Crotty *et al.* [20, p. 213] document some of the issues pertaining to mental health services in rural places including:

> lack of access to psychiatrists and reliance upon GPs to provide primary mental health care; limited availability of non-governmental community services for referral; professional isolation; excessive GP workloads; limited facilities for crisis care and transportation to and management of acute clients by metropolitan tertiary services.

Whilst the recruitment, retention and capacity of mental health professionals are recognized as a major issue impacting upon mental health service provision [20], the way in which services are socially structured through particular discursive constructions of 'health' and 'mental health' can also create tensions in rural communities. For instance, Muir-Cochrane *et al.* [21] found that the separation of mental health and health services, as well as an overly clinical focus and neglect of social support needs, was detrimental in terms of the mental health needs of older people living in rural South Australia. The literature also reveals that rural cultures of stoicism and self-reliance, the close social proximity of community members that inhibit anonymity and the stigma associated with mental illness are considered to prevent help seeking in rural communities [21–24].

7.3 Bridging the rural/urban divide using ICT for mental health service provision

ICT is often advanced as a panacea for delivering mental health services to rural and remote communities [25,26]. This is often because ICT is considered a cost-efficient solution to overcoming social isolation and resource deprivation to reach vulnerable people in order to provide psycho-social services and support drawing on personnel and expertise located in urban centres. However, the advancement of ICT as a potential solution is also an outworking of the expansion and integration of ICT across a multitude of facets of everyday life. Indeed, ICT provides an integral framework for a contemporary form of social organization and social practice coined 'the network' society where 'virtuality becomes an essential dimension of our reality' [27]. In a network society, individuals belong to and participate in virtual communities hosted by social networking apps such as Facebook, Twitter and Instagram and enabled through webpages and e-mail in ways that both overlap with and extend non-virtual communities. Indeed, to differentiate between 'real' and 'virtual' society is increasingly nonsensical as the boundaries and characteristics of the two increasingly intermesh. The principle feature of ICT is that it enables users to communicate and access information without geographical restriction. However, the technologies that constitute ICT have proliferated to such an extent that to use the term 'ICT' conveys little of the exact nature of the technology or communication in question. The definition offered by West and Heath [28, p. 211] captures some of the possibilities;

> Broadly speaking, ICT is the term applied to a range of tools and media that provide the infrastructure for communication and includes devices such as telephones and computers with all of their applications including internet, email, mobile telephones, instant messaging and social networking.

Through technologies that connect users to each other and to the virtual spaces of the internet, ICT includes modes of synchronous interpersonal interaction in real time such as video-conferencing and virtual chat rooms as well as asynchronous modes that do not rely on simultaneous usages such as e-mail and text messages. As Mishna *et al.* [29] observe, modes of ICT shape the possibilities for how users interact and communicate. Webcams are a medium for visual and audio communication that provides the closest approximation to face-to-face inter-personal interaction and can be used to facilitate one-on-one or group discussion. Specialized video-conferencing software can enhance this modality through the inclusion of technologies such as online 'white' boards, break-out rooms and online documents that can be viewed by all. Smart phones not only provide opportunities for audio, textual and visual communication between users but also a platform for access to the wealth of possibilities for information and communication offered through the internet and custom designed software apps and a means for creating and sharing videos and photos. The evolution and permutations of ICT have thus transformed and continues to transform, the geographical, temporal and spatial nature of communication and access to information as well as the possibilities for the ways in which users can connect and communicate using verbal, textual and visual mediums. Taken collectively, ICT, therefore, provides a diverse range of potential applications for social work services to bridge geographical and resource divides between urban and rural places and communities.

7.4 An ambivalent engagement: social work and ICT

A number of professions have adapted readily to some of the possibilities offered by a digitalized world including psychology, nursing, pharmacology and medicine [28]. Disciplines oriented towards physical health including medicine, nursing and allied health specialties have been at the forefront of developing and implementing tele-health applications using ICT to provide consultations, recommend treatment and monitor health information remotely for patients who are socially isolated, unable to travel or who live some distance from the required service [30–33]. Social work, however, appears to have been slow to engage and incorporate ICT as a useful tool in social work practice [34,35]. Historically the social work profession has responded to the technological changes of the Industrial Revolution through the increased use of information exchange and the growing of social organizations, community development approaches and through the beginnings of the Settlement House Movement [36]. Yet the social work profession has been reluctant to embrace rapid technological advancements due to concerns that a managerialist approach has been seen to impose technology use on the profession rather than it being seen as a practice-led approach. The neoliberalist and economic rationalist approaches to the human services and social work sectors in recent decades have incorporated principles of greater efficiencies, risk management strategies and shrinking resources. Hence, social workers are experiencing greater pressures with increased workloads and accountability processes for increased evidence-based outcomes [37–39]. The incorporation of technologies is therefore often seen as an additional approach to provide social work services in a more cost-efficient manner that has been critiqued in terms of 'the Mc Donaldization' of the social services [28]. Mishna [29] has highlighted the dramatic changes that have impacted on traditional social work practices through the use of internet services and cyber net communication. Traditional principles of social work practice including professional boundaries, ethical and legal issues, and the helping relationship are aspects of social work that will become increasingly challenging with the advancement of technology. The use of technology has also been considered by the social work profession to negatively impact on core practice principles through the dehumanization of the therapeutic relationship. Concerns have also been expressed regarding client confidentiality and the ethical challenges regarding informed consent within an online context of intervention and support [34,40,41].

The delivery of treatment services for mental health through ICTs such as video conferencing has been well trialled in the field of psychology and the literature in this field offers a useful evidence base for social work to draw upon [e.g. 26,42–47]. This literature also points to similar professional concerns regarding the impact ICT has on therapeutic relationships. Dunstan and Tooth [42, p. 88] for instance suggest that while a range of studies has shown the therapeutic equivalence of ICT service delivery 'the uptake rate of video-conferencing by Australian psychologists is relatively low'. They argue reasons for this reticence include fears that therapeutic alliance [between client and professional] will be impaired [48,49]; non-verbal messages will be difficult to detect or interpret [50]; and that operating ICT equipment will be troublesome [49]. Yet studies of the therapeutic efficacy of video-conferencing and related tele-psychology initiatives have shown positive outcomes in terms of the subjective well-being of clients equivalent to and in some cases outcomes better than would be expected for face-to-face service delivery [26,42,51–53]. A study of the delivery of cognitive behavioural therapy [CBT] for the treatment of bulimic disorders by video-conferencing to people living in rural and remote areas of Scotland and Shetland by Simpson *et al.* [44] provides a useful insight into what works well in the delivery of services via ICTs. Simpson *et al.* [44] highlight that the alliance, positive attachment and bonding between therapist and client – which is particularly significant in the treatment of eating disorders –

was not at all impeded. Clients in this study reported that while 'different', their relationship with their therapist in the video-conferencing process was 'not necessarily any better or worse than a face-to-face relationship would be' [p. 162]. A recent mixed methods study of psychotherapy delivered by video-conference revealed high levels of client satisfaction, comfort, security and control with telepsychology [54]. Psychology has also been proactive in ways to engage students in the use of ICTs in rural and other settings as a means to increase their confidence and familiarity with working in non-urban contexts [42,52,54].

Despite the reticence of the profession as a whole, there have been some examples of the successful use of ICT in social work practice reported in the literature [55–60]. It has been argued that with the use of technology some clients may feel emotionally safer and able to able to engage around sensitive or emotionally distressing issues given the higher degree of anonymity and confidentiality that is afforded by some ICT platforms [56,61].

Both professionals and clients are expected to adapt and integrate ICT into their ways of being and to be able to use the technology in a competent manner. This poses major challenges particularly in relation to the digital divide [62]. This concept refers to some members of the community who for various reasons may be unable to fully maximize the opportunities to engage in a digital world. This is due to factors including limited or no access to computers or minimal computing skills, limited access to broadband, or simply due to a nominal understanding or awareness of its potential and benefits. In addition, a number of socio demographic factors also impact the use of technology including race, language, ability, age, gender, level of education, employment and income [63].

7.5 Sustainable engagement with ICT to meet rural community mental health needs

ICT offers a potential solution to rural mental health service deficiencies by connecting residents in rural Australia with specialist professionals located in urban centres and information resources available on the internet. Australia like other nations, however, has been subject to ICT projects which have been 'fragmented and uncoordinated, leading to problems of accessibility, scalability, duplication, and lack integration within existing systems' [1,2]. Technology cannot simply be inserted into complex social systems and rural communities with an expectation that if it is installed it will be utilized. This is because, as Kearns [64] work illustrates, mental health care occurs within complex intersections between place, health and social processes embedded in history and cultural contexts. Therefore, it is not only the level of service need or viability of the technology to be used which warrants consideration. As research relating to ICT use in education has demonstrated, the degree of local participation in the development, design, mode, timing, introduction and delivery style are important [65,66]. In addition, aspirations for the deployment of ICTs to improve human service delivery to people living in remote communities in

Australia needs to be understood against the broader cultural-historical and political context of Australia's colonial past and the ensuing struggles of Indigenous people to assume self-management and control over their own affairs [65,67]. In analysing the impact and efficacy of ICT used to provide tertiary education into Aboriginal communities in remote areas of central Australia, a recent study by Wood, Tedmanson, Underwood, Minutjukur and Tjitayi [67] suggests incorporating local context and community relevance are critical factors in gaining successful outcomes from initiatives delivering educational or related services in remote, especially Indigenous, community settings. So rather than simply a technological project, attempts to integrate ICT within complex social systems for mental health services that bridge urban and rural places need to be approached using community collaboration as a platform for decision-making. This will help to ensure community ownership and control over the direction, implementation, and use of ICT so that the technology can be tailored to the needs and requirements of the human operators and service users.

As Crotty [20] observes, relationships between people are important to providing mental health services in rural areas. It is likely, therefore, that the sustainability and success of any technological approach to the provision of mental health services in rural areas will depend on the degree to which it is integrated within human and social relations between urban and rural sites of practice. Professional relationships between psychologists, social workers, mental health nurses and GPs provide a network of mental healthcare to support client's needs with ICT simply the mechanism for communication. A study on the delivery of CBT-based psychology services via ICT to mental health clients in rural and remote Queensland experiencing anxiety and depression demonstrates how this might be accomplished to achieve positive results [26]. In this study, Griffiths *et al.* [26, p. 137] map how a psychologist based in the central regional centre of Cairns delivered the CBT intervention via videoconferencing facilities. The case managers observed the 'role-modelling' of the CBT intervention via video conference and reinforced the intervention in face-to-face sessions with their clients following videoconference sessions. Of interest from a social work perspective is the way that in this study case managers were engaged to follow up on the psychology videoconferencing sessions with local visits and face-to-face support work with clients. Such models of professionals working together to maximize client outcomes through using a mix of ICT-brokered external input and local follow through support, provide clues to exciting future options for social work engagement in this space.

Through modes of communication and information exchange enabled by technology, mental health professionals and resources can become connected to form a virtual 'network' that spans across urban health and rural health spaces to create new hybrid health systems [see 68]. As Bourke *et al.* [4, p. 67] elaborate:

> These hybrid forms extend beyond the [constructed] 'typical' disadvantaged rural town struggling to keep a doctor to include the networks of globally connected health practitioners, local leaders, internet-informed health consumers and actors who contribute to reproducing health [and its determinants] locally in different ways.

These hybrid forms of local and global sites and actors enable a 'glocalized' response to social problems such as the provision of mental health services [69]. Some of the benefits of these systems include increases in sharing of client information and regular contact between clients and mental health professionals, building collaborative practice relationships and integrating services irrespective of geophysical distance [65,66,70], developing quick response protocols in times of emergency or natural disaster, professional and collegial support and development for those practicing in rural places [see 71] and developing virtual communities for social support [see 55].

Not only is the deployment of ICT arguably an efficient and viable way to deliver services to rural and remote communities out of the 'reach' of many services currently, it may also be a means by which to reach those currently underserved such as those with physical, mental health, economic or cultural reasons for not wishing to engage in mainstream face-to-face delivery options. For instance, findings from a study by Simpson *et al.* [44] suggest that particular groups of clients may respond more readily to ICT-brokered interventions than others; for example, clients with a high need for control may benefit from ICT-related delivery where 'clients have more control over what they see on their screen', and similarly those with high levels of shame and an avoidant coping style may find it easier to adjust to a therapeutic interaction that is not facing to face 'due to feeling more protected from outside scrutiny or judgement' [44, p. 164]. The capacity for ICTs to be used as a means for enhancing social justice and community development opportunities is a rapidly developing area of emerging interest to social work which warrants further research [36,72].

To harness the potential offered by ICT for social work practice in relation to rural mental health service delivery research is needed that moves beyond a narrow focus on technology and its practical usage or therapeutic effectives of services delivered via ICT for various mental health needs. Whilst this knowledge is needed, it is particularly important that social work develop practice-led approaches that engage ICT within the context of mental health systems that are networked across rural/urban and local/global spaces. Questions that need to be considered include how to ensure that social work practice drives the utilization of ICT rather than practice being technologically driven. This is important if the values and commitments of the social work profession are to direct the nature of engagement with vulnerable and marginalized members of the community. Social work research also needs to consider how the variety of communication mediums of visual, audio and textual forms be used to enhance social work practice in novel and engaging ways and how service delivery can be tailored to complex needs and different client populations using these forms. This includes developing service-user focused forms of service design and delivery [73]. Research that provides an understanding of how ICT can be successfully implemented in rural communities and an insight into the complexities of the interface between human and technological dimensions of complex mental health systems and how these can be navigated would be particularly useful for guiding future projects. In all efforts to promote and advance the implementation of ICT in rural social work practice the issue of access needs to be problematized and solutions identified to bridge the 'digital divide' in rural and remote places [74].

The uptake of ICT into social work practice is dependent on the willingness of social workers in both urban and rural areas to consider technology as a valuable tool and be comfortable and confident to set up and manage systems that utilize ICT. The social work literature in this area points to the need for ICT training to be embedded within social work education [28,29,36]. Baker *et al.* [36] describe some examples of how ICT can be inserted into social work education. To do so will initiate a cultural shift in relation to professional expectations, enable the development of practice-led models of service design and delivery and innovative means of advocacy, provide a site for examining issues such as human rights and ethical issues in relation to ICT [34] and develop competencies in this and proficiency in technology usage. Overall, this would assist in a more responsive approach to the fundamental changes social work has experienced in the transformation to a virtual society becoming reality [36].

7.6 Conclusion

Through innovative platforms for communication and information exchange across local, national and global networks ICT offers innovative and cost-effective possibilities for tailoring mental health services to complex needs, diverse clients and engaging otherwise 'hidden' populations in under-serviced rural and remote areas of Australia. Whilst a discourse of cost-efficiency has been usefully mobilized to advocate for the uptake of ICT in rural health systems, it also provides a reductionist stance on the possibilities afforded by ICT. Rather than being 'something which is better than nothing', the modalities of service design and delivery afforded by ICT contain elements that surpass traditional face-to-face therapeutic encounters.

Research in tele-psychology is instructive in this regard and points to high levels of client satisfaction with therapy via videoconference, less intimidation and shame, greater freedom of expression and a greater sense of control [44]. In addition, ICT also provides greater anonymity and confidentiality to overcome the stigma of seeking support for mental health issues in close-knit rural communities [61]. In terms of infrastructure ICT also enables the development of new hybrid forms of networked systems for interdisciplinary mental health, suicide prevention and social welfare services and supports drawing on people and resources in disparate locations. However, whilst the technological aspects of ICT provide the medium and possibilities for the nature of communication and connectedness, it is important that these do not overshadow their application in service design and delivery if the uptake of ICT in social work is to be sustainable.

Developing practice-based and end-user focused services delivered using ICT according to appropriate and desirable forms of integration of technology with human systems requires social workers to collaborate with IT professionals and project managers in research and innovation. This will ensure that the core values of social work of reaching out to support vulnerable and marginalized communities through services and advocacy based on community development and empowerment will remain central driving forces underpinning the implementation of ICT in social work practice. If the social work profession is to transform the sub-optimal utilization of ICT what is ultimately needed is for social workers to become excited by the possibilities proffered by ICT for social work practice rather than managerial applications. It is only through experiment and experience of trialling ICT and problem solving the ethical and practical problems posed to practice, that social work will advance its engagement with ICT and develop an evidence base for the benefits it encompasses. This knowledge can then be used to shape social work education and drive culture change, develop competencies and engage ICT champions to work with local communities to develop and implement ICT-based services and supports that benefit rural and remote communities.

References

[1] Liaw ST, and Humphreys JS. 'Rural e-health paradox: it's not just geography!'. *Australian Journal of Rural Health*. 2006;14[3]:95–8.

[2] National Rural Health Alliance. *The Little Book of Rural Health Numbers*. https://ruralhealth.org.au/book/little-book-rural-health-numbers: 2017.

[3] Australian Institute of Health and Welfare. *Rural and remote health*. https://www.aihw.gov.au/reports/rural-health/rural-remote-health/contents/rural-health: 2017.

[4] Bourke L, Taylor J, Humphreys JS, and Wakerman J. '"Rural health is subjective, everyone sees it differently": understandings of rural health among Australian stakeholders'. *Health & Place*. 2013;24[0]:65–72.

[5] Dixon J, and Welch N. 'Researching the rural-metropolitan health differential using the "social determinants of health"'. *The Australian Journal of Rural Health*. 2000;8[5]:254–60.

[6] Pong RW, DesMeules M, and Lagacé C. 'Rural-Urban disparities in health: how does Canada fare and how does Canada compare with Australia?'. *Australian Journal of Rural Health*. 2009;17[1]:58–64.

[7] Smith KB, Humphreys JS, and Wilson MGA. 'Addressing the health disadvantage of rural populations: how does epidemiological evidence inform rural health policies and research?'. *Australian Journal of Rural Health*. 2008;16[2]:56–66.

[8] Bourke L, Humphreys JS, Wakerman J, and Taylor J. 'Understanding rural and remote health: a framework for analysis in Australia'. *Health & Place*. 2012;18[3]:496–503.

[9] Bryant L, and Pini B. *Gender and Rurality*. Hoboken: Taylor and Francis; 2011.

[10] Cloke P, Milbourne P, and Widdowfield R. 'Interconnecting housing, homelessness and rurality: evidence from local authority homelessness officers in England and Wales'. *Journal of Rural Studies*. 2001;17[1]:99–111.

[11] Hughes A. 'Geographies of invisibility: the 'hidden' lives of rural lone parents'. In: Holloway L, and Kneafsey M, editors. *Geographies of Rural Cultures and Societies* Aldershot: Ashgate; 2004. pp. 126–44.

[12] Jelinek GA, Weiland TJ, Mackinlay C, Hill N, and Gerdtz MF. 'Perceived differences in the management of mental health patients in remote and rural Australia and strategies for improvement: findings from a national qualitative study of emergency clinicians'. *Emergency Medicine International*. 2011;2011:7 pages.

[13] Ellis IK, and Philip T. 'Improving the skills of rural and remote generalists to manage mental health emergencies'. *Rural and Remote Health*. 2010; 10[3]:1503.

[14] Lonne B. 'Rural mental health and rural social work'. *Rural Society*. 2009;19[4]:370.

[15] Alston M. 'Forging a new paradigm for Australian rural social work practice'. *Rural Society*. 2005;15[3]:277–84.

[16] Speldewinde PC, Cook A, Davies P, and Weinstein P. 'A relationship between environmental degradation and mental health in rural Western Australia'. *Health & Place*. 2009;15[3]:880–7.

[17] Wheeler SA, Zuo A, and Loch A. 'Water torture: unravelling the psychological distress of irrigators in Australia'. *Journal of Rural Studies*. 2018;62:183–94.

[18] Reifels L, Bassilios B, Spittal MJ, King K, Fletcher J, and Pirkis J. 'Patterns and predictors of primary mental health service use following bushfire and flood disasters'. *Disaster Medicine and Public Health Preparedness*. 2015; 9[3]:275–82.

[19] Brown P. 'Mental health in rural Australia'. *Australian Journal of Rural Health*. 2017;25[5]:258–9.

[20] Crotty MM, Henderson J, and Fuller JD. 'Helping and hindering: perceptions of enablers and barriers to collaboration within a rural South Australian mental health network'. *Australian Journal of Rural Health*. 2012;20[4]: 213–18.

[21] Muir-Cochrane E, O'kane D, Barkway P, Oster C, and Fuller J. 'Service provision for older people with mental health problems in a rural area of Australia'. *Aging & Mental Health*. 2014;18[6]:759–66.

[22] Judd F, Jackson H, and Komiti A *et al.* 'Help-seeking by rural residents for mental health problems: the importance of agrarian values'. *Australian and New Zealand Journal of Psychiatry*. 2006;40[9]:769–76.

[23] Rughani J, Deane FP, and Wilson CJ. 'Rural adolescents' help-seeking intentions for emotional problems: the influence of perceived benefits and stoicism'. *The Australian Journal of Rural Health*. 2011;19[2]:64.

[24] Jackson H, Judd F, and Komiti A *et al.* 'Mental health problems in rural contexts: what are the barriers to seeking help from professional providers?'. *Australian Psychologist*. 2007;42[2]:147–60.

[25] Quinn A, and Phillips A. 'Online synchronous technologies for employee- and client-related activities in rural communities'. *Journal of Technology in Human Services*. 2010;28[4]:240–51.

[26] Griffiths L, Blignault I, and Yellowlees P. 'Telemedicine as a means of delivering cognitive-behavioural therapy to rural and remote mental health clients'. *Journal of Telemedicine and Telecare*. 2006;12[3]:136–40.

[27] Castells M. *The Rise of the Network Society*. 2nd edition. Oxford: Wiley-Blackwell; 2010.
[28] West D, and Heath D. 'Theoretical pathways to the future: globalization, ICT and social work theory and practice'. *Journal of Social Work*. 2011; 11[2]:209–21.
[29] Mishna F, Bogo M, Root J, Sawyer J-L, and Khoury-Kassabri M. '"It just crept in": the digital age and implications for social work practice'. *Clinical Social Work Journal*. 2012;40[3]:277–86.
[30] Chakraborty C. *Mobile Health (m-Health) for Tele-wound Monitoring*, IGI: Mobile Health Applications for Quality Healthcare Delivery, 2019, Chapter 5, pp. 98–116.
[31] Fong B, Fong ACM, and Li CK. *Telemedicine Technologies Information Technologies in Medicine and Telehealth*. Chichester: Wiley; 2010.
[32] Rodrigues J, De la Torre Diez I, and Sainz de Abajo B. *Telemedicine and E-health Services, Policies, and Applications Advancements and Developments*. Hershey, PA: IGI Global, Pennsylvania, USA. 2012.
[33] Mehrotra K, Chand P, and Bandawar M *et al.* 'Effectiveness of NIMHANS ECHO blended tele-mentoring model on integrated mental health and addiction for counsellors in rural and underserved districts of Chhattisgarh, India'. *Asian Journal of Psychiatry*. 2018;36:123–7.
[34] Reamer FG. 'Social work in a digital age: ethical and risk management challenges'. *Social Work*. 2013;58[2]:163–72.
[35] Van Der Tier M, Potting M, and Hermans K. 'Stimulating the problem-solving abilities of users in an online environment. a study of a Dutch online social casework intervention'. *Health & Social Care in the Community*. 2018;26[6]:988–94.
[36] Baker S, Warburton J, Hodgkin S, and Pascal J. 'Reimagining the relationship between social work and information communication technology in the network society'. *Australian Social Work*. 2014;67[4]:467–78.
[37] Chenoweth L, and McAuliffe D. *The Road to Social Work & Human Service Practice*. 4th edition. South Melbourne, Victoria: Cengage Learning Australia; 2015.
[38] Payne M, Askeland GA, Jordan DL, and O'Leary PP. *Globalization and International Social Work: Postmodern Change and Challenge*. Abingdon: Taylor & Francis Group; 2008.
[39] Macgowan MJ, and Vakharia SP. *Evidence-Based Social Work Practice: Challenges and Opportunities in the Global Context*. 2015. pp. 39–56.
[40] Csiernik R, Furze P, Dromgole L, and Rishchynski GM. 'Information Technology and Social Work - The Dark Side or Light Side?'*Journal of Evidence-Based Social Work*. Oxon, UK: Taylor & Francis. 2006;3[3/4]:9.
[41] Reamer FG. 'Evolving ethical standards in the digital age'. *Australian Social Work*. 2017;70[2]:148–59.
[42] Dunstan DA, and Tooth SM. 'Treatment via videoconferencing: a pilot study of delivery by clinical psychology trainees'. *Australian Journal of Rural Health*. 2012;20[2]:88–94.

[43] Simpson S, Deans G, and Brebner E. 'The delivery of a tele-psychology service to Shetland'. *Clinical Psychology & Psychotherapy*. 2001;8[2]:130–5.

[44] Simpson S, Bell L, Knox J, and Mitchell D. 'Therapy via videoconferencing: a route to client empowerment?'. *Clinical Psychology & Psychotherapy*. 2005;12[2]:156–65.

[45] Tremont G, Davis J, and Papandonatos GD *et al.* 'A telephone intervention for dementia caregivers: background, design, and baseline characteristics'. *Contemporary Clinical Trials*. 2013;36[2]:338–47.

[46] Davis JD, Tremont G, Bishop DS, and Fortinsky RH. 'A telephone-delivered psychosocial intervention improves dementia caregiver adjustment following nursing home placement'. *International Journal of Geriatric Psychiatry*. 2011;26[4]:380.

[47] Newman L, Bidargaddi N, and Schrader G. 'Service providers' experiences of using a telehealth network 12 months after digitisation of a large Australian rural mental health service'. *International Journal of Medical Informatics*. 2016;94:8–20.

[48] Rees CS, Stone S, and Kenkel MB. 'Therapeutic alliance in face-to-face versus video-conferenced psychotherapy'. *Professional Psychology: Research and Practice*. 2005;36[6]:649–53.

[49] Rees CS, and Haythornthwaite S. 'Telepsychology and videoconferencing: issues, opportunities and guidelines for psychologists'. *Australian Psychologist.* 2004;39[3]:212–19.

[50] Jerome LW, Zaylor C, Deleon PH, and Kenkel MB. 'Cyberspace: creating a therapeutic environment for telehealth applications'. *Professional Psychology: Research and Practice*. 2000;31[5]:478–83.

[51] Richardson L. *'Can you see what I am saying?': An action-research, mixed methods evaluation of telepsychology in rural Western Australia*. Murdock University; 2012.

[52] Simpson S, Rochford S, Livingstone A, English S, and Austin C. 'Tele-web psychology in rural South Australia: the logistics of setting up a remote university clinic staffed by clinical psychologists in training'. *Australian Psychologist.* 2014;49[4]:193–9.

[53] Griffiths KM, Farrer L, and Christensen H. 'The efficacy of internet interventions for depression and anxiety disorders: a review of randomised controlled trials'. *The Medical Journal of Australia*. 2010;192[11 Suppl]:S4.

[54] Simpson S, Guerrini L, and Rochford S. 'Telepsychology in a university psychology clinic setting: a pilot project'. *Australian Psychologist.* 2015; 50[4]:285.

[55] Dodsworth J, Bailey S, Schofield G, Cooper N, Fleming P, and Young J. 'Internet technology: an empowering or alienating tool for communication between Foster-carers and social workers?' *British Journal of Social Work*. 2013;43[4]:775–95.

[56] Callahan A, and Inckle K. 'Cybertherapy or psychobabble? A mixed methods study of online emotional support'. *British Journal of Guidance & Counselling*. 2012;40[3]:261–78.

[57] Mishna F, Levine D, Bogo M, and Van Wert M. 'Cyber counselling: an innovative field education pilot project'. *Social Work Education*. 2013; 32[4]:484–92.

[58] Baker S, Warburton J, Hodgkin S, and Pascal J. 'The new informational paradigm: developing practice-led approaches to the use of mobile ICT in social work'. *The British Journal of Social Work*. 2018;48[6]:1791–809.

[59] Chan C. 'ICT-supported social work interventions with youth: a critical review'. *Journal of Social Work*. 2018;18[4]:468–88.

[60] Law YW, Kwok CL, Chan PY, Chan M, and Yip P. 'Online social work engagement and empowerment for young internet users: a quasi-experiment'. *Journal of Affective Disorders*. 2019;250:99–107.

[61] Baca CT, Alverson DC, Manuel JK, and Blackwell GL. 'Telecounseling in rural areas for alcohol problems'. *Alcoholism Treatment Quarterly*. 2007; 25[4]:31–45.

[62] Wong Y, Law C, Fung J, Lam J, and Lee V. 'Tackling the digital divide'. *British Journal of Social Work*. 2009;39[4]:754–67.

[63] Bryant L, and Principe I. 'Social Capital and the Gendering of Differential IT Use'. In: Garson GD, and Khosrow-Pur M, editors. *Handbook of Research on Public Information Technology*. New York: IGI Global; 2008. Chapter XXII.

[64] Kearns RA. 'Going it alone: place, identity and community resistance to healthcare reforms in Hoki-anga, New Zealand'. In: Kearns RA, Gesler WM, editors. *Putting Health into Place: Landscape, Identity and Well-being*. Syracuse, NY: Syracuse University Press; 1998. pp. 226–47.

[65] Tedmanson D, Fisher S, and Muirhead M. *Anangu Serving Anangu - Plenty Ninti, The PY Ku Network on the APY Lands*. Ninti One Limited (DKCRC Research Report 68). Alice Springs: 2011.

[66] Chakraborty C, Gupta B, and Ghosh SK. 'A Review on Telemedicine-Based WBAN Framework for Patient Monitoring'. *Int. Journal of Telemedicine and e-Health*, Mary Ann Libert Inc. 2013;19[8]: 619–26.

[67] Wood D, Tedmanson D, Underwood B, Minutjukur M, and Tjitayi K. 'Cultural historical activity theory [CHAT] as a framework for exploring the impact of the anangu tertiary education program in remote northwest South Australia'. In: Bozalek V, Ng'ambi D, and Wood D *et al.*, editors. *Activity Theory, Authentic Learning, and Emerging Technologies: Towards a Transformative Higher Education Pedagogy*. Abingdon: Routledge; 2014.

[68] Heley J, and Jones L. 'Relational rurals: some thoughts on relating things and theory in rural studies'. *Journal of Rural Studies*. 2012;28[3]:208–17.

[69] Kelleher R, Ewert P, Yastrubetskaya O, and Williams M. 'Video conferencing applications in social work: work locally, think globally'. *Australian Social Work*. 2000;53[4]:55–9.

[70] Pollock SL. 'Internet counseling and its feasibility for marriage and family counseling'. *The Family Journal*. 2006;14[1]:65–70.

[71] Meier A. 'Offering social support via the internet: a case study of an online support group for social workers'. *Journal of Technology in Human Services*. 2000;17[2–3]:237–66.

[72] Eickhoff K, Tedmanson D, and Wood D. 'Connecting with new ways…New ICTs in remote Aboriginal community contexts'. Joint World Conference on Social Work, Education and Social Development; 9th–12th July, 2014; Melbourne, Vic.

[73] Parrott L, and Madoc-Jones I. 'Reclaiming information and communication technologies for empowering social work practice'. *Journal of Social Work*. 2008;8[2]:181–97.

[74] Radoll P. 'The Primary determinants of indigenous household information and communication technology adoption: remote, rural and urban'. *Australasian Psychiatry*. 2011;19[1 Suppl]:S49–52.

Chapter 8

Technology-enhanced social work practice and education

Kalpana Goel[1], Lia Bryant[1], Renae Summers[2] and Sophie Diamandi[1]

Tele-social work has the potential to broaden the scope of social work practice by improving the accessibility and flexibility of social work services to individuals and groups. This chapter discusses the creative ways in which tele-social work is being implemented, both in Australian and international contexts; challenges and barriers experienced by practitioners, educators, and students. It adds to the knowledge of teaching tele-social work in a classroom setting to build students' confidence and competence in use of technology for social work practice. It proposes to have a cultural shift in academia towards up skilling undergraduate students in using technology for practice purposes.

8.1 Introduction

Compared to medicine and psychology, social work has been slow to engage with digital methods for service provision [1–3]. However, in recent years tele-social work has begun to gain traction [4,5]. Tele-social work provides an avenue of inclusion for those who are unable to participate physically, geographically, or economically. In Australia, where around one third of the population is living in regional and remote locations, the potential for tele-social work to revolutionise service delivery in innovative, inclusive, and cost-effective ways cannot be overlooked [1,6–9]. This chapter explores the creative ways in which tele-social work is being implemented, both in Australian and international contexts and discusses its potential to increase the accessibility and flexibility of services, thereby improving the health and well-being of service users. Potential risks are also considered. Case studies are provided to show how tele-social work is being integrated into social work education, drawing from the authors' experience teaching at a higher education institution in Australia.

[1]School of Psychology, Social Work and Social Policy, University of South Australia, Adelaide, Australia
[2]College of Education, Psychology and Social Work, Flinders University, Adelaide, Australia

8.2 Tele-social work practice

International literature highlights the potential for tele-social work to transform the profession, enabling greater numbers of people to access services and providing demand driven, timely services [e.g. 10–12]. The American Social Work Association suggests that 'technology integration can create a practice that includes flexible, on-demand, personal, and individually paced service' [12, p. 3]. For example, Ozanne and Rose [13, p. 11] note that service providers are 'providing information, education, early intervention, and linkage to other services via interactive websites that enable 24-h access and include information fact sheets, forums, blogs, digital stories, online support groups and links to social networking sites'. The provision of web-based counselling is also growing in Australia [13, p. 110].

Garcia Vaquez *et al.* [3] have argued that mobile phones have created new ways of offering health services; their review of the literature highlighted several studies on the use of text messaging in delivering drug and alcohol services and mental health services. Similarly, in the discipline of psychology, smart phone features such as text messaging, video recording, chat rooms, and conference calls have been found to be useful in parenting education. In one program, parents received brief videos which modelled parent–child interactions, psycho-social education, daily surveys to record progress, and mid-week video calls with a therapist. Parents also recorded videos of home sessions for the therapist to review and provide feedback on [14]. Smart phones and associated apps such as ecological momentary assessment (EMA) have opened up possibilities of monitoring symptoms and providing real time assessments of the client's behaviour, thoughts, and action [15]. Such trials and research evidence from the discipline of psychology are encouraging.

The benefits of tele-social work include connecting with populations that are harder to reach and less likely to access a service in person. For example, tele-social work has been used to provide specialist services to youth with attention deficit hyperactivity disorder and depression [12]. Other examples involve providing services for people with restricted mobility or verbal communication difficulties and people who are spatially and geo-temporally unable to reach services, such as carers [3]. Tele-social work can be used to provide specialised services and allows service users to work at their own pace. For example, education programs developed by social workers enable service users to engage at times that are suitable to them and without time restriction in digesting and using information. A parenting program in the United Kingdom enables parents to access information and social work support [16]. An additional example is mDad (Mobile Device-Assisted Dad), a tool to help new fathers learn about the needs and development of young children and how to engage with their infants and toddlers [4]. Tele-social work also enables service users to remain engaged in a program and with other service users. For example, in the United Kingdom, a platform has been designed to provide a secure online environment to foster social networking between foster carers and to develop a 'community of fostering practice' [17, p. 775]. Similarly,

Smokowski [18] reports use of video creation and computer simulation can enhance behavioural modelling and rehearsal and replace traditional modelling that requires face-to-face contact. These techniques have potential to increase group participants' experience of mastering strategies for behavioural change and reach out to wider participants Several studies have considered the integration of information and communication technology in social work with groups [19–21], with the potential for computers and advanced technologies first recognised in the 1990s [19,22]. In this early contribution, Bowman [19, p. 429] raised the question of whether it would be possible for group work to be reconceptualised and involve the use of technology. Group practitioners were charged with the responsibility of determining how the two spheres of 'high tech' and 'high touch' could be brought together in ways that are reliable yet still provide a sense of community [19, p. 429]. In the Australian context, for example, service providers are facilitating online support groups, for example, for young people diagnosed with cancer [13]. While there is emerging evidence regarding preference towards online support groups, minimal research has been conducted on the development of interpersonal relationships in online groups, which is critical to therapeutic group work [23].

Tele-social work is also a conduit to rural and remote areas where services remain scant in many parts of the world [e.g. 4,24]. In Australia, Regional Access provides mental health support to rural and remote communities, which includes 24 h, seven days per week online chat and telephone support. Similar to telemedicine and telepsychology, there is a range of tele-social work services that connect rural residents to urban service providers. However, for rural tele-social work to be sustainable it must be integrated with local health services and other service providers; furthermore, community participation in the design of services is essential to ensure services are culturally appropriate to Indigenous and rural cultures [24]. Moreover, practitioners need to feel comfortable and competent with the uptake of technology in the rural health practice [25] and adequate provision of professional supervision and training is recommended especially in a constraint practice environment of rural social work practice [26]. Web-based technology tools such as Webinars, Zoom sessions, videoconferencing provide an answer to meet professional development needs when face-to-face supervision and training is difficult to access [26,27].

The literature suggests that the hesitancy of social workers to engage in tele-social work has largely arisen from concerns about the digital divide and the exclusion of the most marginalised groups in society from accessing information and communication technology [28]. Tele-social work could lead to exclusion if face-to-face services are replaced with online programs since this has the potential to reduce access for some service users and decrease the breadth of services available [28]. Social workers are also concerned that they are unable to develop relationships and rapport with clients through the use of technologies. While social work engagement through telephone use, in particular, has been a long-term dimension to practice, social workers are concerned that tele-social work has the potential to replace or reduce funding for face-to-face service delivery.

Bryant *et al.* [24] argue that tele-social work must be a hybrid activity where face-to-face contact with service providers is always an option and practitioners remain closely aligned with any tele-social work activity. The danger lies in governments and other funding bodies designing online programs for cost efficiency. Social workers need to engage with tele-social work and advocate for the use of technology in order to improve service provision, with tele-social work complementing rather than replacing face-to-face practice.

Moreover, reflexivity and evaluation are key to face-to-face practice and are also essential in tele-social work. It is imperative that on-going evaluation is undertaken and new evaluation tools targeted at tele-social work are developed. There are limited detailed evaluations of the delivery of tele-social work services. Further, for tele-social work to be effective, time is required to train service users and providers in how to use technologies. Unfortunately, similar to psychology field [29], the social work profession is lagging behind in developing standards and guidelines to train students and practitioners in tele-social work. Additionally, rigorous monitoring and adapting technologies are required to meet service users' needs.

8.3 Tele-social work education

Several authors have evaluated the integration of information and communication technologies in social work education, arguing for increased research in this area [2,21,30–35]. More specifically, teaching tele-social work within social work degrees has been proposed, in order to generate a cultural shift towards practice-led, progressive models of tele-social work [1,36–38].

Professional associations, such as the Australian Association of Social Workers (AASW) [39,40], have encouraged the inclusion of tele-social work in social work education. Despite the AASW and other professional bodies such as the National Association of Social Workers (NASW), the Association of Social Work Boards (ASWB) and the British Association of Social Workers (BASW) acknowledging the value of technology in social work practice and education, the rapid advancement of the digital age has meant that teaching practices and the necessary learning environments to support social worker competencies in these areas, although evolving, are still lagging. Ultimately, as Reamer [41] argues, the move to integrate tele-social work at a practice level will grow from social workers' capacity to make thoughtful decisions which evaluate advantages and disadvantages for service users on a case by case basis. This capacity however relies upon the openness of social workers who have been inspired through innovative education in up-to-date learning environments. Research on tele-social work education suggests that it is essential for students to be trained in tele-social work by embedding content into the social work curriculum [2,36,37]. Romano and Cikanek [21] affirm including WebCT in group work counselling course increased in students' knowledge and comfort level in use of technology and argued for its integration in different courses. This integration will not only prevent social workers from graduating with outdated skills but, as Dunlop and Fawcett [2] argue, will also support a holistic approach where students and educators are working towards increased comfort and confidence with information and communication technologies. Experimenting with technology in learning environments is critical to the progression of tele-social work, with resistance to the uptake of information and communication technologies predicted as one of the key barriers to its successful implementation. Therefore, it is crucial that teachers embrace their role as 'electronic advocates' [2, p. 144]. Gelman and Tosone [42] state that the lack of scholarship relating to the education and training of social workers in information and communication technologies is surprising, especially considering the ways in which information and communication technologies have been used by social movements to work towards social change.

Watling [43] argues that while the merging of information and computer technologies and social work education should be welcomed, our knowledge of how these structures will come together is currently limited. Colvin and Bullock [30] have examined some of the potential barriers to implementing tele-social work into the curriculum; key challenges that were identified as potentially inhibiting the acceptance and incorporation of information and communication technologies included 'self-efficacy', 'computer anxiety', 'intrinsic motivation', and 'professional boundaries'. Questions arose over whether or not the inclusion of technology in social work education would actually be of benefit, due to the underlying belief that technology would compromise interpersonal relations and the capacity to form bonds [30,44]. Conversely, opportunities can be found in the rapid and continuous innovation and improvements in technologies; examples of this include ever-increasing internet speeds and the advent of real-time video communications. Colvin and Bullock [30] also point to the way in which technologies are enabling educators to create simulated environments. A small number of studies have explored 'virtual field environments' in social work field education [30,45,46]. Most of the barriers identified have been technology related, such as issues concerning internet access, equipment and a lack of technical support. In spite of these drawbacks, Birkenmaier [45] highlights its potential within the field education curriculum where technology could be used to increase regular communication with students on placement, strengthen student–teacher relationships, and provide external supervision in the absence of onsite supervision. The next section focuses on two examples of the application of tele-social work in social work education.

8.3.1 Teaching tele-social work in group work

Working with groups is central to social work practice and group work is part of the social work curriculum in Australia. This case study focuses on the introduction of tele-social work in a large first year, an undergraduate subject on group work. In this subject, students engage in practice-based learning in order to develop their skills in facilitating groups. Students work together to plan and facilitate one session of a group for their final assessment. Students role play as group leaders and the class role play as group members. The teaching team trialled introducing tele-social work to develop students' skills in using technology and engaging remote participants. Students were required to demonstrate skills in tele-social work as a part of their final assessment.

To design the tele-social work content the teaching team worked with online educational designers to trial different platforms and equipment. It was established that remote participation would be simulated in a room next to the classroom, using Adobe Connect, laptops, and webcams. This enabled synchronous communication via videoconferencing and online chat. Screen sharing and document sharing features also enabled students to share resources with remote participants.

A training video was developed as an educational tool and demonstrated how to use and set up the technology to facilitate remote participation. This was accompanied by a step by step written guide. Staff participated in training sessions prior to the commencement of teaching to enhance their confidence and skill in the use of technology in a group setting. These sessions were useful for troubleshooting and raising teaching questions and concerns.

The video and written guide were also made available to students. Students were briefly introduced to tele-social work in the first week of teaching and were given a brief demonstration of how to set up the technology. A lecture on the use of information and communication technology in group work was delivered, which provided research or evidence base on the use of technology in group work. Following this, students practiced using technology during tutorials. This enabled students to practice and experiment in a simulated environment that was both supervised and supported. It also led to discussions about the implementation of tele-social work and highlighted similarities and differences in facilitating face-to-face and online groups, as well as strategies facilitators can use to enhance group members' experiences.

When facilitating a group session for their final assignment, students used a checklist to ensure technology was appropriately managed; this included room set up, checking the video and audio in both locations, having a backup plan in case internet connection is lost and keeping IT support contact details handy to troubleshoot any technical difficulties faced during the session. A co-facilitator was appointed in each team to facilitate remote participation, for example, by managing chat, monitoring cues from remote participants and including remote participants in activities, while other team members focussed on facilitating the session with face-to-face group members. While students at the metropolitan campus simulated remote participation in a room next to the classroom, students on regional campuses were able to facilitate the remote participation of students on other regional campuses in their group session, using this technology.

Overall, it was found that students were able to apply group work skills to include remote participants in the session and largely felt comfortable using technology. Teaching staff's mixed responses towards using technology in group work at the beginning of the subject dramatically improved towards the end, and they expressed increased confidence in using technology. This trial helped to teach staff to overcome some of their negative perceptions, as well as actual challenges, by embracing alternate strategies in their teaching practice. Similarly, students reported problems with technology and equipment were a source of frustration at times. Some students found this confusing and stated that it complicated their learning experience. There was a strong call from students to receive more training and practice time in using technology.

In terms of applying what students learnt to practice, they identified that specific communication skills are required for effective tele-social work communication, in particular; paying attention to non-verbal cues, the need for louder and clearer speech, improved attending skills, and the ability to communicate cross culturally.

Students also identified concerns about the security of online environments and the risk to service user confidentiality, privacy, and safety. Issues surrounding confidentiality, the discussion of sensitive topics and the possible need for emotional care and support were also identified by teaching staff. In addition, teaching staff recognised that differences in people's comfort levels in using technology, and the availability and reliability of the internet, could disadvantage some service users. Similarly, students saw tele-social work as having the potential to reach certain populations, for example, people in rural and remote locations, people living with disabilities and people experiencing mental illness, while excluding others, for example, people from culturally and linguistically diverse backgrounds as well as disadvantaged groups who may not be able to afford or access the technologies required. These findings echo discussions in the literature about the potential of tele-social work to both narrow and widen the 'digital divide'.

While students recognised the accessibility and flexibility of tele-social work, they expressed concern that it would compromise relationships between service users and providers, which are central to social work practice. Specific issues that were identified in relation to technology use included compromised vision of participants and non-verbal communication and a concern that this would hinder the formation of relationships and trust. The availability of appropriate, effective technology was viewed as crucial to overcoming such issues. Students were concerned that advancing the practice of tele-social work prematurely, without proper systems in place, would impact on the uptake and effectiveness of tele-social work. Hence, the development and integration of appropriate technologies are integral to the success of tele-social work.

8.3.2 Applying tele-social work in field education

The Australian Association of Social Work [40] requires that students complete 980 h of supervised field education in order to qualify as social workers. Field education is a form of work integrated learning and allows students to gain industry experience. Social work students are placed in human service organisations and develop the skills required for professional practice. Students are supported in field placement through social work supervision and fortnightly field education tutorials which are held on the university campus and are facilitated by a qualified field education coordinator.

Universities offering social work degrees have a responsibility to prepare students for practice in both metropolitan and rural areas. Currently, service providers in rural and remote areas are struggling to recruit and retain qualified social workers in various roles including in child protection [47], aged care [48] and small, non-government organisations [49]. Therefore, students' placement in rural and remote areas is considered as one strategy to meet the workforce shortage. Studies have found that students who have had exposure and undertaken a field placement in a rural area tend to stay or return to the region after completion [50]. This also benefits educational institutions who struggle to find sufficient placements in metropolitan areas. However, it is recognised that students need to be well supported to meet the challenges of rural field placements, which can include isolation, lack of professional supervision and visibility in small communities [27, p. 69].

This case study examines the use of tele-social work to provide supervision and education to social work students on field placement and preparation of students for first placement in rural areas of South Australia. While research has investigated the use of information and communication technologies in social work education more generally [2,21,30–35], there has been little attention to the use of information and communication technologies in field education [51].

Each semester, approximately 10 to 15 social work students undertake field placements in rural areas of South Australia. Geographically, the placements are widely dispersed, ranging from 100 to 700 km from a regional campus of the university. In addition, some students who usually attend the metropolitan campus are placed in regional towns in South Australia, making it difficult to attend tutorials. The field education coordinator based at a regional campus facilitates a fortnightly 2-h tutorial for all students on field placement in rural areas. Tutorials are facilitated using web-based videoconferencing, i.e. Skype for Business. This application is purchased by the university and both staff and students can use it from mobile devices such as laptops, mobile phones, and tablets. Some students attend the tutorial in person. Pedagogically, the use of technology helps to facilitate inclusivity and participation. Technically, its usage makes learning accessible to students living and working in rural areas.

Facilitating tutorials using web-based videoconferencing requires planning and preparation; this includes scheduling a meeting, providing instructions on how to use the application and undertaking a test run to ensure that students are familiar with the technology. The field education coordinator also ensures the contact details for each student and for IT support are on hand, in the event that they encounter log in issues. The tutorials start at least 15 min prior to the scheduled time so that everyone can check audio and video functions and seek help if necessary, before the class starts. The use of the chat function is often helpful if there are audio and video issues and instructions can be delivered to suggest alternative ways to mitigate the challenges of technical issues.

Strategies that have been found helpful in facilitating students' participation and engagement include slowing the pace of the conversation, alternating the discussion between online and face-to-face students, regularly checking in with students to ascertain good audibility and monitoring the screen for the call failure. Some of the challenges experienced in web-based videoconferencing include call drop, picture freeze and loss of voice, which can require technical assistance.

Besides such technical difficulties, which are manageable with IT assistance and technical experience, several benefits have been observed. Students placed in rural areas can be part of a learning community, students who participate online and face to face are able to connect with and learn from each other and all students develop an appreciation of the challenges of living and working in rural and remote areas. Students can share their experiences of field education in a safe environment, reflect on their learning, voice any concerns they might have and receive professional support.

Moreover, students are trained in the use of information and communication technologies in social work, through experiencing it in the field education. This prepares students to become professionals who are comfortable and confident in using technology in social work, which is particularly relevant to practice in rural and remote areas due to the lack of accessibility to specialised services and professional supervision.

Students' preparation for their first field education placement is vital for a smooth transition from the classroom to a practice environment. Videoconferencing is also used to teach preparation for field education subjects across two regional campuses. This subject focuses on the integration of theory and practice, developing ethical practice, learning to write case notes and preparing for supervision. One strategy that has been useful in engaging students in learning, using videoconferencing, is to alternate between individual, small group and large group activities. Students require access to a computer to complete individual activities online, enabling the teacher to access their work in real time. Another alternative is to use a collaborative teaching space, purpose built with this functionality. During small group activities, the teacher may be unable to hear discussion at the other location. This has been managed by checking in with students at the remote location and encouraging each student to contribute to the discussion. Time management and having a lead time of 15 min as a buffer is important in facilitating groups through technology. The use of videoconferencing in facilitating educational groups requires special consideration of semi-circular seating arrangements to allow a full camera view at both locations and the minimisation of outside noise in the classroom to experience good sound quality in an online environment.

8.4 Conclusion

In summary, embedding tele-social work in the social work curriculum is crucial as it enables students to develop their skills in tele-social work practice. It also enables students to think critically about the benefits and risks of tele-social work. Furthermore, it increases their digital literacy and confidence in using technology in social work, making students more likely to use tele-social work in their future careers. Teaching staff's familiarity, competence, and confidence in using technology is integral to ensuring that students have a positive experience of tele-social work. Thus, on-going professional development and constant exposure to new innovative technologies will result in positive outcomes in generating interest and confidence amongst students.

Tele-social work has the potential to transform the profession of social work and increase the accessibility and flexibility of services. However, tele-social work must complement rather than replace face-to-face service provision. There are multiple examples of tele-service delivery across disciplines including social work, which have had successful results. It is timely for social work to consider the full potential of tele-delivery in group work, counselling, community development, field education, and other key areas of practice.

8.5 Future work

Embedding tele-social work in the social work curriculum is crucial in generating interest and confidence amongst students.

Research into the successful use of tele-social work in practice can support changes in the curriculum.

More research is required in instructional models and approaches trialled on successful learning outcomes for students.

Institutional support to provide funding, technical support and professional development of staff is warranted for the effective implementation of tele-social work.

References

[1] Bryant, L. *Critical and creative research methodologies in social work.* United Kingdom: Routledge; 2015

[2] Dunlop, J.M. and Fawcett, G. 'Technology-based approaches to social work and social justice'. *Journal of Policy Practice*. 2008;7(2–3):140–54

[3] Garcia Vazquez, Y., Ferrás, C., Aguilera, A. and Rocha, A. 'The present and future of psychosocial therapy for vulnerable people in Spain. The contribution of mobile phones'. *Cuadernos de Trabajo Social*. 2017;31(1): 235–49

[4] Lee, S.J. and Walsh, T.B. 'Using technology in social work practice: The mDad (Mobile Device Assisted Dad) case study'. *Advances in Social Work.* 2015;16(1):107–24

[5] Christson, A. and Adedoyin, A. 'Deploying virtual communities of practice as a digital tool in social work: a rapid review and critique of the literature'. *Social Work Education.* 2016;35(3):357–70

[6] Alston, M. 'Globalisation, rural restructuring and health service delivery in Australia: Policy failure and the role of social work'. *Health & Social Care in the Community*. 2007;15(3):195–202

[7] Barlow, D.M. 'Electronic community networks in rural Australia: A model for social development in the Information Society'. *Australian Social Work.* 1997;50(1):3–8

[8] Regan, S. 'Overcoming the tyranny of distance: Exploring the use of teleconferencing group counselling'. *Australian Social Work*. 1997;50(1):9–14

[9] Warburton, J., Cowan, S., Winterton, R. and Hodgkins, S. 'Building social inclusion for rural older people using information and communication technologies: Perspectives of rural practitioners'. *Australian Social Work*. 2014;67(4):479–94

[10] Dombo, E.A., Kay, L. and Weller, K. 'Clinical social work practice and technology: Personal, practical, regulatory, and ethical considerations for the twenty-first century'. *Social Work in Health Care*. 2014;53(9):900–19

[11] Craig, S.L. and Calleja Lorenzo, M.V. 'Can information and communication technologies support patient engagement? A review of opportunities and challenges in health social work'. *Health Social Work, Social Work in Health Care*. 2014;53(9):845–64

[12] Berzin, S.C., Singer, J. and Chan, C. 'Practice Innovation through Technology in the Digital Age: A Grand Challenge for Social Work, American Academy of Social Work and Social Welfare', Working Paper No. 12. 2015

[13] Ozanne, E. and Rose, D. *The organisational context of human service practice*. South Yarra: Palgrave Macmillan. 2013

[14] Jones, D.J., Forehand, R., Cuellar, J. *et al.* 'Technology-enhanced program for child disruptive behavior disorders: Development and pilot randomized control trial'. *Journal of Clinical Child & Adolescent Psychology*. 2014; 43(1):88–101

[15] Clough, B.A. and Casey, L.M. 'The smart therapist: A look to the future of smartphones and mHealth technologies in psychotherapy'. *Professional Psychology: Research and Practice*. 2015;46(3):147–53

[16] Chan, C. and Holosko, M.J. 'A review of information and communication technology enhanced social work interventions'. *Research on Social Work Practice*. 2015;26(1):88–100

[17] Dodsworth, J., Bailey, S., Schofield, G., Cooper, N., Fleming, P. and Young, J. 'Internet Technology: An Empowering or Alienating Tool for Communication between Foster-Carers and Social Workers?'. *British Journal of Social Work*. 2013;43(4):775–95

[18] Smokowski, P. 'Beyond role-playing: Using technology to enhance modeling and behavioral rehearsal in group work practice'. *Journal for Specialists in Group Work*. 2003;28(1):9–22

[19] Bowman, R.L. 'Life on the electronic frontier: The application of technology to group work'. *Journal for Specialists in Group Work*. 1998;23(4):428–45

[20] Penner, N. and Schulze, M. 'Group work in a technology-rich environment'. *Journal of Interactive Learning Research*. 2010;21(1):111–37

[21] Romano, J.L. and Cikanek, K.L. 'Group work and computer applications: Instructional components for graduate students'. *Journal for Specialists in Group Work*. 2003;28(1):23–34

[22] Horne, S. 'From coping to creating change: The evolution of women's groups'. *Journal for Specialists in Group Work*. 1999;24(3):231–45

[23] Kozlowski, K.A. and Holmes, C.M. 'Experiences in online process groups: A qualitative study'. *The Journal for Specialists in Group Work.* 2014; 39(4):276–300

[24] Bryant, L., Garnham, B., Tedmanson, D. and Diamandi, S. 'Tele-social work and mental health in rural and remote communities in Australia'. *International Social Work.* 2018;6(1):143–55

[25] Moffatt, J. and Eley, D. 'Barriers to the up-take of telemedicine in Australia-a view from providers'. *Rural and Remote Health Journal.* 2011; 11(1581):1–6

[26] Goel, K., Hudson, C. and Cowie, J. 'Building research capacity for social work practitioners: a regional perspective'. *Social Work Education.* 2018; 37(8):1028–43

[27] Zuchowski, I., Hudson, C., Bartlett, B. and Diamandi, S. 'Social work field education in Australia: Sharing practice wisdom and reflection'. *Advances in Social Work and Welfare Education.* 2014;16(1):67–80

[28] Steyaert, J. and Gould, N. 'Social work and the changing face of the digital divide'. *British Journal of Social Work.* 2009;39(4):740–53

[29] McCord, C.E., Saenz, J.J., Armstrong, T.W. and Elliott, T.R. 'Training the next generation of counseling psychologists in the practice of telepsychology'. *Counselling Psychology Quarterly.* 2015;28(3):324–44

[30] Colvin, A.D. and Bullock, A.N. 'Technology acceptance in social work education: implications for the field practicum'. *Journal of Teaching in Social Work.* 2014;34(5):496–513

[31] Chakraborty, C., Gupta, B. and Ghosh, S.K. 'A review on telemedicine-based WBAN framework for patient monitoring'. *Int. Journal of Telemedicine and e-Health, Mary Ann Libert Inc.* 2013;19(8):619–26

[32] Jones, S.J. 'Benefits and challenges of online education for clinical social work: three examples'. *Clinical Social Work Journal.* 2015;43(2):225–35

[33] Phelan, J.E. 'The use of e-learning in social work education'. *Social Work.* 2015;60(3):257–64

[34] Smith, W. 'Relational dimensions of virtual social work education: mentoring faculty in a web-based learning environment'. *Clinical Social Work Journal.* 2014;43(2):236–45

[35] Washburn, M. and Zhou, S. 'Teaching note-technology-enhanced clinical simulations: Tools for practicing clinical skills in online social work programs'. *Journal of Social Work Education.* 2018;54(3):554–60

[36] Baker, S., Warburton, J., Hodgkin, S. and Pascal, J. 'Reimagining the relationship between social work and information communication technology in the network society'. *Australian Social Work.* 2014;67(4):467–78

[37] Mishna, F., Bogo, M., Root, J., Sawyer, J.L. and Khoury-Kassabri, M. '"It just crept in": The digital age and implications for social work practice'. *Clinical Social Work Journal.* 2012;40(3):277–86

[38] West, D. and Heath, D. 'Theoretical pathways to the future: Globalization, ICT and social work theory and practice'. *Journal of Social Work.* 2011; 11(2):209–21

[39] Australian Association of Social Workers. 'Code of Ethics, AASW', viewed 20 December 2018; https://www.aasw.asn.au/document/item/1201

[40] Australian Association of Social Work. *Australian Social Work Education and Accreditation Standards (ASWEAS) Guideline 1.2: Guidance on field education programs.* Canberra, ACT; 2012. 1–12

[41] Reamer, F.G. 'Clinical social work in a digital environment: Ethical and risk-management challenges'. *Clinical Social Work Journal.* 2015;43 (2):120–32

[42] Gelman, C.R. and Tosone, C. 'Teaching social workers to harness technology and inter-disciplinary collaboration for community service'. *British Journal of Social Work.* 2010;40(1):226–38

[43] Watling, S. 'Digital exclusion: potential implications for social work education'. *Social Work Education.* 2012;31(1):125–30

[44] McCarty, D. and Clancy, C. 'Telehealth: Implications for social work practice'. *Social Work.* 2002;47(2):153–61

[45] Birkenmaier, J., Wernet, S.P., Berg-Weger, M. *et al.* 'Weaving a web: The use of Internet technology in field education'. *Journal of Teaching in Social Work.* 2005;25(1–2):3–19

[46] Wolfer, T.A., Carney, M. and Ward, J. 'Acquiring and implementing videoconferencing technology to enhance the field work experience'. *Journal of Technology in Human Services.* 2002;19(4):43–63

[47] Riebschleger, J., Norris, D., Pierce, B., Pond, D.L. and Cummings, C. 'Preparing social work students for rural child welfare practice: Emerging curriculum competencies'. *Journal of Social Work Education.* 2015; 51(sup2):S209–24

[48] Hodgkin, S., Warburton, J., Savy, P. and Moore, M. 'Workforce crisis in residential aged care: Insights from rural, older workers'. *Australian Journal of Public Administration.* 2017;76(1):93–105

[49] Barton, H., Bell, K. and Bowles, W. 'Help or hindrance? Outcomes of social work student placements'. *Australian Social Work.* 2005;58(3):301–12

[50] Smith, T., Cross, M., Waller, S. *et al.* 'Ruralization of students' horizons: Insights into Australian health professional students' rural and remote placements'. *Journal of Multidisciplinary Healthcare.* 2018;11;85–97

[51] Shorkey, C.T. and Uebel, M. 'History and development of instructional technology and media in social work education'. *Journal of Social Work Education.* 2014;50(2):247–61

Chapter 9

Advanced telemedicine system for remote healthcare monitoring

Akash Gupta[1], Chinmay Chakraborty[1] and Bharat Gupta[2]

In this chapter, an advanced telemedicine system has been presented for monitoring remotely located patients suffers from various types of diseases. Telemedicine is a multidisciplinary field, which needs expert physician and staff, which also include high cost and types of equipment to provide quality service to patients. As telemedicine systems are now capable of monitoring remote patients with greater efficiency using numbers of advance computational methods, and researchers showing great interest in this field. Telemedicine systems may support to deal with various types of biomedical signals like EEG (electroencephalography), ECG (electrocardiography), EMG (electromyography), etc. along with the integration of modern techniques. This chapter also deals with standards uses by telemedicine system along with its special features. A cloud-based workflow model for monitoring of remote patients has been proposed here. For the continuous monitoring and analysis of biomedical signals obtained from remote patients, telemedicine system may play a great role for technical, social, and cultural development of society. Here, a discussion has been made on various aspects of the monitoring system and different issues with latest development and improvement in this field.

9.1 Introduction

Epilepsy is a neurological disorder, which is needed to be continuously monitored. Those patients, who suffer from such disease, require proper medicines and suggestions regarding the disease. Telemedicine provides the facility to take care of the patients located in remote/rural areas in distance, which have very limited facilities regarding the problem. Telemedicine can provide consultation and communication with medical experts to such patients [1]. It provides a solution not only for epilepsy care but also for another disease as well. Using telemedicine technology, we

[1]Department of Electronics and Communication Engineering, Birla Institute of Technology, Jharkhand, India
[2]Department of Electronics and Communication Engineering, National Institute of Technology, Bihar, India

can access information about epileptic patients from a remote area [2]. For the telemedicine system, Internet of Things (IoT) also plays an important role in the communication point of view. It helps to take care of patients, delivery of medicines, suggestions, a record of medical data, information transfer, etc. [3,4]. A wireless body area network-based telemedicine system can also be proposed for monitoring of epileptic patients, which will be able to monitor patients continuously in real-time. Such a system can collect information using sensors and this information can be processed to experts/hospitals using various devices like smartphones or others based on the use of different protocols [5].

The monitoring of patients using telemedicine facility is an emerging field in research (Figure 9.1). As, we are now moving towards caring and monitoring of patients in real-time along with, which are located in a remote area too. If this monitoring is possible in a quick way, it will be beneficial for both patients as well as experts. Monitoring of remote patients may be categorized in a different way like monitoring of mobile patients, telehealth, health, etc. in each of the case information can be accessible by hospitals/experts. Using telemedicine system early detection of any disease (epilepsy) and continuous monitoring is possible. It will also help to reduce the cost, a number of hospitalized patients, recording of data, etc. and able to improve the accuracy and efficiency [6]. In the field of remote monitoring, a lot of work is going on with the growth of the IoT. As a problem related to health is increasing in a faster way, it needs to get solved quickly. Telemedicine provides an easier solution to take care of remotely located patients from the hospital

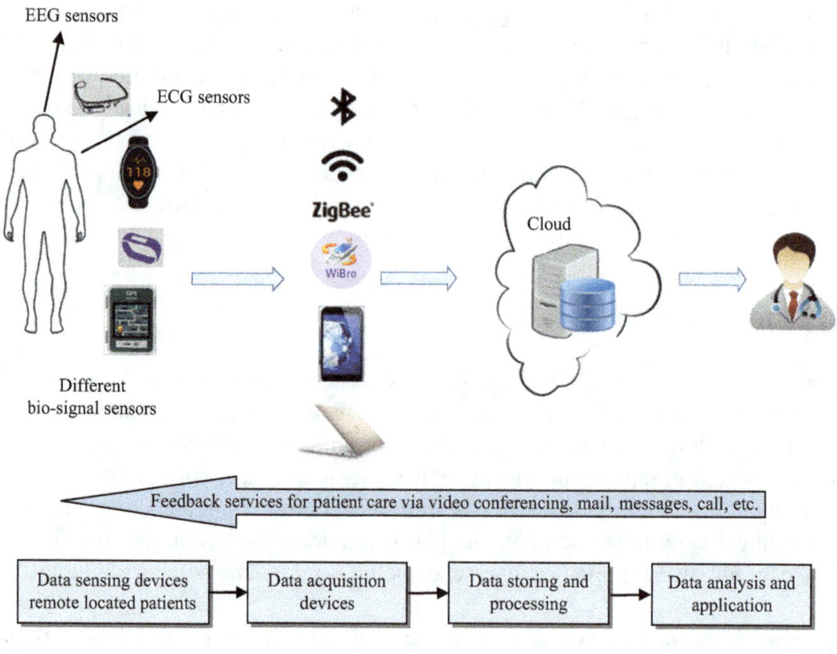

Figure 9.1 Telemedicine systems for monitoring of remotely located patients

itself. Technologies have been evolved in that level of extent, where patients can do their work and still monitoring is possible. The use of current communication technology and use of sensors makes such kind of monitoring possible. Such technologies can monitor patients based on diseases or based on condition. Telemedicine provides comfort to patients with a better cure. Researchers are doing their work continuously regarding epilepsy monitoring with new applications related to remotely located patients. With the use of such applications, patients will be able to do their regular activity with minimum discomfort. These telemedicine systems can provide ambulance service or drug delivery, even in case of emergency.

For remote monitoring of patients or use of telemedicine systems, few basic elements in a system are required given as acquisition of data, the transmission of information to hospital/experts and information transmission medium. Using various types of sensors data may be acquired from the epileptic patients, that sensors may be wireless too. Some of the sensors are such types, which are contactless and have a great impact on prediction too. Wireless sensors may work on correspondence to a given precised network, known as wireless sensor network. The collected information can be processed to a cloud or may directly send to the experts. From the cloud, hospital/expert can access the biomedical information. Based on collected information experts may give their suggestions according to information received. If the patient's condition is serious, then required ambulance service may provide to remotely located patients and may admit in hospitals.

Telemedicine can improve health care services by reducing any vulnerability in analyzing the information and give back suitable health service in terms of quality, cost, etc. to epileptic patients. Telemedicine service based on video EEG data has been presented [7]. In this proposed system high speed of the Internet, data transfer and specialist members are required, which make system costlier. The real-time tele-EEG service has been presented, which helps to get suggestions from the experts in a quicker way [8]. With the concern of cost reduction, work has been presented [9], this article discussed processor to detect epileptic seizures according to the age of the patient. This work has the novelty of a low-cost telemedicine system and able to perform classification of patients. The telemedicine system has been growing very fast and the use of IoT makes it possible. IoT has been included in the telemedicine system. Some of the telemedicine architecture presented here which also deals with security issues [10]. It proposes real-time health monitoring using IoT-based smart home system. The monitoring of remotely located patients is also benefited by this technology.

For monitoring of remotely located patients, telemedicine system is based on the smart health monitoring system. In such a system, security is an issue, which requires verification before getting access for the purpose of different health-related applications [11]. As we know epilepsy is a neurological disorder, with telemedicine, applications of teleneurology have been presented [12]. Teleneurology has great benefits for the patients exist in a rural area or for persons who are working with military or person who have very little movement. It is an application for remote caring of patients even in the locations which are topographically disconnected. Teleneurology can take care of the patients with a disease like epilepsy [13].

9.1.1 Monitoring of remotely located epileptic patients

The monitoring of epileptic patients located in the remote area consists of a system to acquire various sensor data from patients. Here we are mentioned about epileptic patients, so most common data can be gathered from EEG sensors. There are various studies already have been done in which sensors are directly placed on the human brain to collect data. Sometimes it is difficult in terms of mobile patients or in working condition. In this situation data may get affected, hence it does not reflect proper disease. Therefore, for monitoring such patients itself a difficult job and give them proper suggestions and care is also necessary. Some of the monitoring systems presented in various research articles. The various remote monitoring systems have been presented here [14], which also reviews about advancement in remote health monitoring. The development of a machine to machine communication for health monitoring and other various applications has been presented [15]. Various types of sensors have been used for data collection purpose along with its processing and other issues have been presented and deal with the use of mobile computing with wireless body area network has also been presented in regards to the monitoring of remote patients. Tsakalakis *et al.* [16] give a survey report which compares various existing monitoring system based on various movable and implantable sensors, using wearable devices, etc. Baig *et al.* [17] give a comparison over various smart systems related to health monitoring of remote patients and deals with challenges and factors affecting the system. This paper compares the monitoring system based on the existing traditional system and advanced smart system which includes mobile health and wearable health system. For monitoring of remotely located patients, a survey has been presented [18], mainly concentrated on data processing methods, low cost, system accuracy, and especially data privacy and protection.

Epilepsy is a most common neurological disorder and it happens because of abnormal electrical activity in the human brain, due to this, patients may lose their memory power, conscious state, sensing ability, etc. Monitoring of such neurological diseases of remotely located patients is a challenging job; even designing of such a monitoring system is itself a challenge. Designing such a system requires precision, accuracy, analysis of big data, etc. makes the system more complex. For monitoring of patients, based on emotion recognition using automatic nervous system has been presented [19], which will be helpful for the prediction of seizures from epileptic patients based on their behavior. A survey has been presented regarding the monitoring of remotely located patients and telemedicine services to cure neurological disorders [20]. Along with it helps to monitor epilepsy or brain-related disorder. In these various issues related to telemedicine has been pointed and some solution has been given. Prabhakar *et al.* [21] discussed regarding epilepsy classification, a remote monitoring system has been presented. Here, authors actually worked on the data size reduction and their feature extraction classification has been performed with an accuracy of more than 95%.

As we know that for monitoring of epileptic patients, analysis of the EEG signal gives necessary information. For the purpose of analyzing the EEG signal, it requires the transmission of data directly from patients to practitioners through a communication link. Prabhakar *et al.* [22] presented how EEG is used to represent the human condition. For the purpose of finding seizures, spikes in EEG signal usually observed and compared with seizure period EEG signal. Prabhakar *et al.* [23] proposed a system for the purpose of a wireless telemedicine system, a basic framework has been proposed for seizure prediction methods. During recent years, numbers of research are going on for automatic classification and seizure detection. Prediction of epileptic seizures using various features has been presented [24] here based on line length features and artificial neural networks, the seizure detection of epileptic patients has been presented [25], which gives an efficient way for monitoring of remote or hospitalized patients. In this chapter, a used feature is based on wavelet transform multi-resolution decomposition. The Hadamard transform-based PAPR (peak-to-average power ratio) reduction for telemedicine applications used for classification of epilepsy is presented [26]. For wireless epileptic patient monitoring, a PCA-based mapping technique has been introduced which is implemented for reducing PAPR [27].

9.1.2 Motivation

Telemedicine system including IoT plays an important role in monitoring the remotely located epileptic patients and sensing seizures. With the help of various sensors or wearable devices, the system will be able to acquire epileptic data and able to process them. Along with remotely located patients, the telemedicine system works efficiently for mobile patients too. In this telemedicine system, various devices are linked with each other to process information, which follows cloud computation. It became necessary for a very huge amount of EEG data. As we know, to maintain these data with security and privacy cloud computation is necessary.

The telemedicine system has a variety of applications that motivate us to use it. For example, remotely located epileptic patients may get suggestions or advice from health experts using a telemedicine system. This system may include transmission of high-quality images of the remotely located patient and based on patient condition, behavior or emotion expert may provide advice. Along with the suggestion, continuous monitoring of epileptic patients is also possible with the telemonitoring system. Within the system acquiring EEG data and their storing and finally processing it, may possible. There are various methods available to process information, which can process signals, images, videos, etc.

In this chapter, we have discussed various telemedicine systems, their basic architecture, and advancement in this system. Such systems are flexible and can be configured as per requirement. These systems may able to process real-time information and get a response in a secure way. In other terms, we can say that a properly arranged telemedicine system may help to provide emergency services and can optimize the cost by reducing the parameters likes hospitalization, treatment, etc. As the telemedicine system is in the developing stage, it motivates us to work in this direction for social, economic and technical development of the country/world.

9.1.3 Objective

The main objective of this book chapter is to acquire knowledge about the telemedicine system and use it for monitoring of remote-located epileptic patients and prediction of seizures. The telemedicine system is based on some sensors and wearable devices, which help to collect data and transmit them through a medium with maintaining security and privacy. The main objective is to provide quick and accurate service to patients and their caretakers. The telemedicine system is an effective way to provide service to the person, who can not avail the costlier facility and the one who needs care or treatment urgently. This system is most suitable for the patients affected with long term neurological disease. In this chapter, we are going to introduce the framework and various applications of a telemedicine system for monitoring of epileptic seizures of different patients (hospitalized or remotely located). As the telemedicine system is IoT enabled, reflects a variety of applications mentioned below in (Figure 9.2), we have focused on e-health. This telemedicine system can help to monitor several diseases from hospitalized patients/remote-located patients. Using the system diseases like epilepsy, others brain or heart-related disease, allergies, asthma, chronic diseases, conjunctivitis, UTIs, etc. various health-related problems can be monitored and taken care and time to time suggestion can be provided.

9.1.4 Organization of the chapter

The organization of this chapter is presented in the given order: first of all, we provided a brief introduction of a telemedicine system to monitor remotely located

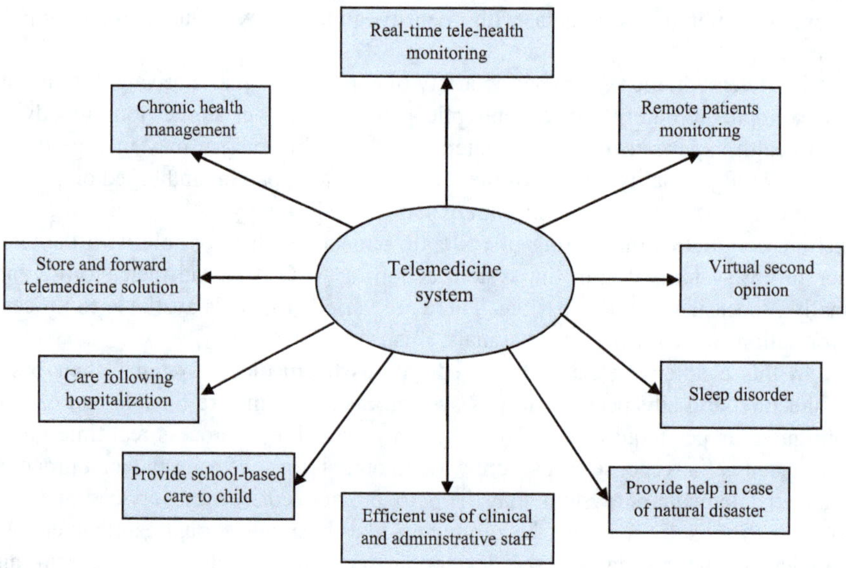

Figure 9.2 Applications of the telemedicine system

patients. Correspondingly we have made a literature survey related to telemedicine systems to monitor various kinds of diseases and gone through various research papers. In continuity, we have presented a general model of telemedicine system to monitor remotely located patients. To monitor remotely located epileptic patients we have presented a brief discussion here. Then, we have presented a discussion in short about motivation and objective behind the writing of this book chapter, which includes some application of remote location patient monitoring telemedicine system too. Further, we have mentioned about monitoring of remote patients to monitor chronic disease, heart-related problems, to monitor diabetic patients, and intensive care unit (ICU) patients, etc. Then, we have presented standards for telemedicine system using which system can perform well. Further, we have briefly described types of telemedicine systems and presented its special features. Then, we have shown the workflow model of the telemedicine system based on cloud to monitor remote patients. In continuity, we have presented the advantage and disadvantages of telemedicine system briefly. Further, we have mentioned about various challenges facing by telemedicine system to monitor remote patients. Finally, we have made some conclusions and presented the future scope of related work.

9.2 Monitoring of remotely located patients

9.2.1 Remote patients' chronic wound monitoring

Chronic wound monitoring is a challenge in telehealthcare technology [28]. As our body covered with skin, which protects us from various causes like extreme sunlight, heat, various chemicals, polluted air, etc. actually it works as a shield. The wound is cause of damage in the skin. The wound is described as, due to any injury or any other cause damage to the skin. Because of this, wound patients may have several problems like pain, infection, swelling in tissues, etc. which may affect other body parts too. Sometimes this wound may be dangerous and become chronic, which may prevent its healing and become the cause of immobility, reduced quality life. Due to extreme wound condition, the patient may suffer from the loss of his stability, mental condition, etc. As we know, the chronic wound may take a longer time to get back normal and may vary patient to patient. A chronic wound not only affects the patient life but also the entire family gets disturbed due to the wound and its caring cost. For the treatment of the wound, proper care and the medical facility must require. These may be categorized in open and closed types. In open wound, usually skin may break; blood came out, etc. whereas in case the close wound skin surface is normal but internal tissues may damage/internal bleeding may possible.

The use of telemedicine provides audio-video communication in two-way interaction, which helps the patients to get treatment in a faster way along with the proper suggestion. The telemedicine system may provide medical facilities to remote patients with the help of a specialist practitioner and can help to transmit/process information through a communication system or using the cloud. The main objective of this system is to provide proper health service to the user. Telemedicine may provide service to various health control purposes like telecardiology, teledermatology, teleoncology, etc. along with monitoring of remotely located patients, which works based on wireless communication platforms with the use of IoT. The telemedicine system may provide accurate, reliable, and secured service with optimum cost. With serious problems and unavailability of medical facilities, patients may use such system; even use of smartphones makes such system very efficient, which can collect information from patients and able to transmit them over the cloud. Telemedicine systems are classified in two ways, the first one is a real-time telemedicine system and another one is a store-and-forward system. In the real-time system, the practitioner may help to collect information and transmit/process them either through the live transmission of data or through video conferencing mode. In store-and-forward telemedicine system captured independent patient data in the form of images, text files, etc. may send through telemedical Agents, which help to transmit information over the Internet to hospitals for further treatment [29]. The telemedicine system provides services to patients located in rural along with urban areas. The system can provide superior performance in case of wound monitoring and for their treatment. There are various sensors help to collect wound data from patients. Oduncu *et al.* [30] describe using digital color image processing, analysis of skin wound images. The system uses cameras or smartphones to collect images and used for transmission and processing. In this image, analysis has been done based on the wound area and color distribution on it. For telemedicine system, the smartphone may play an important role, which helps to improve efficiency. With the use of such devices or mobile apps, patients located in distance may greatly benefit. Kevin *et al.* [31] presented that telemedical agent collects wound data using a smartphone high-quality camera and transmit them to a telemedical hub to get a proper suggestion. Such a system may use messaging or calling only in case of emergency. The telemedicine system may use various features of smartphones to improve the service and may help to store patient data.

To provide proper and successful, telemedicine system requires various like accessibility, reliability, flexibility, security, cost, storage, optimization, ease in upgradation, etc. For better functioning of the system, it requires better communication and security mechanism, so that along with image data, videos of the wound can be transferred for getting a superior medical solution (Figure 9.3) representing wound monitoring of remote patients. In telemedicine system data gathered from patients, processed over the cloud to network-connected hospitals, where data will be further analyzed and according to practitioner opinion suggestion will be provided to the patient through a telemedical agent.

9.2.2 Remote patients monitoring related to heart patients

Telemedicine system may help for monitoring of heart-related disease. As in the case of any problem in the body, there may be some significant signs related to the heart, which gives information about body situation. Monitoring of heart also gives information about unknown diseases like a heart attack, blood clotting, blood pressure, etc. are the most frequent and common problem. There is a need to monitor ECG (electrocardiogram), heart rate, blood pressure, oxygen percentage in blood, respiration

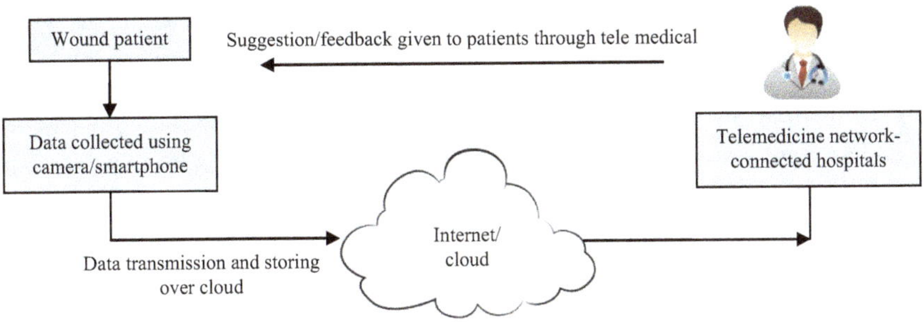

Figure 9.3 Remote patients chronic wound monitoring

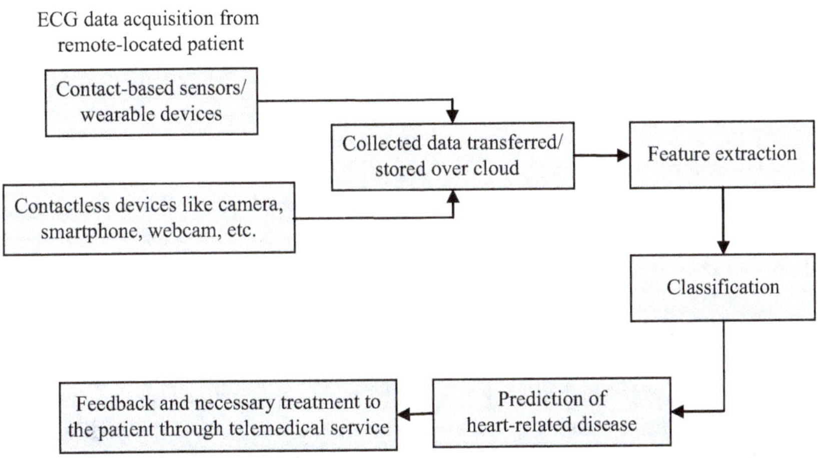

Figure 9.4 Remote patients monitoring of heart patient

rate, etc. Telemedicine system provides the opportunity to local patients or remotely located patients to take care of such facility. In this system, various wearable devices are there which helps to monitor and collect the data with accuracy. There are various mobile phone-based apps, which able to monitor ECG remote patients [32].

To monitor heart-related patients (Figure 9.4), the main challenge is to acquire the signal, so that it can give proper information about the condition of patient health. There are contact-based and contactless methods to acquire the ECG signal, in which the contact-based method is very common. A telemonitoring system has been presented [33], which uses hardware as well as Android-based software methods to monitor heart patients. To monitor variations in heart rate and ECG signal, an autonomous nervous system has been presented [34]. For real-time monitoring and treatment of patients affected with heart disease have been presented [35] and observed that the author uses support vector classification algorithm for decision-making and achieved 85% accuracy. Ferreira *et al.* [36] present a system, which gives an idea to measure ECG, temperature of body, oxygen concentration level in the blood, airflow through lungs, etc. A telemedicine system for the purpose of an emergency health service, a study has been presented [37], which uses shelf medical device for monitoring of biomedical signals. For contactless method, there are various researches already going on and some of the work has been presented here. An approach for estimating heart rate based on camera/facial video has been presented [38]. Based on skin color processing, an estimation of heart rate for remote patients has been presented which uses principal component analysis and empirical mode decomposition classification method [39]. An approach based on machine learning; to monitor heart rate using webcam has been presented and achieved good accuracy [40].

9.2.3 Remote patients monitoring related to diabetic patients

Diabetes is a serious health problem. Due to this, patients may lose this earlier. Hence it is required to monitor blood glucose levels in the body. Maintaining its level not only has reduced risk of diabetes but also provides a healthier lifestyle. To continuously monitor blood, the glucose level in real time is a challenging task. Monkaresi *et al.* [41] discussed self-management of diabetes based on the android application for patients located in urban as well as a rural area. An energy-efficient healthcare system for continuous monitoring of glucose level in blood-based on fog has been presented [42], which is able to provide an alert during an emergency situation. An automatic feedback message system has been presented [43], which provides a way to maintain database for blood pressure, the glucose level in blood, weight, uses of medicine, body activeness, etc. There are various noninvasive techniques to monitor blood glucose levels presented [44], which inform us about various applications and advantages of this method and improvement requires. Some of the contactless methods for monitoring glucose levels have been presented [45,46], which uses time to time, good quality images of retina and foot respectively and analyzed them.

9.2.4 Remote monitoring for intensive care unit (ICU) patients

Monitoring of ICU patients is a difficult task. To monitor such patients, the telemedicine system requires a specialized group of staff along with access control by doctors, which helps to continuous monitoring of patients. The telemedicine system provides an opportunity for patients located in a remote location to get direct assistance from doctors, which increases the efficiency and quality of patient care. Development of a telemedicine system for monitoring of patients in ICU presented [47]. A study about setup cost and their effectiveness of telemedicine system for intensive care unit patients has been presented [48]. Here, the author has made an analysis based on pre-title and post-tele-ICU period patients' care and found it economical. For remote monitoring of Intensive care unit patients, a workflow has been presented [49,50], which uses time and motion study. Paper presented shows that authors have used 9 intensive care units to remotely monitor 132 beds, which involves a team of 13 members.

9.3 Standards for telemedicine system

The telemedicine system works using some standards and follows the guideline. At the time of implementing the telemedicine system for e-health, some guidelines and standards are presented [51], which follows ethical issues standards based on mutual understanding between patients and practitioners, security and privacy. By the author, it is mentioned that there are three types of guidelines for the purpose of clinical, technical, and operational analysis. The main focus of the telemedicine system is to monitor remotely located patients. The guidelines specially focused on teledermatology, telepathology, surgical system, telepsychiatry, and home-based telenursing. For the purpose of remote patient monitoring and in the field of m-health, there is a requirement of well-established standards and set of rules for the whole telemedicine system, which makes telemedicine system more reliable and accurate. For the advancement of a telemedicine system, the health resource and service administration (HRSA), office of the advancement of telehealth and department of defense has been presented a guideline in the United States, to establish reliable and compatible telemedicine system. For the purpose of video consultation in a telemedicine system, standards are defined by the international telecommunication union (ITU). H.320 and H.323 are most common and recent standards for multimedia conferencing, which are using ISDN37 and IP networks (Table 9.1). For the purpose of communication through the medical image, a standard has been provided by digital imaging and communication in medicine (DICOM). These standards are sufficiently able for image acquisition, the transmission of image data supports analysis and able to provide compatibility and long-standing storage.

9.4 Types of a telemedicine system

The telemedicine system provides a range of health services instead of just monitoring patients in real-time. This system includes various clinical services with the help of telecommunication technology. In the classification of the telemedicine

Table 9.1 Standards designed for telemedicine system

Standards for telemedicine system	Formulated by
To get compatibility, interoperability, reliability, accuracy, and scalability of a telemedicine system	Office for the advancement of telehealth, the health resource and service administration and department of defense
For the purpose of video conferencing H.320 and H.323 standard using ISDN and IP network respectively	International Telecommunication Union (ITU)
For the medical image data acquisition, transmission and reception and storing capacity	The Digital Imaging and Communications in Medicine (DICOM)

system, the system is mainly categorized by way of providing healthcare solutions. Store and forward telemedicine solution, remote patient monitoring, and real-time telehealth are an important class of telemedicine system.

Store and forward telemedicine solutions also termed as asynchronous telemedicine. It allows health service providers to transfer the patient's medical information in the form of images, videos or reports, etc. from a different area. The system provides the services with security, reliability, and maintains privacy (email–one of the ways to share information). As in the case of getting suggestions through email, it does not require real-time data processing. It uses to collect reports, store it and transmit it and as there is no direct communication between doctor and patient, it is treated as an asynchronous approach. For example, teleradiology, teledermatology mainly focused on the store and forward telemedicine solution. This method helps to improve the efficiency of the e-health system, as there is no requirement for being patients and experts at the same location at the same time. With the use telemedicine system, provides quicker service, lower waiting time for patients, easy accessibility, etc.

Remote patient monitoring telemedicine system allows healthcare service providers to monitor patients located in a remote area, based on data collected directly collected from the patient's body through sensors (wearable devices). This type of telemedicine system also termed as telemonitoring of home telehealth. The system allows the experts to take care of patients by finding any alert signs from the patient's data during treatment or rehab. The remote patient monitoring system is growing very rapidly and becoming popular as it is very much helpful for long term care. For example, an epileptic patient may get seizures, any time during his working activity. In such case, it is required to monitor patients regularly and collect symptoms and in case of any warning sign, the patient should get alert either through message or by his caretaker, so that any miss happening can be prohibited. The telemedicine system makes easier communication between health experts and patients. The main reason for becoming popular for such a system is that patients can monitor themselves using wearable devices and collected sensors data can be transferred automatically to experts. Patients may get home-based healthcare services at low cost, reliability, and accuracy. A real-time telehealth telemedicine system is another class of telemedicine systems; in which patients can be monitored in real-time through multimedia conferencing. As in this type of system, both doctors and patients can communicate with each other simultaneously; the system is also termed as a synchronous system. It is an easier way for patients located in a remote area to get consult with doctors from anywhere in the world and may get a quicker solution or treatment. It is also convenient for doctors with just good quality of Internet connection, webcam, and microphone facility.

9.5 Special features of the telemedicine system

Telemedicine system is helpful in the e-health field from various points of view like providing ambulance service patient care, consultation with a specialist, monitoring of remotely located patients, providing mobile hospital service, etc. to provide quality service. There is number of specialties of the telemedicine system, which are adopted precisely and provide healthcare solutions with reliability and accuracy (Figure 9.5).

1. *Teledermatology*: It is a popular application of telemedicine systems. Solution for teledermatology is based on the store and forward technology, which allows the provider of health service to transfer health-related information of patients located over long distances using audio, images and video data communication. With this technology service providers may able to send data of diseases like rashes, skin problems, etc. for consultation, analysis and treatment purposes and even can be used for educational purposes.
2. *Telenephrology*: When it is required to monitor remotely located patients related to any problem linked with kidney, telenephrology provides the solution in the form of consultation and treatment.
3. *Teleobstetrics*: Usually for pregnant women, it is required to continuously visit the hospital and a meeting with an obstetrician, for proper guidance and suggestion during pregnancy. Teleobstetrics allows the monitoring of such patients and can help to get time to time suggestions.

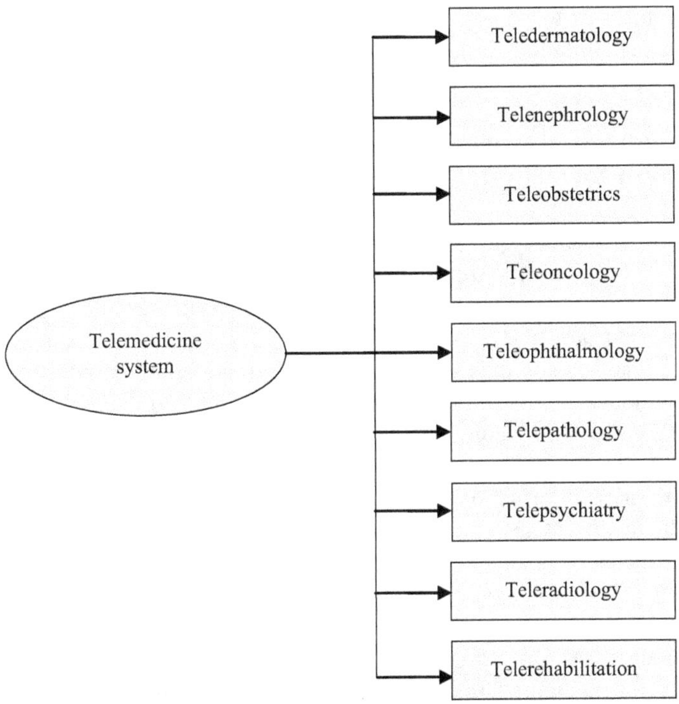

Figure 9.5 Specialties of a telemedicine system

4. *Teleoncology*: This system allows us to taken care and monitoring of remotely located patients affected with cancer. Teleoncology systems can provide a solution based on the store and forward images for the purpose of detection and analysis, even some system supports live video analysis.
5. *Teleophthalmology*: It is another feature of the telemedicine system, which allows monitoring remotely located eye patients. The system can detect and treat any eye-related problem and may provide the solution based on the store and forward method. This system allows experts to collect ocular image data and monitor the patients carefully.
6. *Telepathology*: It uses telecommunication system technology to transmit image pathology data for analysis and detection of any problem. The system uses to store and forward method to share high-quality images and video data.
7. *Telepsychiatry*: It helps the patients for providing remote monitoring and accesses them to health service. It is a popular method for diagnosing the patients as there are limited numbers of experts available for psychiatry.
8. *Teleradiology*: This is one of the oldest fields in the telemedicine system. The system can provide solutions to radiological patients and able to transmit the images like X-ray, CT (computed tomography) scan, and MRI (magnetic resonance imaging) scan to distance located hospitals. With the use of teleradiology, patients can achieve quicker suggestions from experts.
9. *Telerehabilitation*: Telerehabilitation system works based on computer and communication technologies to enhance rehabilitation facility. The system can deliver rehabilitation services to remote patients.

9.6 Cloud-based workflow model of a telemedicine system for remote patient monitoring

IoT cloud-based telemedicine system plays a huge role in the monitoring of patients located in urban as well as rural areas. With the use of various IoT devices like wearable sensors, smartphones, etc., patient's data can be collected easily and stored and using proper processing technologies collected information further can be used for analysis and diagnosis of disease. Using a cloud-based system even a very huge amount of data of any disease can be maintained precisely and used for various applications. In Figure 9.6, we are presenting a cloud-based working model of a telemedicine system for monitoring of remotely located patients. The presented system can share information from patients end to experts end and vice-versa, provides the facility of analyzing, storing, and monitoring user health data securely. The important element of the presented system is data collection, which can be obtained using various wearable sensors and collected information can be stored over a cloud server, where it can be maintained and kept securely. Healthcare experts can access this information and can analyze the patient's data and suggest accordingly for medicines. In case of emergency, the healthcare service provider may bale to provide ambulance service to patients for further necessary action. Over the cloud collected patients signal me be enhanced and further recovered and

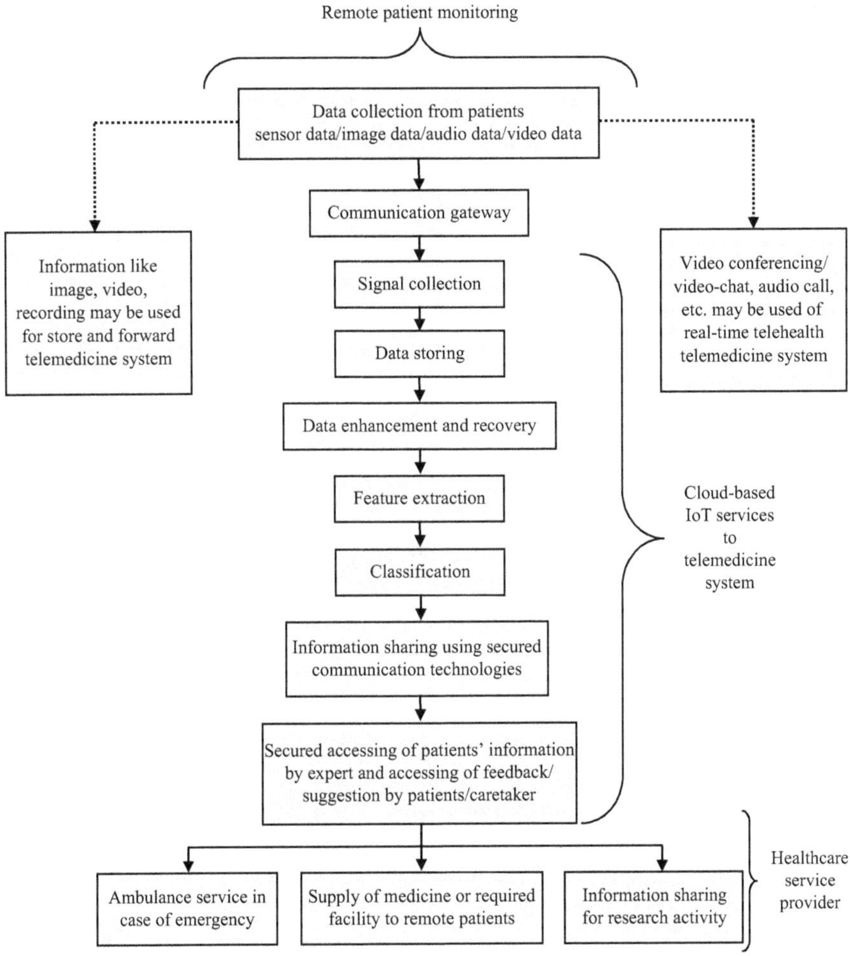

Figure 9.6 Workflow diagram for remote monitoring telemedicine system

necessary steps like feature extraction, classification for disease prediction and diagnosis can be taken. The system will be able to provide patient monitoring continuously to both located in hospital and home.

9.7 Advantage and disadvantage of the telemedicine system

The telemedicine system provides better care in terms of monitoring and cost-effectiveness to users. The system allows users located in remote areas, which need most, to access such a facility. With the use of the telemedicine system, the healthcare sector is evolving continuously. As we know everything has few negative points along with its good features, similarly, the telemedicine system has some advantages as well as a disadvantage too. Mainly telemedicine provides virtual communication between patients and doctors, but with enhancing popularity, it is widely acceptable worldwide. Using cloud-based IoT services/current technologies makes telemedicine system very advantageous in the health care sector.

(a) Time-saving is possible
(b) Improved patient care system
(c) Provide economical healthcare service
(d) Regular and continuous monitoring of patients
(e) Direct consultation from specialist health experts
(f) Patients may able to get the second opinion around the world
(g) Ease in access and provide more convenience for patient care
(h) With the use of proper guideline and standards smooth workflow of the system

The telemedicine system saves time and money for the patients. Most of the time patients may require visiting the hospital continuously, for the patients located in a remote area, it becomes a very hectic job to go the hospital, get appointments and wait for doctors even in case of emergency. Regular visiting of the hospital may kill time and money both, telemedicine system may help to save both and provide a better cure. The telemedicine system provides easy accessibility to doctors as well as patients. Most of the patients around the world are from the older group, which may have a problem even in moving, for such patient's telemedicine may provide health service at their home itself. Most of the times it is possible to monitor patients with the help of their health-related data, reports, etc. but sometimes direct consultation is much needed. For this purpose, through audio or video call patients may get direct suggestions from patients. Telemedicine system works with the use of IoT and the present user are well equipped with IoT devices like smartphone, sensors, etc. using these patients may connect with experts very frequently and able to get feedback quickly. Health service provider linked with telemedicine system ensures that patient condition is good or in case of emergency may able to provide health-related services. The system can monitor patients even after discharge from the hospital and able to keep track of recovery status.

Along with above all number of advantages, the telemedicine system has few drawbacks also. As telemedicine system involves various standards and equipment, to handle and operate them precisely there is a requirement of expert technicians and training. With the use of virtual consultation, direct meetings with doctors may reduce, as we know there is no alternate of meeting with doctors and get back home with confidence. Without direct meetings and physical checkups, it completely looks like an uncompleted diagnosis and treatment. Sometime hospital rules/policies may change and patients may get the unnecessary headache of doing things like fee payments, refunds, etc.

1. Perfect Internet environment
2. The requirement of the number of equipment
3. To follow the change in policies in hospitals

4. The requirement of technical and experienced staff
5. No direct communication with healthcare experts
6. May chance of delay from the healthcare service provider
7. There may be a chance of getting incorrect data through sensors
8. Training of staff to operate telemedicine equipment precisely
9. When it is required to meet directly with doctors and physical checkup is compulsory, in such cases telemedicine system cannot help
10. Battery support is an issue with IoT devices.

9.8 Challenges for designing the telemedicine system

The telemedicine system can monitor remote patient care and able to manage healthcare service providers. The system plays an important role in monitoring the patient who is even not able to move, chronic diseases as well as behavioral illness. There are various factors, which are still a challenge for the telemedicine system and monitoring remote patients. Setup cost for telemedicine system for monitoring the remote patient is higher, even to avail the facility it will be costlier, to attract patients along with paying an extra amount of money itself a challenge. Even after, set up of telemedicine system, way of the utilization of telemedicine system itself a challenge. There may chance of a huge number of patients, out of which some them are such types, to whom it does not require an urgent suggestion, due to this the patient who really needs the quick service may have to wait in quit to get a response. As still there is a need for improvement in the telemedicine system for monitoring patients, sometimes it is possible to wrong prediction of disease by mistake. In such case, patient may suffer from unnecessarily drug dosage or allergy.

As we are aware of the benefits of remote patient monitoring telemedicine systems, there are some other technical issues from which, we have to deal and still a challenge to meet the standards. At present still, most of us and older patients believe that physical meetings with doctors and checkup beneficial. For such a perspective, an educated person may use the facility frequently. Hence education is an issue for the success of a remote patient monitoring system. Another issue is from the healthcare service provider side, the service provider must able to provide cost-effective service to patients. For monitoring of remote patients using telemedicine system, there is some sort of guidelines and standards should be there, to make a possibly effective way of communication. As there are various types of sensors to collect patient information, to transmit them carefully over the cloud, proper standards should be followed. The acquired patient's information must be stored and managed carefully so that accessing information should not be hectic. Analyzing this huge amount of data about patient's health should be proper so that proper care and treatment must be possible [52]. As we know, the IoT is very useful for remote patient monitoring telemedicine systems. IoT-based wearable device is an important part of telemedicine system to acquire patient information, which requires privacy and security, as there may be the possibility of data alteration, hacking, etc. in some of the cases, level of security must meet the requirement

[53,54]. For the set-up of remote patient monitoring telemedicine system, there are various devices which are battery operated like wireless body sensors, etc. as there is the use of battery continuously to the smooth working of the system and various operation like acquisition, enhancing and processing of signal [55]. For above all smartphone can play important role to handle telemedicine systems in terms of acquiring and transmitting patient data [56].

9.9 Conclusion

In this chapter, we have discussed the telemedicine system to monitor the health of remote patients. In the previous few decades, the role of IoT is also getting increased day by day and IoT health network becoming stronger. Monitoring of remotely located patients is still an up growing field and having a huge impact on modern society. Telemedicine system using IoT cloud has shown great effect in the healthcare sector, especially for old age people, who are even not able to move, for those provides home-based health solutions. Currently, the most numbers of the hospital are connected through the network and supplying various types of health services with optimum use of resources. The use of a smartphone with remote patient monitoring telemedicine system is also enhancing health. These devices can provide health solutions in a secured and quick way. This chapter also deals with various social, cultural and technological issues of monitoring remote patients. The telemedicine system can reduce the cost of providing health services with uses of mobility and computation. Including above all we have mentioned various standards of the telemedicine system, which represented some rules and guidelines for the proper functioning of the system. Here, we also have discussed a few challenges of telemedicine system and advantages and disadvantages showing huge benefits in social life. In this chapter, we have discussed remote monitoring of epileptic patients, heart patients, diabetic patients and monitoring of patients belong to the intensive care unit. These telemedicine systems reflect that to improve and providing quality of health service a well-organized structure and standards should be followed, even though till now effective and assured services are not guaranteed. It very much depends on the health service provider and experts.

9.10 Future scope

With the faster advancement of technology, there are very huge and assured positives in the future of telemedicine. It is very much possible that with technological advancement, the telemedicine system will be widely acceptable and easily accessible in the future. There are various wearable devices and smartphone-based application, which can help to monitor the remote patients and able to collect, store and transmit the data from user end to destination end. With continuous upgradation of the IoT-based services, telemedicine system will eliminate all barriers like state-wise or nation wise service. Presently a huge number of patients using and referring to the telemedicine system and even showing great interest in it, represent a bright future of it. For a successful telemedicine system, there is a need for research to solve the query related to challenges like security, home-based solution, quality of services, etc. Still, such systems are in the early stage of monitoring chronic diseases, there is a lot to improve. Along with all these, with predefined guidelines, it is not guaranteed to get assured health service, henceforth change is necessary to get improved remote patient monitoring outcomes.

References

[1] AlDossary S., Martin-Khan M. G., Bradford N. K. and Smith A. C. (2017). A systematic review of the methodologies used to evaluate telemedicine service initiatives in hospital facilities. International Journal of Medical Informatics, 97, 171–94.

[2] Ahmed S. N., Wiebe S., Mann C. and Ohinmaa A. (2010). Telemedicine and epilepsy care — a Canada wide survey. Canadian Journal of Neurology Sciences, 37(6), 814–18.

[3] Abdulnabi M., Al-Haiqi A., Kiah M. L. M., Zaidan A. A., Zaidan B. B. and Hussain M. (2017). A distributed framework for health information exchange using smartphone technologies. Journal of Biomedical Informatics, 69, 230–50.

[4] Alanazi H. O., Zaidan A. A., Zaidan B. B., Kiah M. L. M. and Al-Bakri S. H. (2015). Meeting the security requirements of electronic medical records in the ERA of high-speed computing. Journal of Medical Systems, 39(1), 165.

[5] Hussain M., Zaidan A. A., Zidan B. B. *et al.* (2018). Conceptual framework for the security of mobile health applications on Android platform. Telematics and Informatics.

[6] Malasinghe L.P., Ramzan N. and Dahal K. (2019). Remote patient monitoring: a comprehensive study. Journal of Ambient Intelligence and Humanized Computing, 10(1), 57–76.

[7] Campos C., Caudevilla E., Alesancoc A. *et al.* (2014). Setting up a telemedicine service for remote real-time video-EEG consultation in La Rioja (Spain). *International Journal of Medical Informatics*, 81, 404–14.

[8] Lasierra N., Alesanco A., Campos C., Caudevilla E., Fernandez J. and Garcia J. (2009). Experience of a real-time tele-EEG service. 31st Annual International Conference of the IEEE EMBS. New York: IEEE; 5211–14.

[9] Thangavelu S. K., Kasthuri N., Sundaram V., Aravind N. and Bilakanti N. (2016). A stand-alone EEG monitoring system for remote diagnosis. Telemedicine and e-Health, 22(4), 310–16.

[10] Talal M., Zaidan A. A., Zaidan B. B. *et al.* (2019). Smart home-based IoT for real-time and secure remote health monitoring of triage and priority system using body sensors: multi-driven systematic review. Journal of Medical Systems, 43(3), 1–34.

[11] Zaidan B. B., Haiqi A., Zaidan A. A., Abdulnabi M., Kiah M. L. M. and Muzamel H. (2015). A security framework for nationwide health information exchange based on telehealth strategy. Journal of Medical Systems, 39(5), 1–19.

[12] Wechsler L. R., Tsao J. W., Levine S. R. *et al.* (2013). Teleneurology applications: Report of the Telemedicine Work Group of the American Academy of Neurology. Neurology, 80(7), 670–76.

[13] Ahmed S. N., Mann C., Sinclair D. B. *et al.* (2008). Feasibility of epilepsy follow-up care through telemedicine: a pilot study on the patient's perspective. Epilepsia, 49(4), 573–85.

[14] Malasinghe L. P., Ramzan N. and Dahal K. (2017). Remote patient monitoring: a comprehensive study. Journal of Ambient Intelligence and Humanized Computing. doi:10.1007/s12652-017-0598-x

[15] Chen M., Wan J., Gonzalez S., Liao X. and Leung V. C. M. (2014). A Survey of recent developments in home M2M networks. IEEE Communications Surveys & Tutorials, 16(1), 98–14.

[16] Tsakalakis M. and Bourbakis N. G. (2014). Health Care Sensor- Based Systems for Point of Care Monitoring and Diagnostic Applications: A Brief Survey. 2014 36th Annual International Conference of the IEEE Engineering in Medicine and Biology Society. doi:10.1109/embc.2014.6945061

[17] Baig M. M. and Gholamhosseini H. (2013). Smart health monitoring systems: an overview of design and modeling. Journal of Medical Systems, 37(2), 1–14.

[18] Erden F., Velipasalar S., Alkar A. Z. and Cetin A. E. (2016). Sensors in assisted living: a survey of signal and image processing methods. IEEE Signal Processing Magazine, 33(2), 36–44.

[19] Wac K. and Tsiourti C. (2014). Ambulatory assessment of affect: survey of sensor systems for monitoring of autonomic nervous systems activation in emotion. IEEE Transactions on Affective Computing, 5(3), 251–72.

[20] Schneider R. B. and Biglan K. M. (2017). The promise of telemedicine for chronic neurological disorders: the example of Parkinson's disease. Lancet Neurology, 16(7), 541–51.

[21] Prabhakar S. K. and Rajaguru H. (2017). Development of patient remote monitoring system for epilepsy classification. In: Goh J, Lim CT, Leo HL (editors) The 16th international conference on biomedical engineering: ICBME 2016, 7th to 10th December 2016, Singapore. Singapore: Springer Singapore; 80–7.

[22] Prabhakar S. K. and Rajaguru H. (2015). Analysis of centre tendency mode chaotic modeling for electroencephalography signals obtained from an epileptic patient. Advanced Studies in Theoretical Physics, 9(4), 171–7, HIKARI Ltd.

[23] Winterhalder M., Maiwald T., Voss H. U., Aschenbrenner-Scheibe R., Timmer J. and Schulze-Bonhage A. (2003). The seizure prediction characteristic: a general framework to assess and compare seizure prediction methods. Epilepsy & Behavior, 4(3), 318–25.

[24] D'Alessandro M., Esteller R., Vachtsevanos G., Hinson A., Echauz J. and Litt B. (2003). Epileptic seizure prediction using hybrid feature selection over multiple intracranial EEG electrode contacts: a report of four patients. IEEE Transactions on Biomedical Engineering, 50(5), 603–15.

[25] Guo L., Rivero D., Dorado J., Rabuñal J. R. and Pazos A. (2010). Automatic epileptic seizure detection in EEGs based on line length feature and artificial neural networks. Journal of Neuroscience Methods, 191(1), 101–9.

[26] Prabhakar S. K. and Rajaguru H. (2017). Hadamard Transform Based PAPR Reduction for Telemedicine Applications Utilized for Epilepsy Classification. 3rd International Conference on Movement, Health and Exercise, 33–36.

[27] Prabhakar S. K. and Rajaguru H. (2017). PCA Based Selective Mapping Technique for Reduced PAPR Implemented for Distributed Wireless Patient Monitoring Epilepsy Classification System. 3rd International Conference on Movement, Health and Exercise, 41–44.

[28] Chakraborty C., Gupta B. and Ghosh S. K. (2016). Mobile Telemedicine Systems for Remote Patient's Chronic Wound Monitoring, IGI: M-Health Innovations for Patient-Centered Care, Ch. 11, 217–43, ISBN: 9781466698611.

[29] Chakraborty C., Gupta B. and Ghosh S. K. (2014). Mobile metadata assisted community database of chronic wound images. Wound Medicine, 6, 34–42.

[30] Oduncu H., Hoppe A. and Clark M. (2004). Analysis of skin wound images using digital color image processing: a preliminary communication. Lower Extremity Wounds, 3(3), 151–6.

[31] Kevin H. and Yuan-T Z. (2003). Implementation of a WAP-based telemedicine system for patient monitoring. IEEE Transactions on Information Technology in Biomedicine, 7(2), 101–7.

[32] Nguyen H. H. and Silva J. N. A. (2016). Use of smartphone technology in cardiology. Trends in Cardiovascular Medicine, 26(4), 376–86.

[33] Szydło T. and Konieczny M. (2016). Mobile and wearable devices in an open and universal system for remote patient monitoring. Microprocessors and Microsystems, 46, 44–54.

[34] Lanata A., Valenza G., Nardelli M., Gentili C. and Scilingo E. P. (2015). Complexity index from a personalized wearable monitoring system for assessing remission in mental health. *IEEE Journal of Biomedical and Health Informatics*, 19(1), 132–9.

[35] Otoom A. F., Abdallah E. E., Kilani Y., Kefaye A. and Ashour M. M. S. (2015). Effective diagnosis and monitoring of heart disease. International Journal of Software Engineering and its Applications, 9(1), 143–56.

[36] Ferreira F., Carvalho V., Soares F., Machado J. and Pereira F. (2015). Vital signs monitoring system using radio frequency communication: a medical care terminal for bedridden people support. Sensors and Transducers, 185(2), 93–9.

[37] Thelen S., Czaplik M., Meisen P., Schilberg D. and Jeschke S. (2015). Using off-the-shelf medical devices for biomedical signal monitoring in a telemedicine system for emergency medical services. IEEE Journal of Biomedical and Health Informatics, 19(1), 117–23.

[38] Hassan M. A., Malik A. S., Fofi D. *et al.* (2017). Heart rate estimation using facial video: A review. Biomedical Signal Processing and Control, 38, 346–60.

[39] Bogdan G., Radu V., Octavian F., Alin B., Constantin M. and Cristian C. (2015). Remote Assessment of Heart Rate by Skin Color Processing. 2015 IEEE International Black Sea Conference on Communications and Networking (BlackSeaCom).

[40] Monkaresi H., Calvo R. A. and Hong Yan. (2014). A machine learning approach to improve contactless heart rate monitoring using a webcam. IEEE Journal of Biomedical and Health Informatics, 18(4), 1153–60.

[41] Hood M., Wilson R., Corsica J., Bradley L., Chirinos D. and Vivo A. (2016). What do we know about mobile applications for diabetes self-management? A review of reviews. Journal of Behavioral Medicine, 39(6), 981–94.

[42] Devarajan M., Subramaniyaswamy V., Vijayakumar V. and Ravi L. (2019). Fog-assisted personalized healthcare-support system for remote patients with diabetes. Journal of Ambient Intelligence and Humanized Computing. doi:10.1007/s12652-019-01291-5

[43] Fioravanti A., Fico G., Salvi D., García-Betances R. I. and Arredondo M. T. (2015). Automatic messaging for improving patients' engagement in diabetes management: an exploratory study. Medical & Biological Engineering & Computing, 53(12), 1285–94.

[44] Vashist S. K. (2012). Non-invasive glucose monitoring technology in diabetes management: A review. Analytica Chimica Acta, 750, 16–27.

[45] Askew D. A., Crossland L., Ware R. S. *et al.* (2012). Diabetic retinopathy screening and monitoring of early stage disease in general practice: design and methods. Contemporary Clinical Trials, 33(5), 969–75.

[46] Hazenberg C. E. V. B., Bus S. A., Kottink A. I. R., Bouwmans C. A. M., Schönbach-Spraul A. M. and van Baal S. G. (2011). Telemedical home-monitoring of diabetic foot disease using photographic foot imaging – a feasibility study. Journal of Telemedicine and Telecare, 18(1), 32–6.

[47] Bhagwan V. and Grobbelaar S. S. (2017). Development of a Telemedicine System for Monitoring Intensive Care Patients. Proceedings of the 2017 International Conference on Information System and Data Mining - ICISDM '17.

[48] Franzini L., Sail K. R., Thomas E. J. and Wueste L. (2011). Costs and cost-effectiveness of a telemedicine intensive care unit program in 6 intensive care units in a large health care system. Journal of Critical Care, 26(3), 329.e1–329.e6.

[49] Tang Z., Weavind L., Mazabob J., Thomas E. J., Chu-Weininger M. Y. L. and Johnson T. R. (2007). Workflow in intensive care unit remote monitoring: a time-and-motion study. Critical Care Medicine, 35(9), 2057–63.

[50] Vranas K. C., Slatore C. G. and Kerlin M. P. (2018). Telemedicine coverage of intensive care units: a narrative review. Annals of the American Thoracic Society. doi:10.1513/annalsats.201804-225fr

[51] Loane M. and Wootton R. (2002). A review of guidelines and standards for telemedicine. Journal of Telemedicine and Telecare, 8(2), 63–71.

[52] Raghupathi W. and Raghupathi V. (2014). Big data analytics in healthcare: promise and potential. Health Information Science and Systems, 2(1), 1–10.

[53] Zubaydi F., Saleh A., Aloul F. and Sagahyroon A. (2015). Security of Mobile Health (mHealth) Systems. 2015 IEEE 15th International Conference on Bioinformatics and Bioengineering (BIBE).

[54] Yin Y., Zeng Y., Chen X. and Fan Y. (2016). The internet of things in healthcare: an overview. Journal of Industrial Information Integration, 1, 3–13.

[55] Ghamari M., Janko B., Sherratt R., Harwin W., Piechockic R. and Soltanpur C. (2016). A survey on wireless body area networks for ehealthcare systems in residential environments. Sensors, 16(6), 831.

[56] Gupta A. Chakraborty C. and Gupta B. (2019). Medical information processing using smartphone under IoT framework, Springer: energy conservation for IoT devices, Studies in Systems, Decision and Control, 206, 283–308, ISBN 978-981-13-7398-5.

Chapter 10

Impact of tone-mapping operators and viewing devices on visual quality of experience of colour and grey-scale HDR images

Shaymaa Al-Juboori[1], Is-Haka Mkwawa[1], Lingfen Sun[1] and Emmanuel Ifeachor[1]

Tone-mapping-operators (TMOs) provide a useful means for converting high dynamic (HDR) images to low dynamic range (LDR) images so that they can be viewed on standard displays, but this may influence the visual quality of experience (QoE) of the end-user. There is a need to understand the impact of TMOs to inform the choice of TMO algorithms for different displays, especially for small-screen-devices (SSDs) such as those used in mobile phones. This is important, as mobile devices are becoming the primary means of consuming multimedia contents. However, few studies have been undertaken to assess the impact of TMOs and viewing devices (especially SSDs) on the visual QoE of the user when using. In this chapter, we evaluate subjectively and objectively, the commonly used TMOs in different displays and resolutions for colour and grey-scale HDR images. Our results show that viewing devices have an influence on the TMOs performance, suggesting the need for a careful choice of TMO to enhance the viewing-QoE of the end-user. As expected, the higher resolution, the better HDR-image quality. Surprisingly, there was no significant difference between the Mean of Opinion Score (MOS) scores for colour and grey-scale images in SSDs. The device and TMOs affect QoE for colour and grey HDR-image equally. We found Shannon entropy (SE) to be a good objective measure of quality for colour and grey HDR images, suggesting that entropy may find use in automated HDR quality control assessment schemes, while; HDR-VDP-2 is a good objective measure for colour HDR image only.

10.1 Introduction

With advances in multimedia technology, high dynamic range (HDR) representation of the image content is attracting increased interest as a means of improving visual QoE, especially in imaging applications such as photography, TV and cinema [1,2]. A

[1]Signal Processing and Multimedia Communication, School of Computing, Electronics and Mathematics, University of Plymouth, Plymouth, UK

common problem that is often encountered in practice is how to visualize HDR images on standard display devices that are designed to display LDR images. To overcome this problem, TMOs have been developed to convert HDR to LDR images [1,3–5]. However, tone-mapping procedures inevitably cause information loss, because of the reduction in the dynamic range of the image. With many TMOs proposed in recent years, it is unclear, which TMO faithfully preserves the structural information in the original HDR images, and which TMO produces natural-looking realistic LDR images for different displays [1,6]. In particular, a few TMOs are designed for use with SSDs such as those of mobile phones and tablets [7,8].

As SSDs are rapidly becoming the leading platform for multimedia content consumption, there is a need to ensure an optimal QoE when viewing HDR content on typical mobile device displays [6,9]. This problem is exacerbated by the existence of a large variety of brands and models of mobile devices, with their differing resolutions and sizes, it is also unclear whether existing TMOs can be used directly with SSDs [6]. These issues have recently begun to be addressed [7–12], but only a small number of studies have been reported so far. Urbano *et al.* [8] carried out the first evaluation of TMOs on a mobile device, the authors found that the performance of TMO algorithms on SSDs differed significantly compared to the performance on LDRs. However, the study was based on only one mobile device, making difficult to generalize the findings. Melo *et al.* [4] evaluated six TMOs on HDR video using three different displays including one mobile device (a Tablet) and found significant differences in the TMOs performance between LDRs and SSDs displays. However, only one SSD was used in the study and it was based on HDR video and not HDR image. Akyüz *et al.* [12] investigated how TMOs and exposure fusion performs on SSDs. three HDR images of real scenes were evaluated on 24″ and 3″ displays. They found that the viewing device did not affect the ranking of the image quality significantly. However, the results cannot be generalized to all mobile devices, since the display size of the SSD used was relatively small. In general, the results from previous studies are inconclusive in a number of aspects. For example, Urbano *et al.* and Akyüz *et al.* found differences in the displays while Melo *et al.* did not. In addition, in all previous studies, the visual QoE of the end-user was not considered [6]. Consideration of the QoE of the end-user is important if we are to capture more fully the end-users expectations and viewing experience [13]. HDR should enhance the viewing experience of the end-user and as a result, it is attracting interest both industry and academia as a means of enhancing the viewing QoE in imaging applications. However, it is unclear whether different mobile devices have differing influence on the viewing QoE of HDR images, and if so, to how this compares with LDRs.

In addition, there are concerns about the use of grey-scale HDR images because there are no TMOs for such HDR images at present. We hypothesize the HDR processing techniques used for colour HDR images should give improved visual QoE for the grey HDR images because the local perceptual contrast in a wider range of the scene will be preserved [14]. In this chapter, we have made a number of experiments in order to determine the best TMOs that can be applied to the grey-scale HDR images.

In our recent study [6], we investigated the impact of TMOs and viewing devices on visual QoE for coloured HDR images, subjectively and objectively using ten different TMO algorithms with LDR displays and different sizes and resolutions for SSDs (i.e. mobile and tablet). We found that SSDs' gave better subjective results than the LDR displays with different TMOs. Moreover, for the mobile, higher resolutions gave more favourable MOS results. In this chapter, we extend our previous study to address a number of concerns about the impact of TMOs and SSD on the visual QoE of the end-user. In particular, we investigate the impact of different mobile devices and resolutions and TMOs on the QoE for colour and grey-level HDR images. The chapter provides a new insight into the impact of viewing devices and TMO algorithms on the visual QoE for both colour and grey-scale HDR images and how QoE scores change with the TMO.

The remainder of the chapter is organized into five sections as follows: In Section 10.1, we present a comparison of HDR images with traditional images. In Section 10.3, we present the methodology used to investigate the impact of the TMOs and viewing devices on the HDR quality. In particular, we discuss the subjective and objective methods used to assess the impact. In Section 10.4, we present the results of the investigation and compare the results of both approaches. Section 10.5 discusses the comparison of subjective and objective assessments of HDR image quality. Section 10.6 discusses the results and highlights their implications. Section 10.7 concludes the paper and highlights potential future research directions.

10.2 Comparison of HDR images with traditional images (LDR)

An HDR image can describe a greater range of colour and brightness than can be represented in an LDR image. While a standard LDR image typically uses 8 bits to store each colour of a pixel, an HDR image is most often specified to floating point precision. The difference makes it possible to encode the entire range of colours and luminances visible to the human eye [4,15,16]. Floating-point values can represent values between integers, moreover, because of the scaling factor; they can represent a much greater range of values. On the other hand, floating-point operations usually are slightly slower than integer operations [17].

The luminance of the HDR image in the real world vary from 10^4 cd/m^2 to 10^6 cd/m^2 and can be stored as floating point values [4,15]. On the other hand, the LDR of images/videos store the intensities of the scene as integer pixel values, normally in the range [0 255] which represent colours that should appear on a display device and not necessarily correspond to the scene intensities [3,15]. According to this, the areas that are too dark are clipped to black (0) and areas that are too bright are clipped to white (255). Undoubtedly, this will lead to losses in both contrast and visual details. The representation of a floating point in HDR overcomes this; instead of the bright and dark areas being saturated in an ad-hoc manner as is the case with LDR, they are assigned values proportional to the actual scene intensity [3,11,18]. Therefore, HDR content is scene-referred; as a result, an HDR still image can capture very high contrasts, which in turn permits it to incorporate details that the human eye can recognize [19].

Although HDR imaging offers recognizable advantages over the traditional LDR content in terms of the enhanced visual QoE, its large-scale deployment at consumer levels is severely held back due to two major issues [20,21]. The first one stems from the certainty that an HDR file requires larger storage space in comparison to an LDR file. For instance, an HDR still image may occupy 4 times the needed space for an LDR version of the same image [15]. Thus, as a result, effective compression algorithms are needed for HDR images/video. It should be noted that compression of LDR content has been a keen research area in any case and the occurrence of HDR images provides an additional impetus to this field. The second issue is that HDR content cannot be directly displayed on traditional display devices as these cannot provide the required luminance range, which is needed [3].

HDR image rendering algorithms can be generally classified according to the spatial processing techniques into two categories: global and local operators [15,22–26]. The global operator applies the same transformation to every pixel in the image based on the global image content, while for local operators a specific mapping approach is used for every pixel according to its spatially localized content [18,19]. It is significant to stress that in global operators, for every image it is unnecessary for the same operator applied congruently, such as the histogram; the global operator can be a function of image information. Furthermore, the local operators take various approaches to determine the spatial extent of the operator, for example, low-pass filters, edge-preserving low-pass filters, or multi-scale pyramids [27].

In both the global and local tone-mapping approaches, there are strengths and weaknesses. The global operators have a tendency to be computationally simple and as a result, can be easy to perform and faster to implement. The spatial processing of the local operators tends to be computationally more expensive but can permit for a considerable reduction in the general dynamic range [18,24].

In the other hand, processing, an HDR image only globally can lead to losing contrast, which is clearly making a loss in the visibility of detail. Local operators allow increasing the local contrast, which increases the visibility of several parts of the image whereas the global dynamic range Scales the dynamic range of the image to the output devices [15,16].

The choice of the best tone-mapping operator, weather it is global or local depends on the content, display type and size, and other environmental parameters such as back lit lighting, environment illumination, etc. These parameters (context and content) need to be explicitly taken into account when building support for HDR images in existing LDR-based applications and display systems [3,9,11,28].

10.3 Characteristics of SSDs

There are a wide variety of electronic or computing devices, these devices may come in a variety of sizes. Some of these devices may have a full-size screen, such as a desktop computer or a laptop. Mobile computing devices (or simply mobile devices), such as cell phones, PDAs (personal digital assistants), and other hand-held or highly portable computing devices may typically have a screen size that is smaller than a full-size screen offered by most desktop and laptop computers. Problems may arise when attempting to display text, images and other information on a mobile device or other small-screen devices that were formatted for display on a full-size (or larger) screen device.

The popularity of mobile devices is growing daily and as a result, mobile-cellular penetration is reaching nearly 100%. This means that, on average, there will soon be one mobile device per person [9].

Mobile devices have limitations that are not typical of desktop computers and the mobility context is different in many ways from that of traditional visualization. Compared to desktop computers, SSDs are characterized by the following differences:

1. Displays are very limited (smaller size, lower resolution, fewer colours, . . .).
2. The width/height ratio is very different from the usual 4:3.
3. The hardware (CPU, memory, buses, graphic hardware, . . .) is much less powerful.
4. The input techniques are different, e.g. handwriting and pattern recognition on a small surface, one-hand thumb-based input, point-and-tap with a stylus.
5. Slower connectivity, affecting the interactivity of applications when a significant quantity of data is stored on remote databases.

Because of these limitations, visualization applications developed for desktop computers do not scale well to mobile devices. Unfortunately, some of these limitations are not likely to disappear in the near future because mobile devices need to remain compact in size [10,29,30].

One of the goals of this chapter serves to investigate further the possibilities of differences in HDR images tone mapping across displays and, to clarify, whether different sizes and resolution shave an impact on TMO and to what extent. Knowing if there are certain TMOs that perform better under specific circumstances can be also important to further study their battery usage and optimize the impact of visualization of HDR on mobile devices.

10.4 Methodology

In this chapter, we investigated the impact of viewing devices and TMOs on colour and grey-scale images using subjective and objective methods. Subjective methods provide a measure and an insight into user-perceived quality [31,32]. However, they are time-consuming and expensive and as a result, cannot be used for automated quality monitoring or control [32–34]. Objective methods are based on theoretical models, often based on some characteristics of the Human Visual System and/or image processing techniques [6,33]. The two approaches are complementary and should enable us to find out how different devices (LDR/SSD) affect the viewing experience and the TMO algorithms. The results of subjective tests often serve as ground truth for benchmarking objective measures of perceived quality [31,33,35].

10.4.1 Subjective assessment of the impact of TMOS and viewing devices

Subjective quality assessments provide a good basis for evaluating the strengths and weaknesses of the TMOs and viewing devices and their impact on the QoE. The most common methods used to measure subjective quality are those recommended by the International Telecommunications Union (ITU-R) [36]. These methods generally require human participants to rate the image quality, individually, on a specified rating scale. The Mean Opinion Score (MOS) (i.e. the mean of the individual quality scores) is taken as the final quality rating [32–34,37].

In this chapter, a five-point quality scale was used to rate the quality of the HDR images based on the ITU-R BT.500-11 quality rating (see Table 10.1). This scale is suited to naïve observers, i.e. non-experts in HDR image analysis, as it is relatively easy to rate the quality of an image based on an adjective ('Excellent', 'Good', 'Fair', 'Poor' and 'Bad') [36]. In the chapter, we carried out the subjective visual quality assessments in different environments and under different viewing conditions, including outdoor and indoor and with artificial and natural lights.

10.4.1.1 Experimental set-up

Two main experimental set-ups were designed for the study (see Figure 10.1); one of LDR displays and the other for SSDs. Three colour and three grey HDR images were processed by 10 TMOs, giving a total of 60 colour and 60 grey-scale images. The images were then stored in a database accessible from two assessment websites, one website for LDR and one for SSDs. For the LDR assessments, the images were assessed using conventional LDR displays. For SSD assessments, the images were assessed from tablets or mobile phones. The dataset was created using freely available HDR toolbox in MATLAB with, using default settings [15,38]. All the images used in the study represent natural scenes and were selected based on their dynamic range, visual quality and content. The original Images and luminance histograms are shown in Figure 10.2. As a final step, gamma correction of 2.2 was applied to compensate for the image luminance of the viewing device [15]. Most of the LDR image or video formats use so called gamma correction to convert luminance or RGB spectral colour intensity into integer numbers, which can be later

Table 10.1 Five-level scale-rating table

Rating	Definition	Description
5	Excellent	Perfect image quality
4	Good	An image with very good quality
3	Fair	Image with good quality, some loss, but the overall image is acceptable
2	Poor	Poor quality, low image distortion, but understanding the details
1	Bad	Bad quality, high image distortion, hard to understand the details

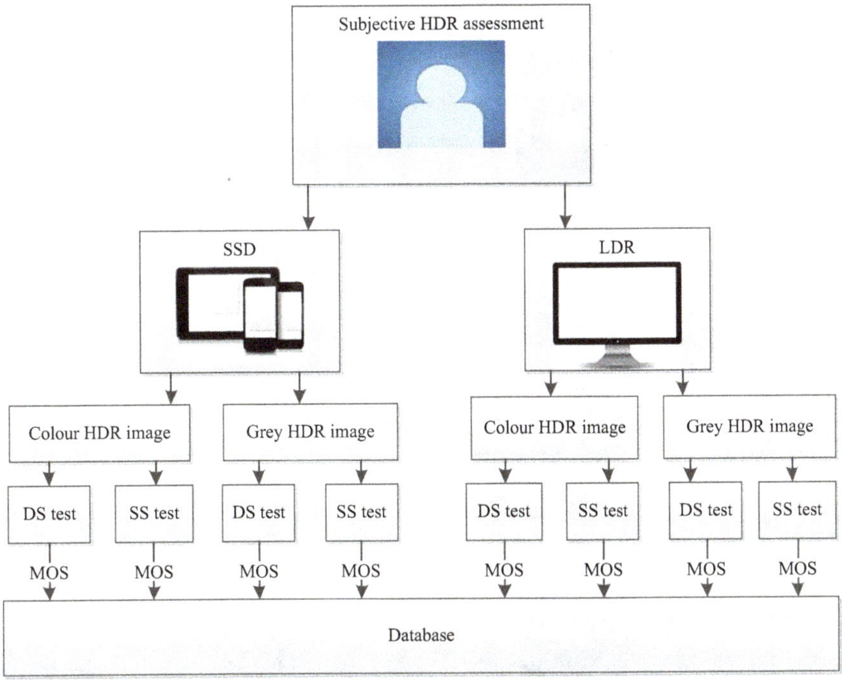

Figure 10.1 Experimental set-up for the subjective assessment

encoded. Gamma correction is usually given the value between 1.8 and 2.8. Gamma correction was originally intended to reduce camera noise and to control the current of the electron beam in CRT monitors (for details on gamma correction, see [1,26]).

10.4.1.2 The TMOs used in the study

Ten well-known local and global TMOs were used in the study [1,24–31,39,40]. Table 10.2 summarises the features of the different TMO algorithms that were used in the investigation. The abbreviations in italics indicate the name we will use for convenience to refer to the operators in this chapter.

10.4.1.3 Participants

Sixty participants were involved in subjective assessments. The age of the participants was between 20 and 50 years. They all had normal or corrected vision and no experience of HDR imaging. The assessments had two tests, a Double Stimuli (DS) and a Single Stimuli (SS). In the DS tests, the quality of tone-mapped images was evaluated in relation to the original HDR image. According to ITU-T P.910 recommendations [41], in the SS test, we used the ACR (Absolute Category Rating). Each sequence is rated individually on the ACR scale. The labels on the scale are 'bad', 'poor', 'fair', 'good' and 'excellent', and they are translated to the values 1, 2, 3, 4 and 5 when calculating the MOS [31] in the DS test used in this

Abbreviation	Original images	Luminance histograms ($\log_{10}$)
Church/colour	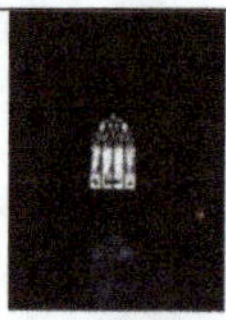	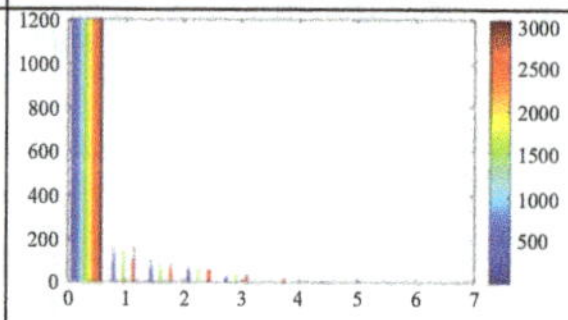
Warwick/colour		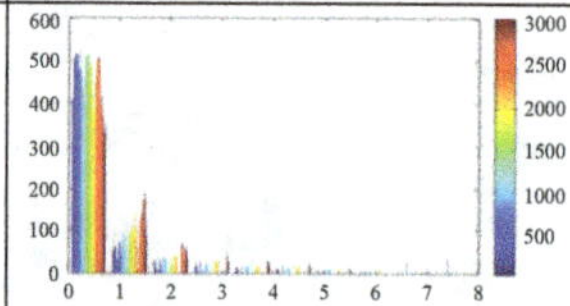
Office/colour	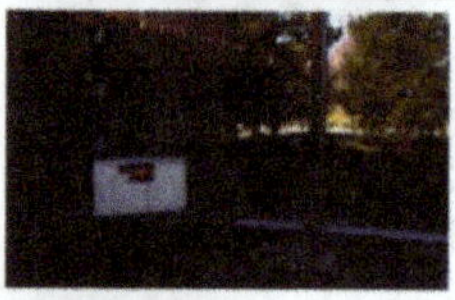	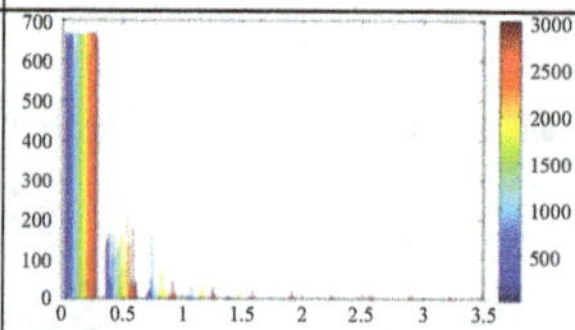
Church/grey	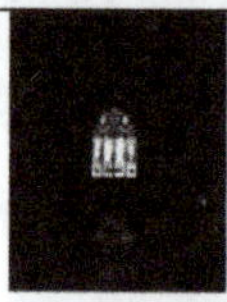	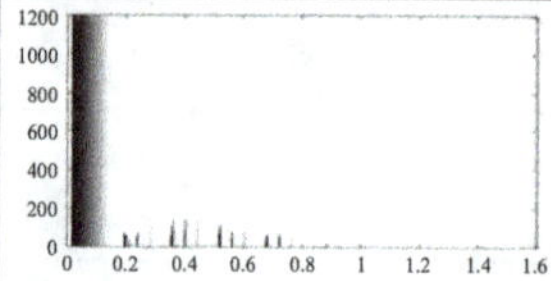
Warwick/grey	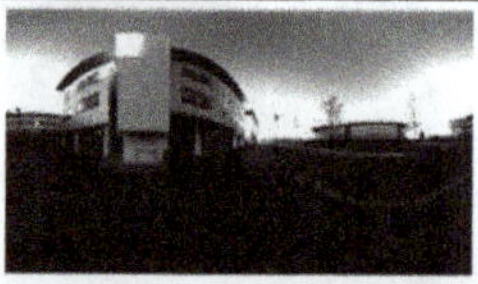	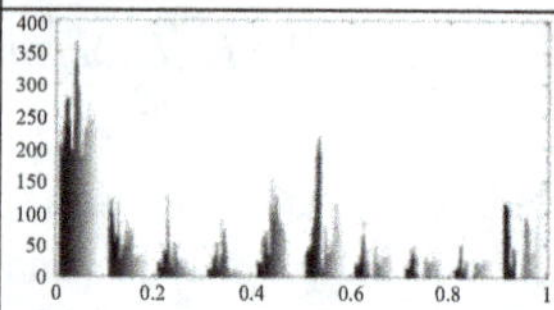
Office/grey	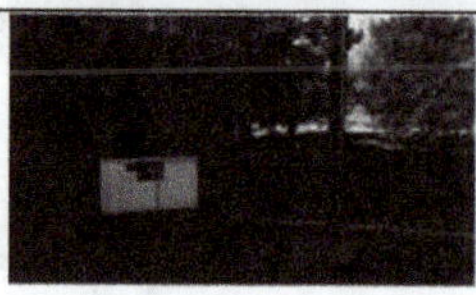	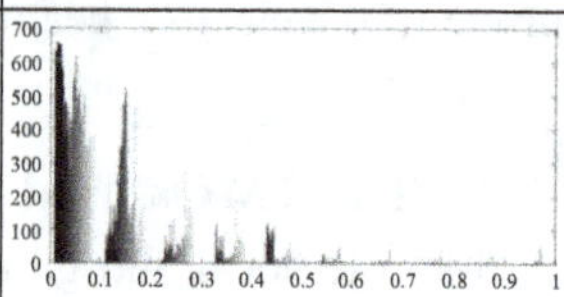

Figure 10.2 Original images and luminance histograms

chapter, we used, DSCQS (Double Stimulus Continuous Quality Scale). The viewer sees an unimpaired reference and the impaired sequence in random order. They are allowed to re-view the sequences, and then rate the quality for both on a continuous scale labelled with the ACR categories. While. At the end of each assessment, the participants submit their individual scores, which are stored in a database for the set-up.

10.4.1.4 Devices used in the study

For the SSDs experiments, five different mobile devices were used and involved 30 participants (see Table 10.3). The devices represented popular mobile devices,

Table 10.2 Summary of the features of the TMOs used in the study

TMOs	Author	Abbreviation	Method description	Process
Ashikhmin	Ashikhmin	AL1	A tone mapping algorithm for high contrast images, the method considers two basic characteristics of the human visual systems (HVS) [51].	Local
Ferwerda	Ferwerda	AL2	This operator is based on a model of visual adaptation from psychophysical experiments that considered various aspects of the HVS such as visibility, visual acuity and illumination changes adaptation [52].	Local
Adaptive logarithmic mapping	Drago	AL3	This is a fast algorithm suitable for interactive applications, which automatically produces realistically looking images for a wide variation of scenes exhibiting an HDR of luminance [26].	Global
iCAM06	Fairchild–Johnson	AL4	Modified ICAM operator, which is based on the physiology of the human's eye photoreceptors. The output of the operator is a combination of a locally adapted value around each pixel of the image and a globally adopted value based on the image averages [25].	Local
Fattal	Fattal	AL5	Compressing the gradient of the image luminance component and then constructing the LDR image by solving a Poisson equation on the compressed gradient image [53].	Gradient domain/ Local
Pattanaik	Pattanaik	AL6	This is a new time-dependent tone-mapping operator, which is based on psychophysical experiments and a photoreceptor model for luminance values. This algorithm briefly can be decomposed into two models: the visual adaptation model and the visual appearance model.	Global
Photographic reproduction	Reinhard	AL7	This is based upon dodging-and-burning in traditional photography. It automatically applies various scales for luminance mapping to the prorated regions of highlights and shadows [54].	Local

(Continues)

Table 10.2 (Continued)

TMOs	Author	Abbreviation	Method description	Process
Tumblin–Rushmeier	Tumblin and Rushmeier	AL8	This TMO preserves brightness relationships, by using a psychophysical model of brightness perception [55].	Global
Ward	Ward	AL9	A visibility matching tone reproduction operator for HDR scenes [56].	Global
Bilateral filtering	Durand and Dorsey	AL10	Fast bilateral filtering for the display of HDR images conserving local details in the image. They argued that an image might be thought of as being composed of an HDR component for low frequencies and an LDR component with a high spatial frequency [57].	Frequency domain/ local

Table 10.3 Mobile devices used for the subjective test

Devices	Participants/ device	Features	Resolution/ pixels
iPhone 6	9	4.7″ Retina HD display	1334×750
iPhone 5S	7	4″ Retina	1136×640
Samsung Galaxy Note II	5	5.5″ Super AMOLED	1280×720
Samsung Galaxy S4	3	5″ HD Super AMOLED	1920×1080
iPad mini 3	6	7.9″ IPS LCD	2048×1536

which are used to consume multimedia contents. For the LDR experiments, a display for personal computers was used. In particular, the Philips Brilliance 221P3LPYES display (21.5″, LED-backlit, LCD panel display, 1920 × 1080 resolution) was used.

10.4.2 Objective assessment of the impact of TMOs and viewing devices

Subjective evaluation is a reliable way to assess image quality, but it is expensive and time consuming. It is further complicated by many other factors such as viewing angle/distance, the device, the vision of the subject, and subjects' mood. Thus, there is a need for objective approach to predict image quality. As there is no established model to evaluate the quality of the HDR image at present [2,15,16,35], we used objective quality metrics which have shown promise in other applications in the study. In particular, we have used the following four metrics: SE, mean square error (MSE), the multi-exposure peak signal-to-noise ratio (mPSNR) and high dynamic range visual-difference-predictor-2 (HDR-VDP-2).

Tone mapping produces images that are different from the original HDR images [3]. In order to fit the resulting image within the dynamic range of the display, tone-mapping algorithms compress, contrast and adjust brightness. Therefore, the tone-mapped image may lose some quality when compared to the original HDR images. However, the images would look very similar and the degradation in quality is not very well predicted by most quality metrics [2,42].

HDR-VDP-2 can predict whether differences between two images are visible to the human observer or not, and can work within the complete range of luminance the human eye can see [2]. mPSNR gives a prediction of the error in the compressed image and is based on the popular PSNR metric [1,15]. The MSE is the simplest and most widely used metric for image quality [32]. SE is widely used to evaluate grey-scale images and has proved to be efficient [43], but has not hitherto been used to evaluate HDR image quality for both colour and grey images.

Shannon entropy: SE provides a statistical measure of the information content of a signal and may be used to characterize the texture of the input image. Low entropy images, such as those containing a lot of black skies, have very little contrast and large runs of pixels with the same values. An image that is perfectly flat will have an entropy of zero. Consequently, they can be compressed to a relatively small size. On the other hand, high entropy images such as an image of heavily cratered areas on the moon have a great deal of contrast from one pixel to another and consequently cannot be compressed as much as low entropy images [43,44]. SE may be defined as in (10.1),

$$H(A) = -\sum_{i=1}^{n} p_i \log_2 p_i \tag{10.1}$$

where $H(A)$ is the SE for the image A, n represents the number of bins (256), and pi is the normalized histogram counts returned from the image histogram for the bin number i.

Mean square error (MSE): The MSE is a measure of signal fidelity which enables us to compare two signals by providing a quantitative score that describes the degree of similarity/fidelity or, conversely, the level of error/distortion between them [32,45–47]. The MSE between the images x and y may be obtained using (10.2):

$$\mathrm{MSE}(x,y) = \frac{1}{N}\sum_{i=1}^{N} (x_i - y_i)^2 \tag{10.2}$$

Multi-exposure peak-to-signal noise ratio (mPSNR): The mPSNR metric works by converting the original HDR image into multiple LDR images at different exposures and then computing the average of the peak signal-to-noise ratios (PSNR) of each individual exposure. This takes into account both the highlights and the shadows of the image. The resulting mPSNR gives us a prediction of the error in the compressed HDR image, but of course, does not consider properties of the human visual system [1,15]. The higher the mPSNR the better the quality of the reproduction is. mPSNR may be computed as in (10.3):

$$\text{mPSNR} = 10\log_{10}\left(\frac{3\times 255^2}{\text{MSE}}\right) \tag{10.3}$$

High dynamic range visual-difference-predictor 2 (HDR-VDP-2): HDR-VDP-2 is a calibrated visual metric for visibility and quality predictions in all luminance. Although the metric originates from the classical Visual Difference Predictor and its extension HDR-VDP, the visual models are very different from those used in earlier metrics. The HDR-VDP extends Daly's visual difference predictor to predict differences in HDR images [31,33,48]. The HDR-VDP-2 was designed to predict visibility rather than quality. In this study, the MATLAB implementation of HDR-VDP-2 was used, but it is also possible to run the metric using an online web service. For the HDR-VDP-2 metric, the parameters were set according to the set-up of the subjective evaluations and only the quality value was used [32].

10.5 Results

10.5.1 Results from subjective assessments

The first step after individual subjective assessments is to determine the overall MOS score, for each image sequence. The raw individual scores were used to obtain the corresponding overall MOS score with 95% confidence interval (CI).

Colour HDR images: In this section, the results of subjective rating are described with the aim of understanding the characteristics of QoE of the tone mapped coloured HDR images and factors that affect QoE in different devices. The results for the SSD experiments for different TMOs are shown in Figure 10.3(a) and (b). For the DS tests (see Figure 10.3(a)), the TMOs AL4 and AL10 (i.e. iCAM06 and Bilateral Filtering) gave the best MOS scores for all the images. These two TMOs preserve image details in relation to the reference image. The worst TMO for all the images was AL6, which had a MOS score of 1 in all cases. For the SS tests (Figure 10.3(b)): AL4 and AL10 again had the best MOS score. AL3 and AL1 achieved a MOS score of between 3.5 and 4, which is good. *AL6* had a MOS of 1 which is the lowest.

The results for the LDR display experiments are shown in Figure 10.4. In the DS tests (Figure 10.4(a)), AL7 gave the highest MOS score for all images, with a MOS score of about 4.5, followed by AL3 and AL4 with MOS scores of around 4. It is worth noting that AL7 is based on luminance's logarithmic compression, while AL3 and AL4 are based on an efficient way of reducing halo artefacts by compressing the dynamic range of the HDR image, which results in a very good HDR image quality [49]. On the other hand, the TMOs AL5 and AL6 gave the worst MOS scores of all the TMOs. The poor MOS results for AL6 are thought to be because after tone mapping with the AL6, the images may still present halos and this affects the overall quality. In the SS test (Figure 10.4(b)), the performance of

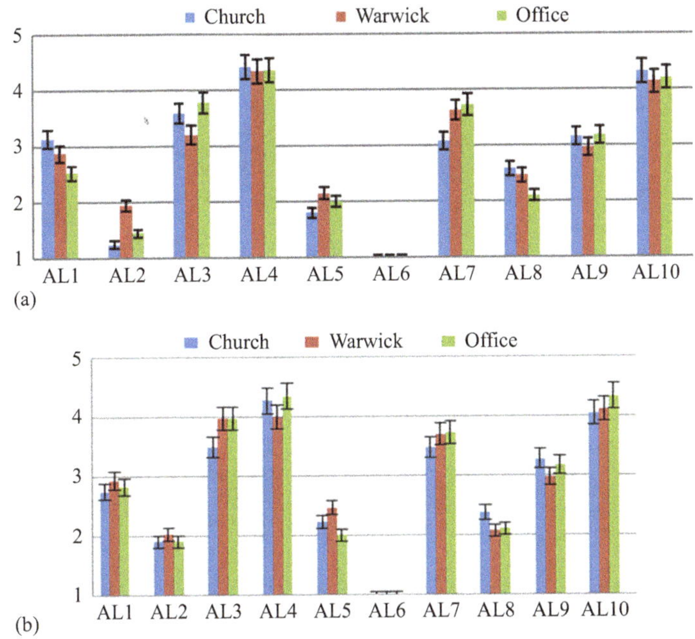

Figure 10.3 Impact of TMOs on MOS for different coloured HDR using SSD: (a) DS test and (b) SS test

the TMOs follows a similar pattern to those in the DS tests, but with minor differences for the best and the worst TMOs [6]. In both SSD and LDR tests AL6 had the lowest MOS score (MOS score of 1) compared to other TMOs. The SSDs used in the study have different display features (including different screen sizes and screen resolutions, see Table 10.3) and these are thought to impact on the perceived viewing quality.

Figure 10.5 shows the results of the influence of the SSDs in uncontrolled viewing conditions in both SS and DS tests. In both tests, the results suggest that the size and resolution of the screen have the most impact on the MOS values achieved. The best results were achieved with the iPad mini 3 followed by iPhone 6 and then iPhone 5S. Samsung Galaxy Note gave the lowest MOS score. In conclusion, we found that QoE is affected mostly by the resolution of the SSDs. However, we found that there is no significant difference in the performance of SDDs for HDR images for both SS and DS tests.

Grey HDR images: In this section, the results of subjective rating of tone mapped grey-scale HDR images are presented to provide an understanding of the impact of viewing displays and TMOs on perceived quality. The results for the LDR display experiments are illustrated in Figure 10.6(a) and (b) for three tone-mapped images. From the figure, it can be seen that the best performance was achieved with the two TMOs AL7 and AL3, with MOS scores of around four. Figure 10.7(a) and (b) shows the impact of TMOs on MOS for different grey-scale HDR images using SSDs for DS

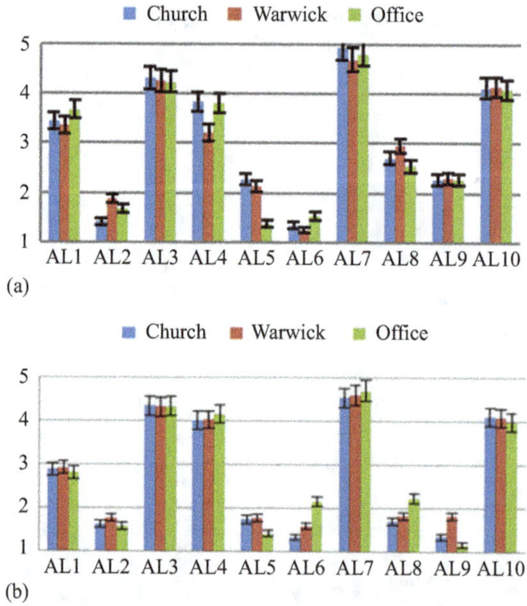

Figure 10.4 Impact of TMOs on MOS for different coloured HDR using LDR: (a) DS test and (b) SS test

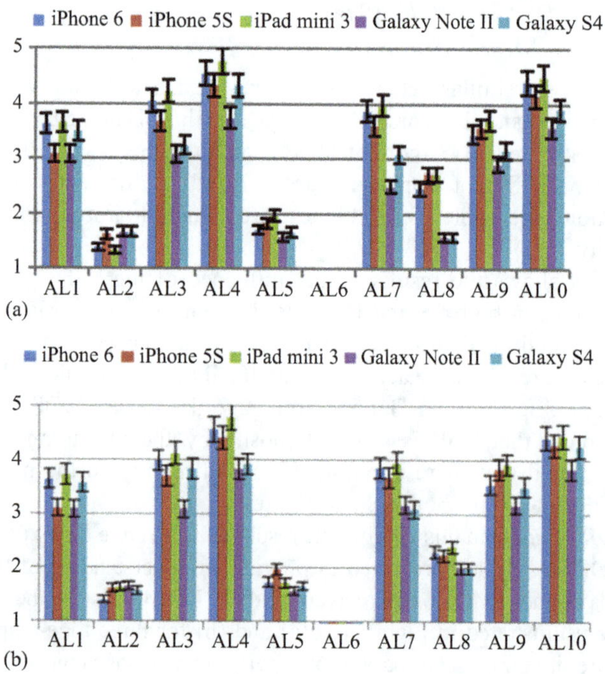

Figure 10.5 Impact of SSDs on TMO quality for coloured HDR: (a) DS test and (b) SS test

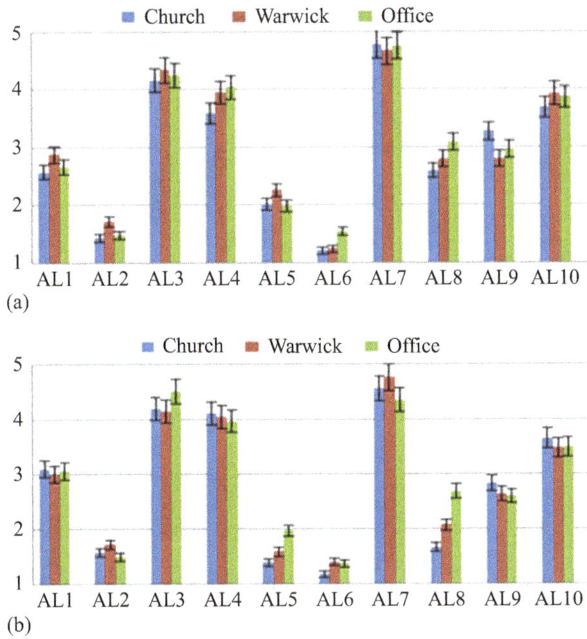

Figure 10.6 Impact of TMOs on MOS for different grey-scale HDR using LDR: (a) DS test and (b) SS test

and SS tests, respectively. Examination of the results shows that AL4 and AL10 had the best performance, with very good MOS scores for all the images, while AL6 was the worst TMO, with the lowest MOS score.

Figure 10.8 shows the results of subjective tests for SSDs for grey-scale images using DS and SS tests. The results show that the best result was achieved with using iPad mini 3 compared to other devices. This is followed by iPhone 6 and then iPhone 5S. In both the SS and DS tests, the results suggest that the SSDs resolution have an impact on the perceived viewing quality.

10.5.2 Results from objective assessments

Entropy: The entropy values for the original images (i.e. Office, Church and Warwick) are 6.2457, 4.5064 and 6.5698, respectively. Figure 10.9(a) and (b) shows the results of entropy for colour and grey-scale images, respectively the results show that AL4 had the highest MOS score, with entropies of 8.0117, 7.3216 and 7.9902 for Office, Church and Warwick, respectively. AL3 was second in performance with the entropies of 7.3225, 6.8097 and 7.3234 for Office, Church and Warwick, respectively. AL3 (Drago) and AL4 (modified iCAM) had the best performance because they give good contrast images while recovering the details of the saturated regions. Therefore, the outputs of these algorithms have a wide histogram and less saturated pixels. Both algorithms use entropy to define the details in the input images [10,24,25,50].

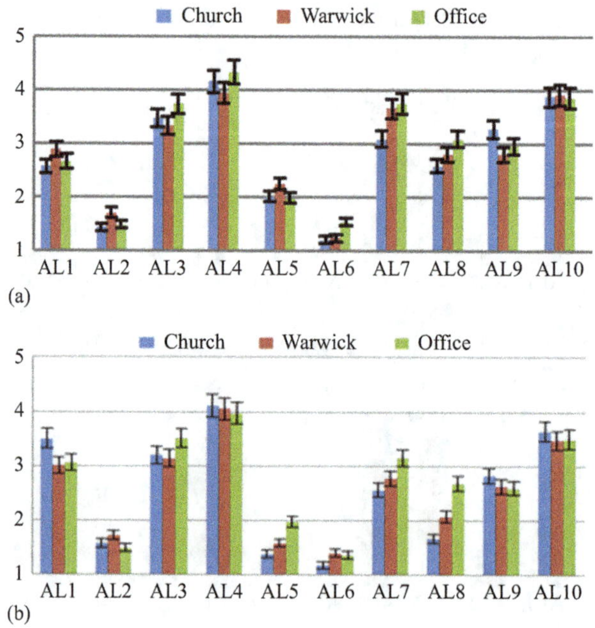

Figure 10.7 Impact of TMOs on MOS for different grey-scale HDR using SSD: (a) DS test and (b) SS test

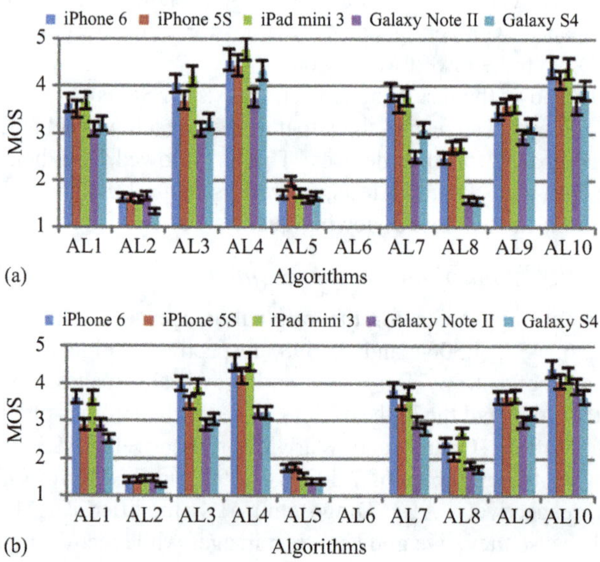

Figure 10.8 Impact of SSDs on TMO quality for grey-scale HDR: (a) DS test and (b) SS test

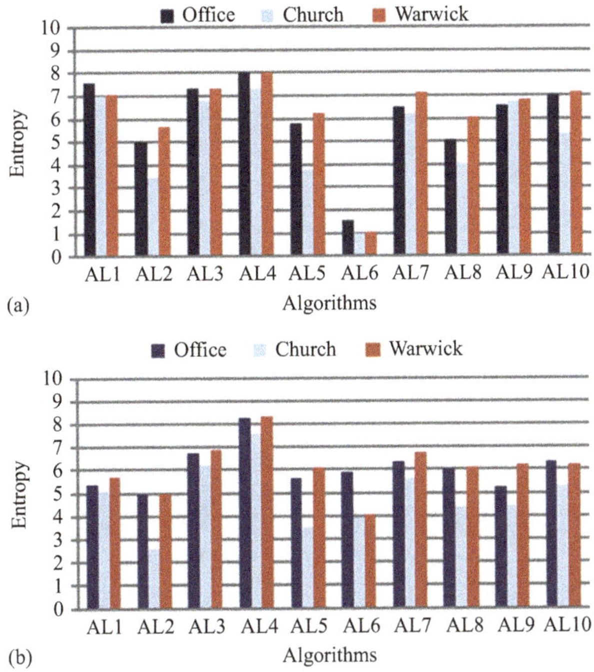

Figure 10.9 Entropy results: (a) colour and (b) grey

The worst entropy result was for AL6 and AL2 for Church image. This is because in the Church image the only source of light was natural light coming in from the windows, while the rest of the Church was relatively dark. It spans a wide dynamic range and has many detailed features that will result in a very wide histogram as we can see from Figure 10.2. As SE is a count of histogram returned from the image, the entropy for Church is less than for the other coloured and grey images.

HDR-VDP-2: The results for HDR-VP-2 are depicted in Figure 10.10. They show that AL7, AL1 and AL10 have the highest scores while AL6, AL8 and AL2 have the lowest score. It is noteworthy that the high-performing operators follow HVS functionality [10]. The HDR-VDP-2 is a map of probability for perceiving visible changes between an HDR image and the corresponding LDR image, i.e., the position of each pixel has a corresponding probability that any visual change can be detected [16,18]. On the other hand, comparison of Figure 10.10(a) and (b) shows that there is a significant difference between the results for AL1 for grey and colour images. Ashikhmin operator (AL1) computes a measure of the surround luminance for each pixel. This measure is then used for the definition of the tone-mapping operator [7]. To conclude, an algorithm that produces better image quality if its HDR-VDP-2 maps contain more pixels with a lower probability of detecting a visible change [16].

mPSNR: The results for the Multi-Exposure Peak Signal-to-Noise Ratio (mPSNR) are shown in Figure 10.10. For colour images, Figure 10.11(a), AL7 gave the best results. The two images, Office and Church, had the best results for

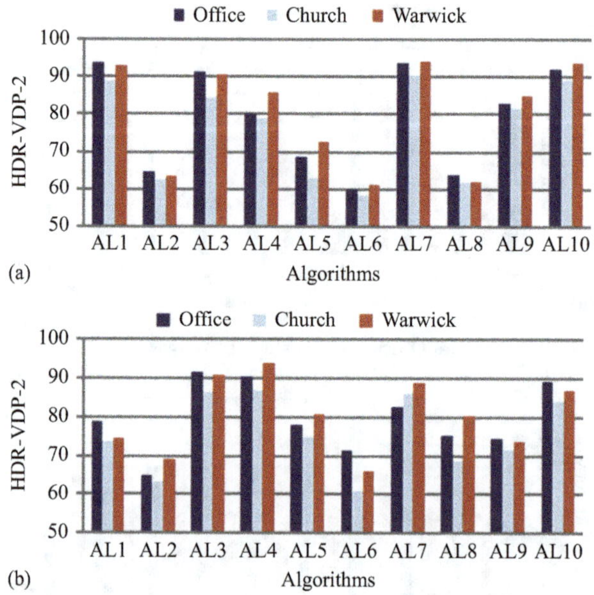

Figure 10.10 HDR-VDP-2 results: (a) colour and (b) grey

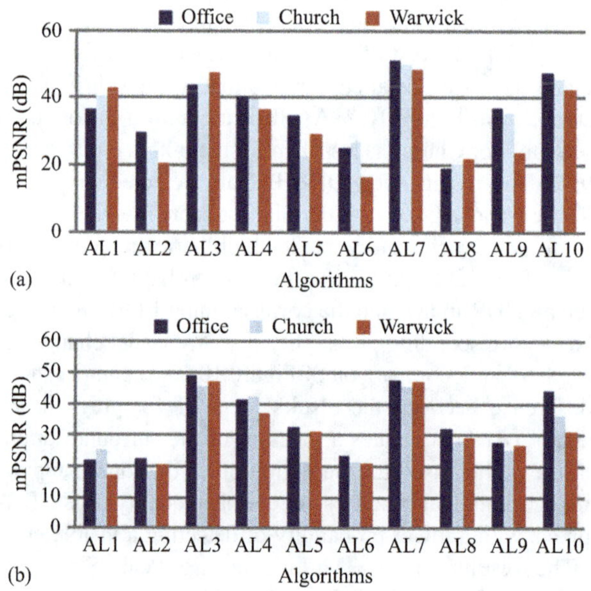

Figure 10.11 mPSNR results: (a) colour and (b) grey

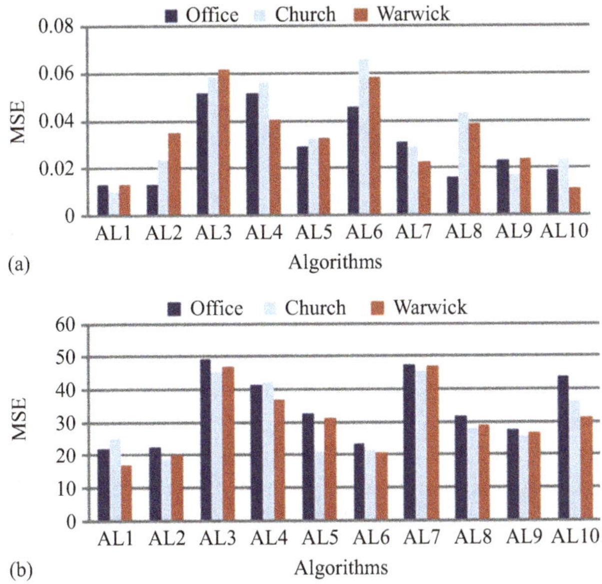

Figure 10.12 MSE results: (a) colour and (b) grey

mPSNR (>50 dB), while, the image, Warwick, was second with an mPSNR of 48 dB. AL10 had mPSNR values of 47, 45 and 42 dB for the three images Office, Church and Warwick, respectively. The worst TMO was AL8 with mPSNR of less than 21 dB for all the images, AL6 was also poor for the three images with mPSNR values of less than 26 dB. In Figure 10.11(b), it is seen that AL3 gave the best mPSNR values (close to 50 dB) for the three images.

MSE: The results for the MSE are shown in Figure 10.12, AL1 performed best with an MSE of less than 0.02, followed by AL9 with an MSE of around 0.02. The worst performance was for AL3, AL4 and AL6. For grey images, Figure 10.12(b), the best performing TMOs were AL6 and AL5, which had MSE values of around 0.005. The worst performance came from AL3, AL4 and AL7. MSE and mPSNR simply quantify the error signal and do not model the human visual system. They have low computational complexities compared to image similarity measures, which model the HVS [14].

10.6 Comparison of subjective and objective assessments of HDR image quality

Three performance indices were used in the study to assess the results of the subjective and objective quality assessments—the Pearson linear correlation (PLC), Spearman rank order correlation (SRC) and Kendall rank correlation (KRC). PLC is a measure of the degree of association between two variables, whilst SRC measures the prediction monotonicity and KRC evaluates the similarity between

Table 10.4 Correlation between the subjective experiments

Group	PLC	SRC	KRC
DS colour/SS colour	**0.9209**	**0.9152**	**0.7778**
DS colour/SS grey	0.7293	0.7697	0.6000
DS grey/SS grey	**0.8910**	**0.8303**	**0.6444**
SS colour/SS grey	0.7113	0.7939	0.6444

Note: Bold values represents the highest values in each set.

two variables. The performance indices may be used to determine the best method for viewing HDR images using SSD from the user's perspective.

Subjective tests: Table 10.4 summarizes the correlations between the perceived quality (MOS values) for colour and grey images in the DS tests with those in the SS tests and all the TMOs. The first row in the table gives the correlation coefficients between the perceived quality in the DS tests and the perceived quality in the SS tests for colour HDR images across all the TMOs. The high correlation coefficients for PLC and SRC suggest that the perceived quality for DS and SS tests are closely related, implying that it may not matter whether we use DS or SS tests to assess the quality. Similar results were obtained between the DS and SS tests (third row) for grey images. The second row gives the correlation between the perceived quality for colour HDR images in the DS tests and those for grey images in the SS tests. The high correlation here and in the fourth row (correlation between the perceived quality for colour and grey images) suggests that the same TMOs may be used for both colour and grey images. However, in general participants preferred colour HDR images to grey images.

Table 10.5 summarizes the correlation coefficients and hence the relationships between subjective and objective quality assessments for different objective quality metrics. They show that for colour HDR images, HDR-VDP-2 gives the best objective quality measures (in both DS and SS tests). For grey images, the entropy is the best. Overall, HDR-VDP-2 and entropy are the best objective metrics for predicting perceived quality and MSE the worst. Entropy performed better for grey images than for colour images. This is because a grey-scale image is a simple image in which the only colours are shades of grey. A 'grey' colour is one in which the red, green and blue components all have equal intensity in the RGB spaces and so it is only necessary to specify a single intensity value for each pixel as opposed to the three intensities needed to specify each pixel in a full-colour image [10]. In both colour and grey images the MSE, which is a full reference metric, was the worst metric. This is because the MSE does not consider the characteristics of HVS and, so it's may not always be significantly correlated with subjective visual quality.

10.7 Discussion

The aim of this chapter is to investigate the impact of viewing devices and TMO algorithms on the visual QoE. We found differences in the visual quality between LDRs and SSDs in the tests. For SSDs, the best TMO was AL4 (iCAM06) and for

Table 10.5 Correlation between MOS and objective quality metrics

	PLC	SRC	KRC
DS colour			
mPSNR	0.7552	0.6848	0.4666
HDR-VDP-2	**0.9398**	**0.8545**	**0.6889**
Entropy	0.8548	0.8061	0.6444
MSE	0.3112	0.2193	0.1794
SS colour			
mPSNR	0.7665	0.7024	0.6444
HDR-VDP-2	**0.9051**	**0.7455**	**0.5111**
Entropy	0.8236	0.6848	0.4667
MSE	0.3716	0.2044	0.1392
DS grey			
mPSNR	0.7913	0.5879	0.3333
HDR-VDP-2	0.8043	0.7376	0.5156
Entropy	**0.8842**	**0.7533**	**0.5511**
MSE	0.4147	0.3863	0.3212
SS grey			
mPSNR	0.509	0.5394	0.3778
HDR-VDP-2	0.682	0.7333	0.6001
Entropy	**0.791**	**0.8182**	**0.6444**
MSE	0.391	0.4911	0.2252

Note: Bold values represents the highest values in each set.

Table 10.6 Ranking of the algorithms from best to worst for colour images

DS SSD		SS SSD		DS LDR		SS LDR	
AL4	4.274194	AL4	4.274194	AL7	4.633939	AL7	4.591061
AL10	4.134409	AL10	4.182796	AL3	4.252381	AL3	4.333333
AL3	3.650538	AL7	3.483871	AL10	4.060606	AL4	4.032051
AL7	3.629032	AL3	3.419355	AL4	3.809965	AL10	4.010606
AL9	3.370968	AL1	3.408602	AL1	3.675414	AL1	2.876923
AL1	3.193548	AL9	3.139785	AL8	2.705202	AL8	1.944545
AL8	2.715054	AL8	2.727599	AL9	2.348485	AL6	1.682323
AL5	2.039147	AL5	1.915995	AL2	1.767898	AL2	1.630769
AL2	1.655914	AL2	1.639785	AL5	1.669048	AL5	1.538462
AL6	1	AL6	1	AL6	1.359848	AL9	1.515152

LDR it was AL7 (Photographic Reproduction) as shown in Tables 10.6 and 10.7, respectively. Both iCAM06 and Photographic Reproduction preserve the edges, which improves the grey level distribution of the generated LDR image during tone mapping which helps to provide better QoE for the end-user by avoiding contouring and retaining more details. For the different TMOs, we found that subjective results for SSDs were better than those for LDR. Moreover, there was no significant

Table 10.7 Ranking of the algorithms from best to worst for grey-scale images

DS SSD		SS SSD		DS LDR		SS LDR	
AL4	4.357527	AL4	4.341086	AL7	4.50060602	AL7	4.391061
AL10	4.134409	AL10	4.149462	AL3	4.12619025	AL3	4.033333
AL3	3.650538	AL7	3.483871	AL1	3.80996472	AL4	3.792692
AL7	3.629032	AL3	3.419355	AL10	3.7393941	AL10	3.125465
AL9	3.237634	AL1	3.275269	AL4	3.546721	AL1	3.254547
AL1	3.060215	AL8	3.060932	AL8	2.5223198	AL8	1.944545
AL8	2.048387	AL9	3.039785	AL9	2.1239863	AL6	1.745433
AL5	2.039147	AL5	1.915995	AL2	1.8344667	AL2	1.577676
AL2	1.489247	AL2	1.473118	AL5	1.537766	AL5	1.465613
AL6	1	AL6	1	AL6	1.2546567	AL9	1.451023

difference in the subjective quality using mobile devices to view HDR images in both the DS and SS tests.

Similar results were obtained for grey HDR images even though colour images may lose important information when transferred to a grey-scale image [21]. We found that the impact of colour has less impact on HDR images than in conventional digital image technology. HDR imaging captures illumination in a higher range, which provides more detail and edge information and better view experience [1–4,6–10,20]. In the SSD experiments, we found that iPad mini 3 and iPhone 6 for both coloured and grey images gave the best-perceived quality. We found that better subjective results are associated with larger SSD resolution. Moreover, the results indicate that SSD size and resolution have an influence on the tone-mapped image reproduction for both coloured and grey HDR images. Mobile devices are now widely used as a platform to consume multimedia information. The rapid growth in the number of mobile devices in use will bring about a demand to optimize the end user QoE when viewing HDR content.

10.8 Conclusions and future work

We have evaluated, subjectively and objectively, the most widely used TMOs in different displays and resolutions to provide an understanding of the impact of viewing devices and TMOs on the visual QoE for both colour and grey-scale HDR images. Our results suggest that the user's QoE of tone-mapped images were significantly different on LDR compared to SSDs. SSDs have an influence on the TMOs performance compared to LDRs. In general, better subjective results are related to size and resolution of SSD. We found that iCAM06 performed the best TMO for SSD and Photographic Reproduction for LDR it was performed the best TMO for both colour and grey-scale HDR images. In addition, we found that there was no significant difference between the subjective score for colour and grey images in SSD, while there is a difference between LDR and SSD. The device and the TMOs appear to affect the quality of both colour and grey equally. For the objective metrics, SE was found to be a good measure of the QoE for both colour and grey HDR images, suggesting that it may find use in automated quality control assessment schemes for HDR images. For future work, we will focus on extensive subjective tests with larger datasets.

References

[1] Banterle F, Artusi A, Debattista K, and Chalmers A. Advanced high dynamic range imaging. CRC Press; 2017.

[2] Mantiuk RRK, Myszkowski K, and Seidel H-P. High Dynamic Range Imaging. John Wiley & Sons, Inc., 2015.

[3] Narwaria M, Perreira Da Silva M, Le Callet P, and Pepion R. Tone mapping based HDR compression: does it affect visual experience? Signal Process Image Commun [Internet]. 2014;29(2):257–73.

[4] Banterle F, Debattista K, Artusi A, *et al.* High dynamic range imaging and low dynamic range expansion for generating HDR content. Comput Graph Forum. 2009;28(8):2343–67.

[5] Valenzise G, De Simone F, Lauga P, and Dufaux F. Performance evaluation of objective quality metrics for HDR image compression. 2014;92170C.

[6] Al-Juboori S, Mkwawa IH, Sun L, and Ifeachor E. Impact of tone-mapping operators and viewing devices on visual quality of experience. 2016 IEEE International Conference on Communication ICC 2016.

[7] Melo M, Bessa M, Debattista K, and Chalmers A. Evaluation of HDR video on small form factor displays. First Int Conf SME Work HDR imaging 2013. 2013;(3):4–7.

[8] Urbano C, Magalhães L, Moura J, Bessa M, Marcos A, and Chalmers A. Tone mapping operators on small screen devices: An evaluation study. Comput Graph Forum. 2010;29(8):2469–78.

[9] Melo M, Bessa M, Debattista K, and Chalmers A. Evaluation of tone-mapping operators for HDR video under different ambient luminance levels. Comput Graph Forum. 2015;34(8):38–49.

[10] Melo M, Bessa M, Debattista K, and Chalmers A. Evaluation of HDR video tone mapping for mobile devices. Signal Process Image Commun. 2014; 29(2):247–256.

[11] Akyüz AO, Fleming R, Riecke BE, Reinhard E, and Bülthoff HH. Do HDR displays support LDR content? ACM Trans Graph [Internet]. 2007;26(3):38.

[12] Akyüz AO, Eksert ML, and Aydin MS. An evaluation of image reproduction algorithms for high contrast scenes on large and small screen display devices. Comput Graph. 2013;37(7):885–95.

[13] Mantiuk R, Daly SJ, Myszkowski K, and Seidel H-P. Predicting visible differences in high dynamic range images: model and its calibration. Human Vision and Electronic Imaging X. Proc SPIE. 2005;5666:204–14.

[14] Park SH, and Montag ED. Evaluating tone mapping algorithms for rendering non-pictorial (scientific) high-dynamic-range images. J Vis Commun Image Represent. 2007;18(5):415–28.

[15] Banterle F, Artusi A, and Debattista KCA. Advanced High Dynamic Range Imaging: Theory and practice. A.K. Peters Inc; 2011.

[16] Eilertsen G, Mantiuk RK, and Unger J. A comparative review of tone-mapping algorithms for high dynamic range video. Computer Graphics Forum. 2017;36(2):565–92.

[17] Kainz F, and Bogart R, and Stanczyk P. Technical introduction to OpenEXR. Ind Light magic. 2009;1–21.

[18] Salih Y, Bt. Md-Esa W, Malik AS, and Saad N. Tone mapping of HDR images: A review. ICIAS 2012 - 2012 4th Int Conf Intell Adv Syst A Conf World Eng Sci Technol Congr - Conf Proc. 2012;1:368–73.

[19] Al-Juboori S, Mkwawa I-H, Sun L, and Ifeachor E. Investigation of relationships between changes in EEG features and subjective quality of HDR images. In: Multimedia and Exposure (ICME), 2017 IEEE International Conference on. IEEE; 2017. pp. 91–6.

[20] Narwaria M, Perreira M, Callet P Le, and Silva D. High Dynamic Range Visual Quality of Experience Measurement: Challenges and Perspectives To cite this version: High Dynamic Range Visual Quality of Experience Measurement: Challenges and Perspectives. 2015.

[21] Arndt S, Brunnström K, Cheng E, Engelke U, Möller S, and Antons JN. Review on using physiology in quality of experience. J Electron Imaging, 2016;2016(16):1–9.

[22] Yoshida A, Blanz V, Myszkowski K, and Seidel H-P. Perceptual evaluation of tone mapping operators with real-world scenes. Proceedings SPIE, Human Visual Electronic Imaging X [Internet]. 2005;5666:192–203.

[23] Drago F, Martens WL, Myszkowski K, and Seidel H-P. Perceptual evaluation of tone mapping operators with regard to similarity and preference. Tech. Rep. MPI-I-2002-4-002, Max Plank Institut für Informatik.

[24] Duan J, Bressan M, Dance C, and Qiu G. Tone-mapping high dynamic range images by novel histogram adjustment. Pattern Recognit [Internet]. 2010; 43(5):1847–62.

[25] Kuang J, Johnson GM, and Fairchild MD. iCAM06: A refined image appearance model for HDR image rendering. J Vis Commun Image Represent. 2007;18(5):406–14.

[26] Drago F, Myszkowski K, Annen T, and Chiba N. Adaptive logarithmic mapping for displaying high contrast scenes. Comput Graph Forum. 2003; 22(3):419–26.

[27] Kuang J, Yamaguchi H, Liu C, Johnson GM, and Fairchild MD. Evaluating HDR rendering algorithms. ACM Trans Appl Percept [Internet]. 2007;4(2):9–es.

[28] Korshunov P, and Ebrahimi T. Influence of context and content on tone-mapping operators. First International Conference on SME Work HDR imaging [Internet]. 2013;(2).

[29] Gelfand N, Adams A, Park SH, and Pulli K. Multi-exposure imaging on mobile devices. Proceedings of the International Conference on Multimedia - MM '10 [Internet]. 2010;823.

[30] Castro T, Chapiro A, Cicconet M, and Velho L. Towards mobile HDR video. 2011;1(July 2010).

[31] Hanhart P, Bernardo MV, Korshunov P, Pereira M, Pinheiro AMG, and Ebrahimi T. HDR image compression: a new challenge for objective quality metrics. 2014 Sixth International Workshop on Quality of Multimedia Experience (QoMEX) (pp. 159–164). IEEE.

[32] Yeganeh H, and Wang Z. Objective quality assessment of tone-mapped images. IEEE Trans Image Process. 2013;22(2):657–67.

[33] Hanhart P, Bernardo MV, Pereira M, Pinheiro AMG, and Ebrahimi T. Benchmarking of objective quality metrics for HDR image quality assessment. EURASIP J Image Video Process. 2015;2015(1):1–18.

[34] Khan A, Sun L, and Ifeachor E. QoE prediction model and its application in video quality adaptation over UMTS networks. IEEE Trans Multimed. 2012;14(2):431–42.

[35] Selmanovic E, Debattista K, Bashford-Rogers T, and Chalmers A. Enabling stereoscopic high dynamic range video. Signal Process Image Commun [Internet]. 2014;29(2):216–28.

[36] RECOMMENDATION ITU-R BT.500-11. Methodology for the subjective assessment of the quality of television pictures [Internet]. 2013. Available from: https://www.itu.int/dms_pubrec/itu-r/rec/bt/R-REC-BT.500-11-200206-S!!PDF-E.pdf

[37] Anegekuh L, Sun L, and Ifeachor E. A screening methodology for crowdsourcing video QoE evaluation. 2014 IEEE Glob Commun Conf GLOBECOM 2014. 2014;1152–7.

[38] F. Banterle HT. HDR toolbox [Internet]. Available from: https://github.com/banterle/HDR_Toolbox

[39] Meylan L, Süsstrunk S, and Susstrunk S. High dynamic range image rendering with a Retinex-based adaptive filter. Image Process IEEE Trans [Internet]. 2006;15(9):2820–30.

[40] Meylan L. Tone Mapping for High Dynamic Range Images. 2006; 3588.

[41] ITU-T International Telecommunication Union. ITU-T Recommendation P.910, "Subjective video quality assessment methods for multimedia applications," International Telecommunication Union, Geneva, 2008.

[42] Mantiuk RK, Myszkowski K, and Seidel H-P. High dynamic range imaging. Wiley Encycl Electr Electron Eng. 2015;6:1–42.

[43] Shannon CE. Prediction and entropy of printed English. Bell Syst Tech J. 1951;30(1):50–64.

[44] Wu Y, Zhou Y, Saveriades G, Agaian S, Noonan JP, and Natarajan P. Local Shannon entropy measure with statistical tests for image randomness. Inf Sci (Ny). 2013;222:323–42.

[45] Chakraborty C, and Gupta B. Adaptive filtering technique for chronic wound image analysis under tele-wound network, Int. Journal of Communication, Navigation, Sensing and Services. 2016;1:57–76.

[46] Rerabek M, Hanhart P, Korshunov P, and Ebrahimi T. Subjective and objective evaluation of HDR video compression. 9th International Workshop on Video Processing Quality Metrics Consumer Electronics. 2015.

[47] Koz A, and Dufaux F. Methods for improving the tone mapping for backward compatible high dynamic range image and video coding. Signal Process Image Commun [Internet]. 2014;29(2):274–92.

[48] Mantiuk R, Kim KJ, Rempel AG, and Heidrich W. HDR-VDP-2: A calibrated visual metric for visibility and quality predictions in all luminance conditions. ACM SIGGRAPH 2011 Pap - SIGGRAPH '11. 2011;1(212):1.

[49] Čadík M, Wimmer M, Neumann L, and Artusi A. Evaluation of HDR tone mapping methods using essential perceptual attributes. Comput Graph. 2008;32(3):330–49.

[50] Fathima E, and Kaliyamoorthie KP. Implementation of gray level images based on the Shannon entropy. Middle - East J Sci Res [Internet]. 2014;19(6): 811–16.

[51] Ashikhmin M. A tone mapping algorithm for high contrast images. In: 13th Eurographics Workshop on Rendering: Pisa, Italy. Citeseer; 2002.

[52] Ferwerda JA, Pattanaik SN, Shirley P, and Greenberg DP. A model of visual adaptation for realistic image synthesis. Proceedings of the 23rd Annual Conference on Computer Graphics and Interactive Techniques; 1996. pp. 249–58.

[53] Fattal R, Lischinski D, and Werman M. Gradient domain high dynamic range compression. ACM Transactions on Graphics (Proc. SIGGRAPH). 2002;21(3): 249–56.

[54] Reinhard E, Heidrich W, Debevec P, Pattanaik S, Ward G, and Myszkowski K. High dynamic range imaging: acquisition, display, and image-based lighting. Morgan Kaufmann; 2010.

[55] Tumblin J, Hodgins JK, and Guenter BK. Two methods for display of high contrast images. ACM Trans Graph. 1999;18(1):56–94.

[56] Ward G, and Simmons M. JPEG-HDR: A backwards-compatible, high dynamic range extension to JPEG. ACM SIGGRAPH 2006 Courses (pp. 3-es).

[57] Durand F, and Dorsey J. Fast bilateral filtering for the display of high-dynamic-range images. Proceedings of the 29th Annual Conference on Computer Graphics and Interactive Techniques - SIGGRAPH '02 [Internet]. 2002;257.

Chapter 11

Modeling the relationships between changes in EEG features and subjective quality of HDR images

Shaymaa Al-Juboori[1], Is-Haka Mkwawa[1], Lingfen Sun[1] and Emmanuel Ifeachor[1]

Quality of experience (QoE) is a human-centric paradigm, which produces the blueprint of human-behavioral-states such as perception, emotion, cognition, and expectation. Recent advances in neurophysiological monitoring tools have facilitated the study of frequency, time, and location of neuronal activity to an unprecedented degree, as well as opened doors to a better understanding of human overall behavioral systems. Physiological signals, such as the electroencephalogram (EEG), have shown promise in revealing the subject's emotion or attention in quality assessment and the correlation of this with media service quality. This chapter proposes a novel objective QoE model for high dynamic range (HDR) images and is based on the relationship between objective (i.e. delta-beta coupling) and subjective measures (i.e. mean opinion score MOS). The analysis of the results indicate that the proposed QoE model has a strong correlation with MOS scores, hence can be effectively used in predicting the overall HDR image quality. An advantage of the model is that it is lightweight and it provides a measure of user-perceived quality, but without requiring time-consuming subjective tests. The model has potential applications in several other areas, including QoE control and optimization. Future mobile providers can benefit from applying the proposed QoE-based model to optimize users' acceptability and satisfaction for different HDR image scenarios.

11.1 Introduction

The introduction of HDR imaging in the last two decades by the community of computer graphics has revolutionized the field and other areas, such as virtual reality, visual effects, photography, and the video-games [1]. The aim of digital

[1]Signal Processing and Multimedia Communication, School of Engineering, Computing and Mathematics, University of Plymouth, Plymouth, UK

cameras is to represent the scene as similar, and as realistic as the scene observed by the human visual system. The luminance, contrast, and all the other parameters related to digital images are gradually getting closer to the parameters experienced by a human observer [2]. There are two separate approaches to acquire HDR images, namely; hardware and software approach [1]. The hardware approach tries to resolve it in the image acquisition pipeline of digital cameras. The digital cameras have been improved in terms of quality and performance yet; photography is still having difficulties with storing and displaying a wide range of radiance variations in the real world. The scenes in the real world comprise of harsh lightening conditions that cause shadows (underexposed regions) or highlights (overexposed regions) in digitally captured images. The reason is that the dynamic range for sensors of camera is not high enough for capturing the overall dynamic range. For this reason, camera sensors, which have the ability to capture a wide dynamic range, have been developed [1–3]. On the other hand, most of the cameras and monitors are LDR, so we need to find a way to use the LDR devices to get the HDR images.

In the software approach, the problem had been defined by post processing techniques. Since the hardware solutions are considered to be expensive and need advance developments in this field which are not preferred by companies or researchers. The software solutions are easy, inexpensive compared to the hardware solutions and generally independent from hardware platforms [1]. The too dark areas are clipped to black (0) and too bright areas are clipped to white (255). Undoubtedly, this will lead to losses in both contrast and visual details [1]. The representation of floating point in HDR conquers this; instead of the bright and dark areas being saturated in an ad-hoc manner as is the case with LDR, they are being assigned values proportional to the actual scene intensity.

To improve the quality of HDR image services, research from academics and industry service providers have focused on developing the QoE models to predict overall user-perceived quality for optimizing quality provision [1]. However, modeling QoE is challenging due to the complex influences of user experience and diverse conditions of image content, context, and mobile devices. QoE is necessary to understand how humans perceive quality from visual stimuli as this can be potentially exploited for developing and optimizing images and video processing algorithms [3,4].

The primary trend in mobile services today is towards HDR as seen with the introduction of the streaming-based services, e.g. mobile TV and photo applications [5]. More the HDR content is being produced and its imminent adoption by the broadcast community means that there will soon be a demand for model HDR content on mobile devices [6]. One of the most critical issues in mobile HDR image delivery services is how to maximize the QoE of the users for the delivered content. An open research question is how HDR images with different contents perform on mobile phones [7]. Mobile devices, however, have certain differences compared to traditional viewing devices from QoE point of view. In particular, they are usually used "on-the-go", making the context variables such as ambient lighting levels, or reflections important variables that need to be considered. Furthermore, despite their evolution so far, mobile devices usually have additional hardware limitations such as power supply, display features, or local storage availability [8,9].

Traditionally, evaluation of the perceived quality of multimedia content is done using subjective opinion tests, such as MOS [4]. However, it is difficult for the user to link the experienced quality to the quality scale [10]. Moreover, MOS does not give an insight into how the user really feels, at the physiological level, in response to dislikes or satisfaction with the perceived quality [4,8,9,11]. To address this issue, measures which can be taken directly (implicitly) from the participant have attracted interest. The EEG is a promising approach that may be used to assess quality-related processes implicitly [11].

At present, there is no standard for using electrophysiology to assess QoE, but contributions are being made to the Telecommunication standardization sector of International Telecommunication Union (ITU-T) on the use of physiological measures for QoE (e.g. ITU-T Contribution COM 12-(039, 112, 103, and 202)) [12]. However, limited research has focused on establishing models to predict the user acceptance of mobile devices [3,13]. The work could be improved by involving more influencing factors of user experience such as device characteristics, content and use context. In addition, previous research on user's acceptance threshold may become inadequate in reflecting user experience for pleasant viewing [12,13].

On the other hand, modeling QoE is challenging due to the variability and complexity of human behavior, as not all humans have similar preferences, feelings or perceptions about a particular service or product [3,14]. Furthermore, user perceptions and preferences continuously change over time. The challenge is how to better understand human behavioral states and transform them into meaningful data [14]. Generally, QoE models are constructed in three steps: (i) collecting subjective evaluation data; (ii) identifying critical elements influencing the subjective value; and (iii) determining the relationship between the subjective value and these elements [3].

EEG features have shown to provide useful insights for QoE characterization. For example, the P300 event-related potential (ERP) signal, which occurs 300 ms post-stimulus presentation, has shown to be a useful EEG feature in characterizing the quality of text-to-speech (TTS), video, and audio-visual systems [13,15]. EEG activity contains oscillations at a variety of frequencies. In EEG, five main different frequency ranges are ascribed to specific states of the brain: delta band (1–4 Hz)),theta band (4–8 Hz), alpha band (8–13 Hz), beta band (13–30 Hz), and gamma band (36–44 Hz) [16,17]. The delta band is present during deep sleep; the theta band occurs during light sleep and is an indicator of decreased alertness. Activity in the alpha band is related to relaxed wakefulness with eyes closed and a decrease in alertness. Beta and gamma bands are ascribed to high arousal and focused attention [9,11].

The clinical research has suggested to us cross-frequency coupling as a mean of characterizing human emotions, mental activation status, and cognition [14,18–22]. As such, motivated by these promising insights, in this chapter, we propose a novel electrophysiology-based QoE model of human behavioral for mobile HDR Images which can be used to predict perceived image quality. We adopted the statistical technique to find the QoE models that can generate the best-fitting estimate of the true acceptability curves.

This aim is achieved through the following objectives:

1. Subjective (explicit) tests, such as mean opinion scores (MOS) during HDR images quality assessment.
2. EEG (implicit) test to understand the frequency components are related to HDR image quality perception in terms of QoE.
3. Investigate the relationships between the coupling between delta and beta frequency sub-bands to characterize human emotions such as anxiety and dissatisfaction.
4. Different natural HDR image content with different tone-mapping algorithms have been used in HDR images quality assessment.

The rest of the chapter is organized as follows. In the next section, we describe the related work; in Section 11.3 we will explain the dataset generation. in Section 11.4 presents the analysis of the results. In Section 11.5 the mobile EEG-based QoE model is presented. Section 11.6 is the limitations and finally, Section 11.7 is the summary.

11.2 Related work

Over the past years, there have been significant research efforts in the domain of QoE modeling aimed at studying the relationships between end-user QoE and psychophysical factors. Modeling QoE is challenging due to the difficulties in representing a complex subjective measure of user experience in a simple and objective way [13].

In [18–22], the delta and the beta frequency sub-bands have been linked to behavioral inhibition states (anxiety and frustration). In Gray's theory [18], the authors suggested that delta-beta coupling appears only in a frustrating situation, that is, it should be state-dependent. Another important point is that for anxiety generation, there must be concurrent and equivalent activation of fear and approach systems. In Knyazev *et al.* [17,21], it is shown that the correlation between mid-frontal delta and beta spectral power increased in healthy male subjects with an increase in anxiety and behavioral inhibition. It has also been found that there is higher positive correlation between delta and beta powers in subjects with higher baseline levels of salivary cortisol (the steroid hormone directly associated with anxiety) [14]. A hypothesis is that coupling reflects higher cortical arousal in frustrating situations [20], the authors found that coupling is very sensitive to external influences since it allowed detection between good and bad performance conditions. Al-Juboori *et al.* [22] explored the usefulness of combining explicit and implicit features in viewing HDR images from the mobile device. The authors suggest that increased EEG delta-beta coupling promotes behavioral inhibition states. Thus, increases in the degree of coupling are associated with decreases in HDR quality

The Video Quality Experts Group (VQEG) [23] is an international consortium of partners that work toward a better understanding of video quality perception as well as related psychophysical experiment design and prediction tools. The recently founded Psychophysiological Quality Assessment (PsyPhyQA) project extends VQEG's scope to investigate psychophysiological measurements. The aim of the PsyPhyQA project is to establish novel psychophysiology-based techniques and methodologies for video quality assessment and real-time interaction of humans with advanced video communication systems. Specifically, some of the aspects that the project is looking at include the definition of experimental methodologies, development of computational prediction models, and the correlates of psychophysics and psychophysiology. The current focus is on the development of an EEG-based experimental test plan and a cross-lab experiment evaluating professional grade with consumer grade EEG equipment for video quality assessment.

Chen *et al.* [24] developed a 3DTV model, the authors investigated 2DTV and 3DTV viewing visual fatigue, by using 16-channel EEG measurements. Significant decreases in gravity frequency and power spectral entropy were observed in several brain regions after viewing 3DTV, which is related to alertness level decline. Based on these findings and psychophysical responses, an accurate evaluation model for 3DTV fatigue was established. All bands changed significantly except the rhythm when subjects were viewing 3DTV. In particular, the energy decreased in and frequency bands while activity increased significantly. Their model is limited to 3DTV visual fatigue.

Politis *et al.* [25] proposed an objective QoE model for predicting 3D stereoscopic video quality using 2D objective quality metrics (PSNR) during video streaming over lossy networks. Subjective quality evaluation results indicate that 3D MOS is a linear combination of left and right view subjective results, while objective measurements based on PSNR for different packet loss conditions have demonstrated that the proposed 3D quality metric is related to the 2D left and right view PSNR. It has been shown that both measured MOS ratings and estimated MOS are strongly correlated, thus the proposed model can be effectively used for estimating the perceived 3D video quality during streaming over IP networks.

Yan Gong *et al.* [26] developed a QoE model with quantifiable metrics for QoE-based evaluation of service usage. They defined five QoE factors (usability, availability, service instantaneousness, service integrity, service retainability); however, they only focus on the relationship between quality of service (QoS) and QoE, considering neither the contextual nor the business domain. In addition, they do not differentiate QoE requirements based on various human roles and characteristics.

The ITU-T's G.1080 [27] proposes a QoE model that classifies QoE factors into two parts: subjective human components and objective QoS parameters. This model classifies the technical QoS parameters as part of the human objective QoE factor; whereas we believe that QoS could influence human behavior like any other business factor (pricing), but it is not an inherent part of the human domain. QoE is set of human centric factors, not technology-centric parameters [54].

Building on these prior works in QoE modeling, we propose a computationally simple model, which is based on the delta-beta coupling and correlates closely with subjectively measured MOS.

11.3 Dataset generation

In this chapter, explicit subjective tests and implicit tests using the EEG were conducted. The explicit subjective experiment has involved several participants viewing and rating the quality of HDR images with different tone-mapping operators (TMOs) while their EEG data were recorded at the same time.

11.3.1 Tone-mapping operators

There is no universal tone-mapping operator that always stands out when compared to others [8]. The choice of the best TMO not only depends on the content, but also on the device used, and other environmental parameters such as backlighting, display type and size, environment illumination, etc. [5,6]. These parameters need to be explicitly taken into account when viewing HDR images. In our experiment, we applied the best four TMOs from previous studies [8,27–29]: *adaptive logarithmic mapping AL1*, *iCAM06 AL2*, *photographic reproduction AL3*, and *bilateral filtering AL4*.

AL1: Adaptive logarithmic: It is a global TMO, which gives a medium quality tone mapped image, it is a fast algorithm suitable for interactive applications, which automatically produces realistically looking images for a wide variation of scenes exhibiting a HDR of luminance. It is based on logarithmic compression of luminance [30].

AL2: iCAM06, Fairchild and Johnson: It is a local TMO, it gives a very high-quality tone mapped image, and it is based on the physiology of the human's eye photoreceptors. The output of the operator is a combination of a locally adapted value around each pixel of the image and a globally adapted value based on the image averages [31].

AL3: Photographic reproduction: It is a global TMO, it gives a medium quality tone mapped image, it is based upon dodging-and-burning in traditional photography. It automatically applies various scales for luminance mapping to the prorated regions of highlights and shadows [32].

AL4: Frequency domain/local TMO: It gives a high-quality tone mapped image, fast bilateral filtering for the display of HDR images conserving local details in the image. They argued that an image might be thought of as being composed of an HDR component for low frequencies and an LDR component with a high spatial frequency [33].

The images used for the validation were computed using a MATLAB® HDR toolbox [34]. We used default settings for operators' performance as presented in the respective papers. The test images in the original "Radiance" format were resized to fit the resolution of the iPhone, then, all the selected four tone-mapping operators were run on each image with default settings to produce LDR versions in JPEG format, which were used in the experimental website.

11.3.2 Test stimuli

Five natural HDR scenes have been selected for this chapter, Church (Indoor, no artificial lighting), Warwick (Outdoor, daytime), Office (Indoor, artificial lighting), Night (Outdoor, nighttime), Lighthouse (Outdoor, sunset time) as in Table 11.1,

Table 11.1 Original HDR image description

Image	Description	Original image	Dimension	Histogram
Church	Indoor, no artificial lighting		670 × 757	55.33
Warwick	Outdoor, daytime		1189 × 598	117.095
Office	Indoor, artificial lighting	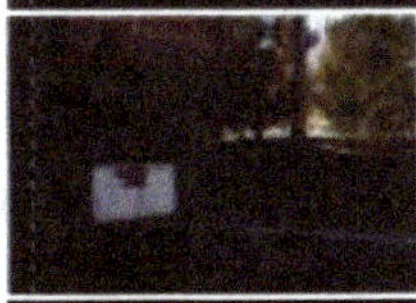	1165 × 751	115.65
Night	Outdoor, nighttime	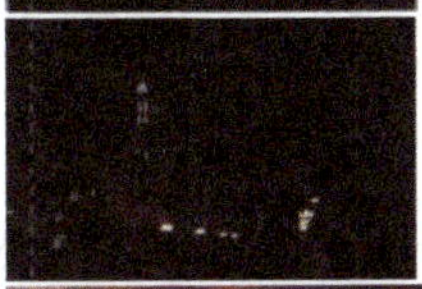	1200 × 798	43.3375
Lighthouse	Outdoor, sunset time	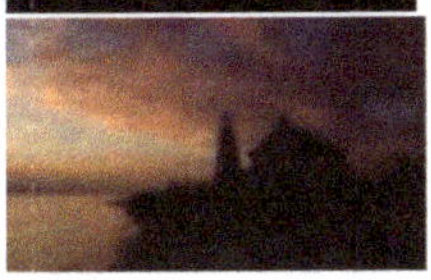	1440 × 980	144.86

based on their visual content and quality, the dynamic range of the content was also among the selection criteria. These five images were processed by four TMOs. Twenty HDR images have been viewed from a website that have been built specifically for the experiment [35]. The images were selected in such a way to have different representations in terms of content type (indoor or outdoor) and luminance range (night and day shots).

11.3.3 Participants

The subjective experiment was conducted in order to analyze if the proposed QoE-EEG in SSDs, it involved a number of participants viewing and rating the quality of HDR with different TMOs while wearing EEG device headset. Table 11.2 shows an overview of the subjective experiment.

Twenty-eight subjects, 13 females, 15 males (mean = 33.6 years old, SD = 3.890, range 25–45 years old) right-handed. In our experiment we based on ITU-R BT.500-13-section 2.5-recommendations, at least 15 observers should be used in the subjective test. All subjects had a normal or corrected vision and non-experts in HDR, but have a

Table 11.2 Overview of the subjective experiment

Participants	
Participants number	28
Male/female	15/13
Occupation	Staff/postgraduate students
Average age	33.6
Environment	Laboratory setup room
Device	
Monitor type	iPhone 8
Size	4.7″
Resolution	1334 × 750 with 326 pixels per inch
Stimuli presentation	
Number of images	20
Presentation order	Randomly
Viewing time	33 s

clear understanding of the test and they all are staff and postgraduate students at Plymouth University. All participants provided written consent forms. Before each experiment, a training session was organized to allow participants to familiarize themselves with the procedure. The content shown in the training session was selected by the experimenters in order to include various examples. The Research Ethics Committee at Plymouth University approved the experiment protocol.

11.3.4 Test setup

The evaluation test-bed is illustrated in Figure 11.1. An iPhone 8 device running on IOS 11.0 operating system was used for displaying the HDR images. An Intel Core™ i7 PC running Microsoft Windows 7 Enterprise operating system was used to process the EEG data. The iPhone and the EEG recording PC were time synchronized to facilitate the data analysis.

11.3.5 Test methodology

The experiment consisted of two sessions, during each session, 10 stimuli were visualized on the device. Half an hour break is done between the two sessions to prevent lack of attention and fatigue of subjects and ensure their comfort. Each session lasted approximately half an hour, excluding the training and the setup of the EEG devices. Each trial consisted of a 30-s baseline phase, an HDR stimulus period and a rating phase is shown in Figure 11.2. During the baseline periods, subjects were instructed to remain calm and focus on a 2D white cross on a grey background presented on the screen in front of them. The physiological signals recorded during the baseline period were used to remove stimulus-unrelated variations of the signals acquired during the stimulus period. Once the baseline period was over, an HDR image stimulus was presented for 30 s. After each stimulus was over, subjects were asked to provide their ratings for the particular HDR image stimulus within 60 s.

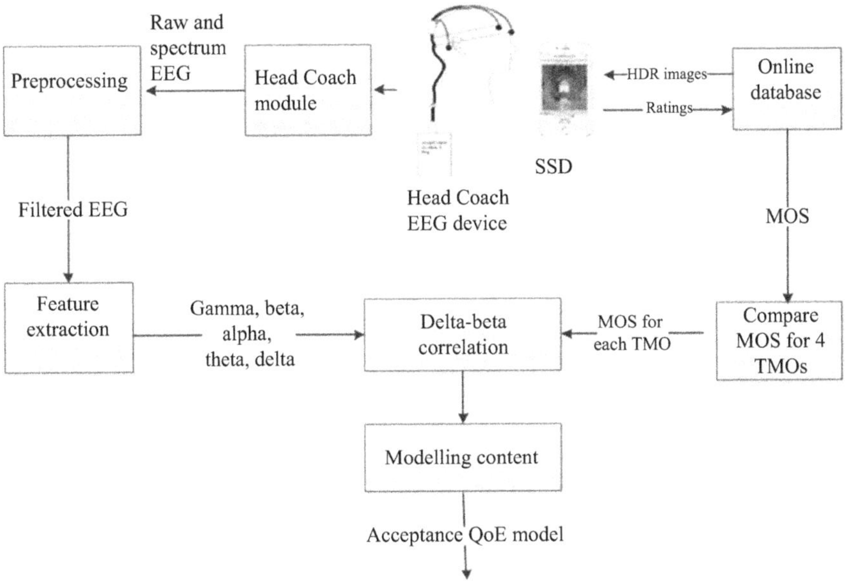

Figure 11.1 The test-bed for HDR image quality assessment

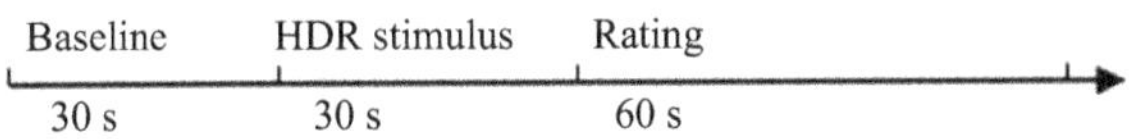

Figure 11.2 Trial timeline

After participants give the rating, the next stimulus appears on the SSD, the order of the sessions and trials were randomized. A website was developed for displaying the test sequences and quality ratings. Subjects were asked to evaluate the HDR stimuli. We chose a discrete five-level scale rating table for ITU-R quality ratings [36], it is more suitable for naïve (non-experts in image processing) observers, and it is easier for them to quantify the quality based on an adjective ("5 = Excellent" and "1 = Bad"). Figure 11.2 illustrates an example of one test trial, including baseline, stimuli, and rating period.

11.3.6 Preprocessing

For the EEG analysis, the MATLAB toolbox EEGLAB was used. The recorded EEG signals are down-sampled to 127.5 Hz, the acquired data were filtered using an IIR Chebyshev-II filter for all the frequency bands between 0.5 and 55 Hz. Thirty-three seconds have been recorded for each subject, only the last 30 s of all signals were used in our analysis, considering that stabilization and adaptation of the HDR contents may take some time.

11.3.7 Feature extraction

Off-line signal processing was performed using a custom written script and EEGLAB toolboxes for MATLAB. The baseline power was subtracted from the trial power, yielding the change of power relative to the pre-stimulus period. The following frequency bands were determined a priori and then extracted: Total bandwidth (0.5–60 Hz), delta (0.5–3 Hz), theta (4–8 Hz), alpha (8–13 Hz), beta (13–30 Hz), and gamma (30–60 Hz). All the further EEG analysis was performed clustering Fp1 and Fp2 channels. RP density was computed for each frequency band in each participant, using the following (11.1):

$$RP(\lambda) = AP(\lambda)/MP(TB) \tag{11.1}$$

where RP = relative power, λ = frequency band, AP = absolute power peak, MP = mean power spectra. RP values were then natural log normalized. The analysis of ERPs was not performed because of the naïve triggering approach and the use of a low-density EEG device.

Delta activity is present during sleep and continuous attention; theta activity occurs during light sleep and provides an indicator of decreased alertness and for encoding new information. Activity in the alpha band is related to alertness and good quality images and is a function of age. Beta activity is related to cognitive thinking and visual attention and is significantly increased in a 3D environment. Finally, gamma band is related to visual information process, brain activity and good quality image [10,11].

11.4 EEG signal acquisition

Most EEG devices are large, expensive, complicated-to-use, mains-powered devices which require the user to be lying down. Alpha-active real-time compact EEG brainwave monitors have been used in the test. It consists of two channels for the left and right side of the head with five electrodes and leads placed at the standard positions on the scalp while the participants were viewing the stimuli, as in Figure 11.3.

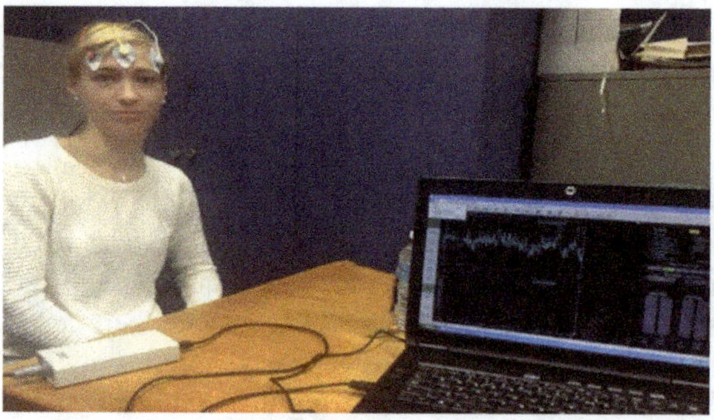

Figure 11.3 A participant preparation before the experiment

A key aspect of the Alpha-Active EEG device is the ability to view and save EEG data in real time in time-domain and frequency-domain in CSV format. It is pocket-sized, robust, cost-effective, simple-to-use, laptop-powered. It can record sound simultaneously with EEG data and samples the raw EEG signal at 127.5 Hz. Head-Coach^{TM} product overcomes the noisy data, by employing a patented efficient and stable algorithm for processing the signal and by making use of cutting-edge hardware for handling the noisy EEG data. This EEG system, developed in the UK in collaboration with academic partners and clinicians [37].

11.5 Analysis of results

11.5.1 Subjective rating analysis

In this section, the results of subjective rating are described with the aim of providing an understanding of the characteristics of QoE of the tone mapped HDR images and factors that affect QoE. The first step was to detect and remove outliers in the subject MOS results so that they do not influence the results. The Outlier detection procedure was applied to the results obtained from the 28 subjects and performed according to the guidelines described in Section 2.3.1 of Annex 2 of ITU-R BT.500-13 [38]. MOS representing the average subjective quality ratings across all participants are usually represented on nominal scales and associated 95% confidence intervals (CI) were presented for the four quality level algorithms [39]. Figure 11.4 shows the average MOS for AL1, AL2, AL3, and AL4 respectively; Bilateral Filtering AL4 had the best performance from the observer's point of view.

11.5.2 EEG signal analysis

It is known that high gamma power corresponds to high brain activity and that the brain is highly activated when the perceived quality is low. This indicates that the perception of low quality is related to negative emotions [40,41]. It also implies that higher gamma means lower quality for the HDR image as shown in Figure 11.5(a).

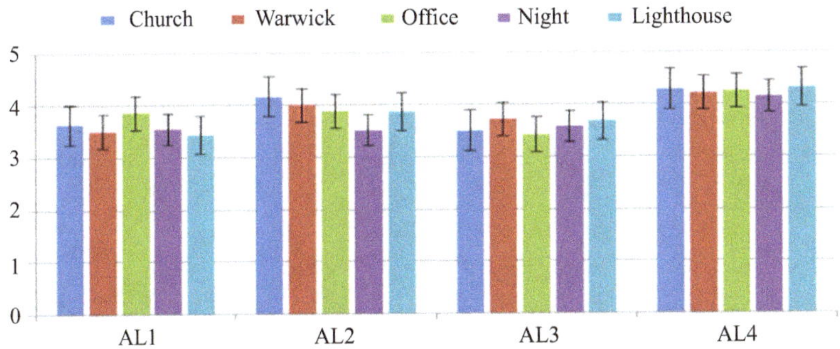

Figure 11.4 MOS and CIs for experienced TMOs

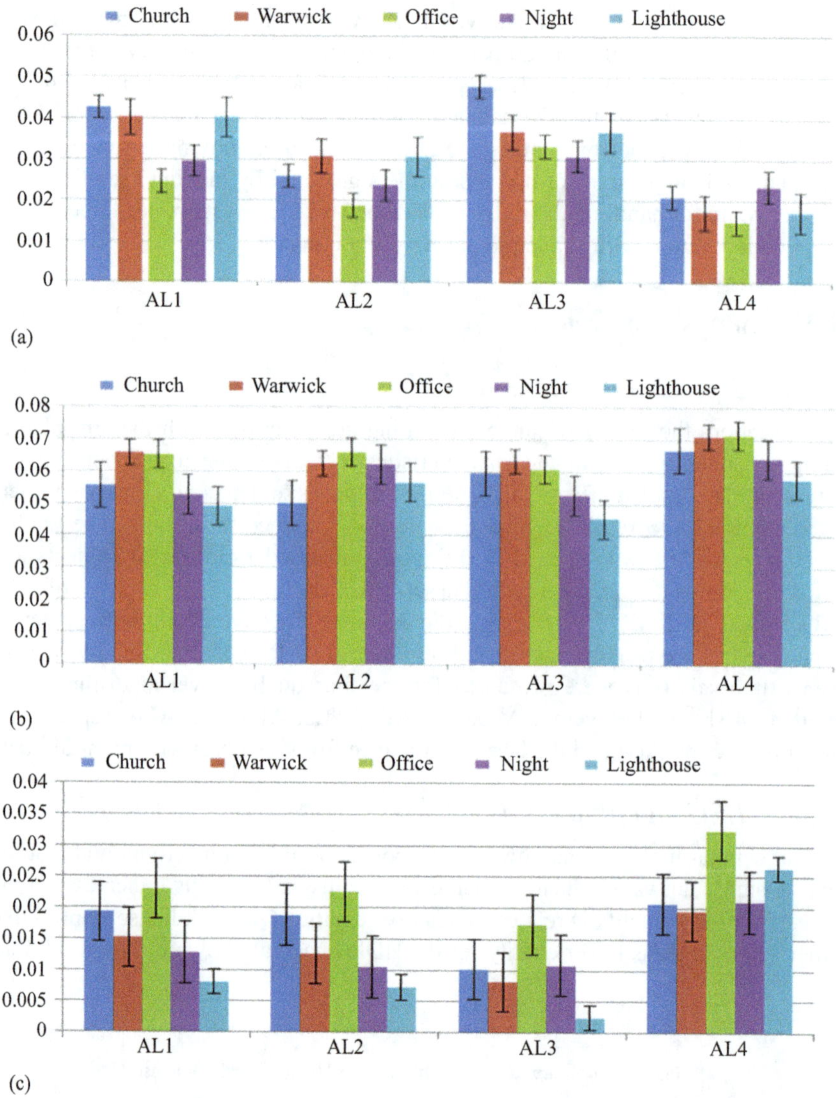

Figure 11.5 Mean power for (a) gamma, (b) beta, (c) alpha, (d) theta, and (e) delta

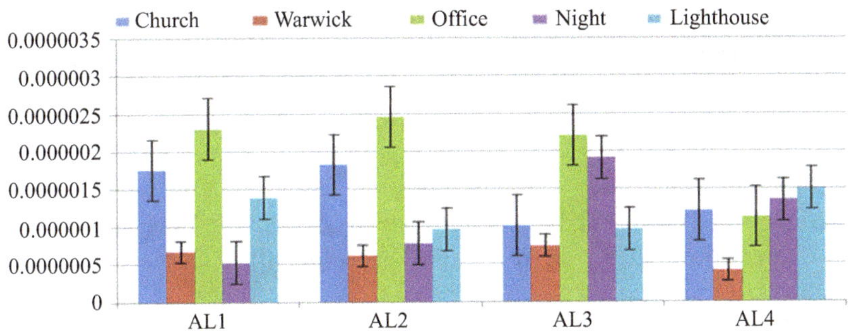

(d)

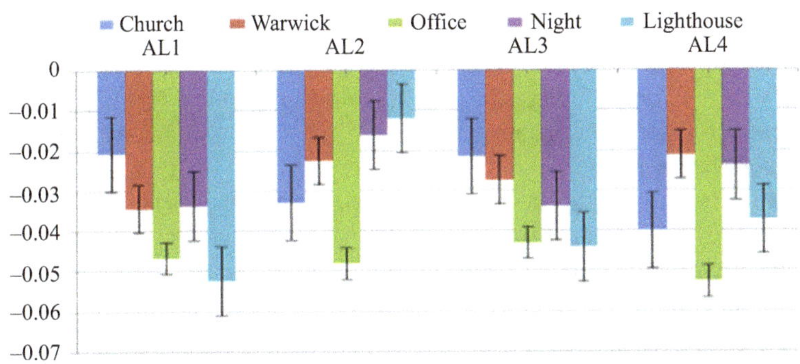

(e)

Figure 11.5 (Continued)

AL4 gave the lowest results, which indicates that it has the highest quality. In accordance with [42,43], we also found a significantly higher beta for positive emotional tasks (high perceived HDR quality in our case) compared to other frequency bands results. Therefore, cognitive and emotional processes seem to take place during quality perception of HDR images. From the beta results, Figure 11.5(b), there is no large variance in the mean power level.

This suggests that the brain reacted cognitively and emotionally with the HDR images in the same way. Furthermore, higher alpha power indicates brain activation when overall perceived quality is high, whereas the alpha power in the brain is deactivated when overall perceived quality is low [11,19,42,44,45]. In Figure 11.5(c), AL4 gave the highest Alpha result, i.e. best-perceived quality. In the theta frequency band, Figure 11.5(d), EEG power is negatively related to cognitive performance and brain maturity, theta synchronization is positively correlated with the ability to encode new information [11,46,47]. From the results, we can see that theta mean power amplitude is very low ($\sim 10^{-5}$) compared with all other frequencies.

11.5.3 Correlation and analysis of variance

To estimate the correlation between changes in the EEG and subjective scores, the mean of all power in the frequency band across subjects was calculated. The Pearson linear Correlation Coefficient was calculated between the mean power values and the MOS for subjective ratings, per frequency bands as in Table 11.3. From Table 11.3 we can see that the highest correlation is between MOS and gamma frequency band [48], but this is negatively correlated; Thus, higher gamma means more a low quality of the HDR image [30,40], AL4 gave the highest correlation.

The results also show that Alpha is positively correlated with MOS and that AL4 gave the highest correlation. The correlation values for the beta band, however, were not high, but they followed the hypothesized inverse relationship trend. This is probably because the subject's judgment may not always follow the objective Neuro-physiological facts [9–11,49]. Additionally, it is likely due to the neutrality of the content utilized for the HDR stimuli, which may not have evoked strong enough emotional characteristics [14]. Theta and Delta correlate positively, but the correlation is weak.

The Pearson correlations were estimated between the mean power values for each frequency band and the subjective ratings, for all image contents (Table 11.4). We found significantly higher beta in *Night* and *Lighthouse* compared to *Church*, *Warwick*, and *Office* for positive emotional tasks (preferred content in our case). Hence, cognitive and emotional processes seem to take place during the quality

Table 11.3 Pearson correlation between MOS and the frequency oscillations for each algorithm (quality)

Frequency band	AL1	AL2	AL3	AL4
Gamma	−0.6605	−0.8132	−0.5660	**−0.8747**
Beta	−0.6005	−0.6492	−0.6012	**−0.6820**
Alpha	0.5320	0.7523	0.5004	**0.7830**
Theta	0.2648	0.2592	**0.3336**	−0.1039
Delta	0.0637	**0.2211**	0.0477	0.0814

Note: Bold values represents the highest values in each set.

Table 11.4 Pearson correlation between MOS and the frequency oscillations for each content

	Church	Warwick	Office	Night	Lighthouse
Gamma	−0.7301	−0.7971	−0.808	−0.362	−0.4675
Beta	−0.5632	−0.4345	−0.443	−0.739	−0.8091
Alpha	0.5857	0.4155	0.6622	0.1765	0.1144
Theta	0.4328	0.4774	0.5769	0.1976	0.1649
Delta	0.1264	0.1109	0.0846	0.0109	0.0116

Table 11.5 ANOVA analysis

Source	*dF*	*F*	*P*-value
Delta	3	5.092	0.001668
Theta	3	5.342	0.001178
Alpha	3	5.356	0.001155
Beta	3	5.470	**0.000984**
Gamma	3	5.292	0.001263

Note: Bold value represents the highest values in each set.

perception of the HDR image. An increase in alpha and theta level is the result of a reduction in quality. This increase may be due to an increased level of anxiety, fatigue, and drowsiness [19]. We found significantly lower alpha and theta in *Night* and *Lighthouse* compared to *Church*, *Warwick*, and *Office*. This finding implies that subjects rated perceived quality by taking into account how pleasant or annoying the content was [50,51]. Moreover, high gamma power corresponds to high brain activity and suggesting that the brain is highly activated when perceived quality is low [40,44,52].

We found significantly lower gamma in *Night* and *Lighthouse* compared to *Church*, *Warwick*, and *Office*; this indicates that low perception of quality is related to negative emotions [14,25]. Methodologically, our results indicate that Theta and Alpha frequency bands offer a means of studying cortical activation patterns during both cognitive and emotional information processing.

To investigate quantitatively whether the HDR image quality has a significant influence on the EEG frequency bands, an ANOVA analysis was performed on the subjective ratings, with a significance *P*-value threshold of 0.001. Table 11.5 summarizes the ANOVA results and beta gave a significant $P\text{-value} < 0.001$. Overall, the results of the ANOVA analysis revealed that beta has an impact on HDR's perceived quality.

However, the other interactions were not significant, $P > 0.001$. It has been established that the beta band is highly associated with cognitive thinking and reflects emotional behavior. Our finding parallels that of Kroupi *et al.* [53] which found that beta frequency band significantly increased in the 3D environment, which received a significantly higher score in comparison to 2D video.

11.5.4 The coupling measurements

To understand human behavioral states at the neural level, the coupling between delta and beta frequency bands was computed as the correlation coefficient between the mean powers in the frequency bands. This is linked with negative behavioral characteristics (anxiety, frustration, dissatisfaction). Clinical literature [14,20,21,24] indicates that increased EEG delta-beta coupling promotes behavioral inhibition states. This means that the closer the coupling (or correlation) is to 0, the more the subject would be satisfied with the test. On the other hand, as coupling or correlation approaches 1, the less the subjects like the HDR image (or

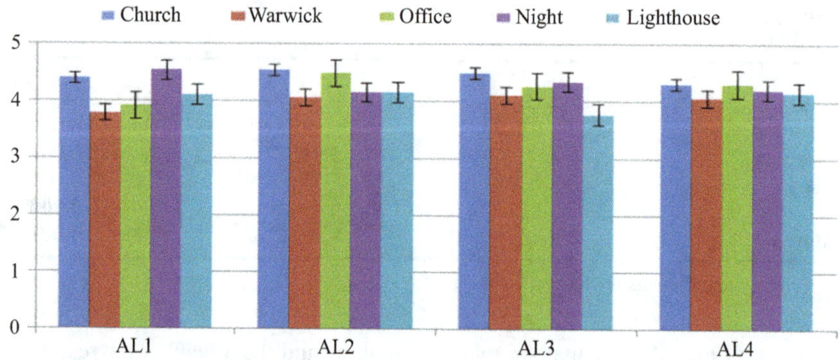

Figure 11.6 MOS and CIs for experienced TMOs after coupling

the more frustrated they are frustrated by the test). By calculating the coupling values between delta and beta for each tone-mapped HDR image quality of the results, high coupling values (e.g. greater than 0.5) would be considered to represent unsatisfied subjects (or subjects who had an unpleasant experience).

To explore this point, the scores for subjects who were unsatisfied were removed (7 out of 28) from the dataset. Figure 11.6 shows the MOS for the four quality levels for the five contents after removing those subjects. By comparing Figures 11.4 and 11.6, we can see the MOS values per algorithm per content have increased. On the other hand, the standard deviation and 95% confidence interval have decreased. The results suggest that it is sometimes difficult for participants to link the experienced quality to the quality scale in explicit tests and that EEG-based measure provides additional and complementary information, which aids understanding of the human perception of the contents.

11.6 A mobile EEG-based QoE model

11.6.1 EEG-based QoE model based on regression technique

We used the generated dataset to highlight the main challenges in developing an EEG-based QoE model of human behavioral for mobile high dynamic range images. We show a novel process to collect user acceptance data through an iPhone, and adopt a nonlinear regression technique to produce mathematical QoE content dependent models for acceptability prediction based on the nature of the data fit curve. We adopted the statistical technique to find the QoE models that can generate the best-fitting estimate of the true acceptability curves. After removing the unsatisfied subjects from the delta-beta coupling, the remaining dataset has been divided into 60% and 40% for training and testing, respectively. The key aspect behind this ratio is that we will have a high probability chance of getting all the target class detailed observation into the training dataset; this will be helpful in the modeling. When we split the dataset by considering the 50:50 ratio, we will not be much confident to capture all the target classes' related observation into the training dataset.

After dividing the dataset, we applied the 60% training data in the MATLAB curve-fitting tool. The remaining 40% of the testing for the entire five image scenarios is used for evaluation. The best fitting equation worked on the five content scenarios was exponential with high R-square values. General exponential model with coefficients (with 95% confidence bounds): Based on the results, the MOS HDR values for HDR images can be modeled as in (11.2) and (11.3):

$$\text{MOS} = f(\text{CT}, \text{CP}) \tag{11.2}$$

where CT is the content type and CP denotes coupling.

$$\text{MOS} = ae^{bx} + ce^{dx} \tag{11.3}$$

where $f(x)$ = MOS, a, b, c, and d are the coefficients (as in Table 11.6) obtained from the regression fittings

11.6.2 Model evaluation

In order to evaluate the EEG-based QoE model, we used 40% for the dataset for validation for the entire five image scenarios. The accuracy of the model was determined by computing the R^2 and the RMSE. The R^2 correlations and RMSE for both training and validation datasets are illustrated in Tables 11.7 and 11.8, respectively. Figure 11.7 depicts the scatter graph of subjective MOS values against the proposed model in (11.3).

Table 11.6 Coefficients of proposed QoE model-based content

Image	**Coefficients**			
	a	***b***	***c***	***d***
Indoor (no artificial lighting)	−1876	−.535	1881	−2.528
Outdoor (sunset)	3.615	5.375	1.986	0.937
Outdoor (night)	5.184	−1.17	5.16e−06	25.19
Indoor (artificial lighting)	644.4	−0.1816	−639.7	−0.178
Outdoor (day)	0.8005	−33.12	4.551	−0.851

Table 11.7 Evaluation of proposed QoE model-based content (training dataset)

	Indoor (no artificial lighting)	**Outdoor (sunset)**	**Outdoor (night)**	**Indoor (artificial lighting)**	**Outdoor (day)**
R^2	0.914	0.834	0.908	0.809	0.912
RMSE	0.170	0.259	0.171	0.211	0.197

Table 11.8 Evaluation of proposed QoE model-based content (validation dataset)

	Indoor (no artificial lighting)	Outdoor (sunset)	Outdoor (night)	Indoor (artificial lighting)	Outdoor (day)
R^2	0.8858	0.7798	0.8782	0.7458	0.8839
RMSE	0.1629	0.1184	0.1440	0.1192	0.1551

The proposed QoE models can achieve high prediction accuracy (RMSE < 0.25, $R^2 > 0.82$), and can be applied to the mobile HDR system to benefit consistent user perception and effective resource allocation.

11.7 Limitations

There are a number of limitations in the project and program of work reported in the thesis. These include the following:

11.7.1 Experimental set-up

While our current experimental setup provides new and relevant information, there are also several limitations and challenges in our method that need to be addressed.

1. TMOs and HDRs: the TMOs arising in our HDR stimulus do not cover the full range of possible qualities as these were only were ten of the most well-known TMOs. Thus, several experiments must be conducted to examine different combinations of TMO qualities.
2. Dataset: the relatively small size of the dataset meant that it was limited to natural scenes; this should be expanded to cover other types of content.
3. In particular, the dataset for the CVD is only 28 subjects; the number should be increased to about 50 in order to evaluate this model sufficiently.
4. Displays: HDR images still need to be presented on HDR displays. They cannot be displayed easily on the current SSD or LCD monitors as these have dynamic range limitations of about 100:1, which is very low compared to HDR displays.

11.7.2 Limitations using mobile devices

The main limitations encountered when using mobile devices in our experiments are listed below:

1. Mobile devices usually have limited memory available for running applications. Moreover, they must run several applications in parallel, which further decreases the memory available for imaging applications.
2. Computational power is also limited which has a twofold impact on the implementation of an HDR system. Firstly, the fusing process must be implemented through simple arithmetic operations to keep the processing time as

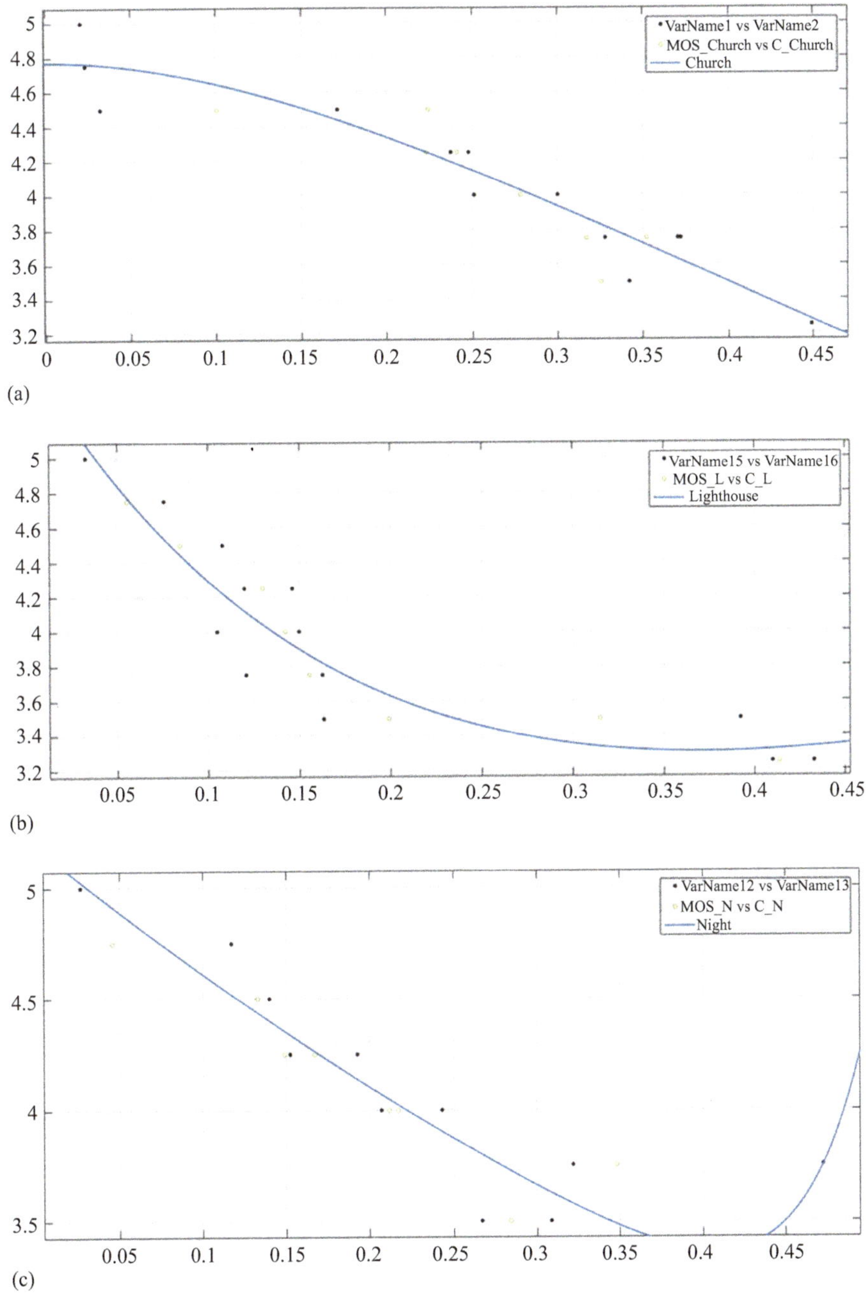

Figure 11.7 The scatter graph of subjective MOS values against the proposed model: (a) indoor (no artificial lighting), (b) outdoor (sunset), (c) outdoor (night), (d) indoor (artificial lighting), and (e) outdoor (day)

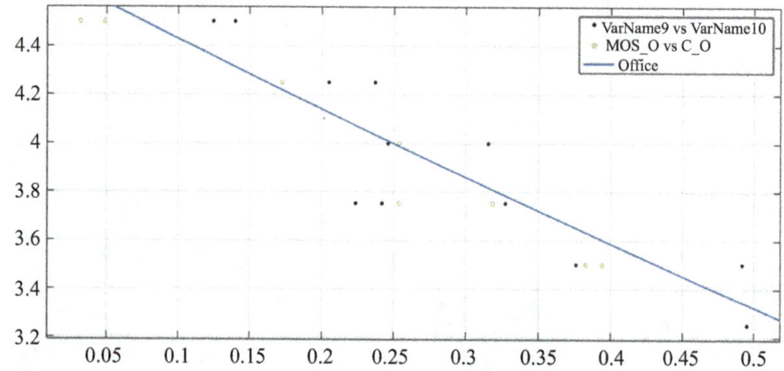

(d)

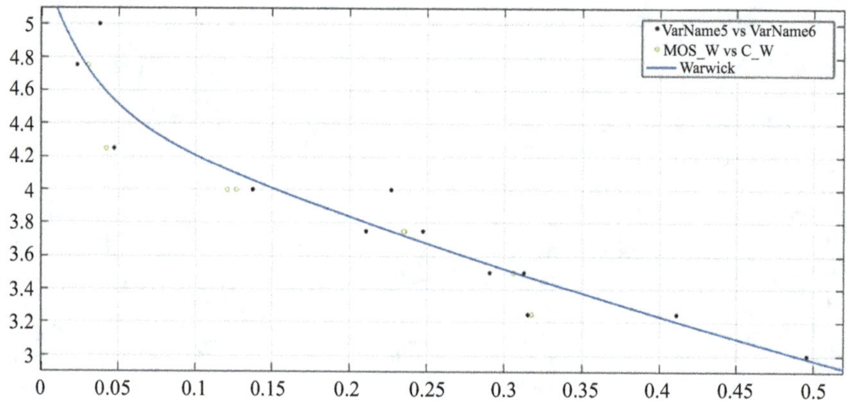

(e)

Figure 11.7 *(Continued)*

short as possible. Secondly, the number of captured images must also be limited.

3. Another limitation of mobile devices is the lack of support they provide for floating point operations. This complicates the implementation of multi-frame approaches that transform the input images in the radiance map (radiance map computation usually results in floating point variables).
4. A notable limitation of the SSD is that the original resolution and aspect ratio of the images were maintained so that a straight comparison could be made between the reference and the tone-mapped sequence of the mobile device. This guarantees that no information was lost when the content was converted to a lower resolution. Small screen sizes would have required the content to be retargeted. Additionally, participants were not allowed to adjust the brightness of the SDD.

11.7.3 Limitations using the EEG device

The main limitations we encountered when using an EEG device are listed below:

1. We used a portable 2-channel EEG device for multimedia quality assessment which was suitable for the lab environment. The 2-channel EEG is a consumer-grade EEG device that is low-cost, lightweight, and inexpensive. However, such devices were not originally intended for research, although they are becoming increasingly popular due to their flexibility and the wide range of suites they offer.
2. Physiological differences between individuals when using the EEG may generate systematic errors between participants or groups. Another key challenge is to design a QoE assessment so that it is applicable to a general population.
3. Attaching sensors to participants can cause a certain degree of discomfort or result in them changing their natural behavior. Moreover, experiments requiring attached sensors are often considerably more complex. Such factors can have a direct impact on the duration of the experiment and, consequently, on the availability of participants.

11.8 Summary

In this chapter, we proposed a novel approach based on content-based HDR image quality prediction model using EEG features. QoE is a promising solution for mobile service providers, however, QoE measurement is challenging due to the variability and complexity of human behavior, as not all humans have similar preferences, feelings or perceptions about a particular service or product. Furthermore, user perceptions and preferences continuously change over time. The challenge is how to better understand human behavioral states and transform them into meaningful data. Twenty HDR images were viewed by 28 subjects, during informal subjective tests and the subjects' EEG data were also recorded and subsequently processed. We proposed a model that has the potential to predict MOS from EEG signal classification, based on the coupling between delta and beta frequency bands. Delta-beta coupling provides information about user anxiety, frustration, and dissatisfaction. As such, if content and service providers want to ensure a rich quality of user experience, the coupling should not be strong enough to incite negative behavioral characteristics in end users.

In our future work, we will focus not only on the limitations for covering the full range of possible qualities to examine the different types of TMO quality combinations but also in increasing the dataset size and content.

References

[1] Banterle F, Artusi A, Debattista K, and Chalmers A. Advanced high dynamic range imaging. Boca Raton, FL: CRC Press; 2017.

[2] Banterle F, Artusi A, and Debattista K CA. Advanced High Dynamic Range Imaging: Theory and practice. Natick, MA: A.K. Peters Inc. (CRC Press); 2011.

[3] Song W, and Tjondronegoro DW. Acceptability-based QoE models for mobile video. IEEE Trans Multimed. 2014;16(3):738–50.

[4] Narwaria M, Perreira M, Callet P Le, and Silva D. High dynamic range visual quality of experience measurement: challenges and perspectives to cite this version: high dynamic range visual quality of experience measurement: challenges and perspectives. 2015.

[5] Melo M, Bessa M, Debattista K, and Chalmers A. Evaluation of HDR video tone mapping for mobile devices. Signal Process Image Commun. 2014;29 (2):247–256.

[6] Melo M, Bessa M, Debattista K, and Chalmers A. Evaluation of tone-mapping operators for HDR video under different ambient luminance levels. Comput Graph Forum. 2015;34(8):38–49.

[7] Al-Juboori S, Mkwawa IH, Sun L, and Ifeachor E. Impact of tone-mapping operators and viewing devices on visual quality of experience. 2016 IEEE Int Conf Commun ICC 2016. IEEE. pp. 1–6.

[8] Mantiuk RK, Myszkowski K, and Seidel H-P. High dynamic range imaging. Wiley Encycl Electr Electron Eng. 2015;6:1–42.

[9] Moon SE, and Lee JS. Perceptual experience analysis for tone-mapped HDR videos based on EEG and peripheral physiological signals. IEEE Trans Auton Ment Dev. 2015;7(3):236–47.

[10] Moon SE, and Lee JS. Implicit analysis of perceptual multimedia experience based on physiological response: a review. IEEE Trans Multimed. 2017; 19(2):340–53.

[11] Moon S, and Lee J. EEG connectivity analysis in perception of tone-mapped high dynamic range videos. Proceedings of the 23rd ACM International Conference on Multimedia. 2015;987–90.

[12] ITU-T International Telecommunication Union. ITU-T Contribution COM 12-039, Investigating the subjective judgment process using physiological data. International Telecommunication Union. 2013.

[13] Engelke U, Darcy DP, and Mulliken GH *et al.* Psychophysiology-based QoE assessment: a survey. IEEE J Sel Top Signal Process. 2017;11(1):6–21.

[14] Laghari KUR, Gupta R, Antons JN, Schleicher R, Möller S, and Falk TH. Objective characterization of human behavioural characteristics for QoE assessment: a pilot study on the use of electroencephalography features. 2013 IEEE Globecom Work GC Workshops 2013. IEEE. 2013;1168–73.

[15] Antons J-N, Cheng E, Engelke U, and Arndt S. Scientific C. Review on using physiology in quality of experience. Hum Vis Electron Imaging. 2016;1–9.

[16] Al-Nuaimi AH, Jammeh E, Sun L, and Ifeachor E. Changes in the EEG amplitude as a biomarker for early detection of Alzheimer's disease. In: Proceedings of the Annual International Conference of the IEEE Engineering in Medicine and Biology Society, EMBS. 2016.

[17] Al-Nuaimi AH, Jammeh E, Sun L, and Ifeachor E. Tsallis entropy as a biomarker for detection of Alzheimer's disease. In: Proceedings of the Annual International Conference of the IEEE Engineering in Medicine and Biology Society, EMBS. 2015.

[18] McNaughton N. Gray's neuropsychology of anxiety: an enquiry into the functions of septohippocampal theories. Behav Brain Sci. 1982;5(03):492.

[19] Knyazev GG, Savostyanov AN, and Levin EA. Alpha oscillations as a correlate of trait anxiety. Int J Psychophysiol. 2004;53(2):147–60.

[20] Sravanth KR, Anudeep P, Sudha S, and Chinmay C. Comparison of attention and meditation based mobile applications by using EEG signals, IEEE: Global Wireless Summit (GWS-SS), 2018, 260–265.

[21] Knyazev GG, Schutter DJLG, and van Honk J. Anxious apprehension increases coupling of delta and beta oscillations. Int J Psychophysiol. 2006; 61(2):283–7.

[22] Al-Juboori S, Mkwawa I-H, Sun L, and Ifeachor E. Investigation of relationships between changes in EEG features and subjective quality of HDR images. In: Multimedia and Expo (ICME), 2017 IEEE International Conference on IEEE; 2017. pp. 91–6.

[23] Huynh-thu Q, Webster A, Brunnström K, and Pinson M. VQEG: Shaping Standards on Video Quality. 2015;17–20.

[24] Chen C, Li K, Wu Q, Wang H, Qian Z, and Sudlow G. EEG-based detection and evaluation of fatigue caused by watching 3DTV. Displays. 2013;34(2):81–8.

[25] Muller MM, Keil A, Gruber T, and Elbert T. Processing of affective pictures modulates right-hemisphere gamma band activity. Clin Neurophysiol. 1999;110(11):1913–20.

[26] Gong Y, Yang F, Huang L, and Su S. Model-based approach to measuring quality of experience. In: 2009 First International Conference on Emerging Network Intelligence. IEEE; 2009. pp. 29–32.

[27] ITU-T International Telecommunication Union. ITU-T G.1080: Transmission systems and media, digital systems and networks. 2008.

[28] Narwaria M, Perreira Da Silva M, Le Callet P, and Pepion R. Tone mapping based HDR compression: does it affect visual experience? Signal Process Image Commun [Internet]. 2014;29(2):257–73.

[29] Čadík M, Wimmer M, Neumann L, and Artusi A. Evaluation of HDR tone mapping methods using essential perceptual attributes. Comput Graph. 2008;32(3):330–49.

[30] Drago F, Myszkowski K, Annen T, and Chiba N. Adaptive logarithmic mapping for displaying high contrast scenes. Comput Graph Forum. 2003;22 (3):419–26.

[31] Kuang J, Johnson GM, and Fairchild MD. iCAM06: A refined image appearance model for HDR image rendering. J Vis Commun Image Represent. 2007;18(5):406–14.

[32] Drago F, Martens WL, Myszkowski K, and Seidel H-P. Perceptual evaluation of tone mapping operators with regard to similarity and preference. Tech. Rep. MPI-I-2002-4-002, Max Plank Institut für Informatik.

[33] Durand F, and Dorsey J. Fast bilateral filtering for the display of high-dynamic-range images. Proc 29th Annu Conf Comput Graph Interact Tech - SIGGRAPH '02 [Internet]. 2002;257.

[34] F. Banterle HT. HDR toolbox [Internet]. Available from: https://github.com/banterle/HDR_Toolbox

[35] Al-Juboori S. Processed HDR images [Internet]. Available from: https://www.fose1.plymouth.ac.uk/spmc/staff/ssal-juboori/eeg/index.html

[36] ITU-T International Telecommunication Union. ITU-T contribution, BT 500-13. Methodology for the subjective assessment of the quality of television pictures. 2010.

[37] Alpha-Active. Alpha-Active Ltd [Internet]. Available from: http://www.alpha-active.com/

[38] RECOMMENDATION ITU-R BT.500-11. Methodology for the subjective assessment of the quality of television pictures [Internet]. 2013. Available from: https://www.itu.int/dms_pubrec/itu-r/rec/bt/R-REC-BT.500-11-200206-S!!PDF-E.pdf

[39] Hanhart P, Bernardo MV, Pereira M, Pinheiro AMG, and Ebrahimi T. Benchmarking of objective quality metrics for HDR image quality assessment. EURASIP J Image Video Process. 2015;2015(1).

[40] Demiralp T, Bayraktaroglu Z, and Lenz D *et al.* Gamma amplitudes are coupled to theta phase in human EEG during visual perception. Int J Psychophysiol. 2007;64(1):24–30.

[41] Muller MM, Gruber T, Keil A, and Muller M. Modulation of induced gamma band activity in the human EEG by attention and visual information processing. Int J Psychophysiol. 2000;38(3):283–99.

[42] Ray WJ, and Cole HW. EEG alpha activity reflects attentional demands, and beta activity reflects emotional and cognitive processes. Science (80). 1985; 228(4700):750–2.

[43] Nemoto H, Korshunov P, Hanhart P, and Ebrahimi T. Visual attention in LDR and HDR images Multimedia Signal Processing Group (MMSPG) and Ecole Polytechnique Fédérale de Lausanne (EPFL), Lausanne, Switzerland. 2015.

[44] Babiloni C, Del Percio C, and Vecchio F *et al.* Alpha, beta and gamma electrocorticographic rhythms in somatosensory, motor, premotor and prefrontal cortical areas differ in movement execution and observation in humans. Clin Neurophysiol. 2016;127(1):641–54.

[45] Klimesch W. EEG alpha and theta oscillations reflect cognitive and memory performance: a review and analysis. Brain Res Rev. 1999;29(2):169–95.

[46] Moretti DV, Fracassi C, and Pievani M *et al.* Increase of theta/gamma ratio is associated with memory impairment. Clin Neurophysiol. 2009;120(2):295–303.

[47] Moretti DV. Theta and alpha EEG frequency interplay in subjects with mild cognitive impairment: evidence from EEG, MRI, and SPECT brain modifications. Front Aging Neurosci. 2015;7:31.

[48] Perez J, and Delechelle E. On the measurement of image quality perception using frontal EEG analysis. In: Smart Communications in Network

Technologies (SaCoNeT), 2013 International Conference on IEEE; 2013. pp. 1–5.

[49] Moon S-E, and Lee J-S. Classifying Perceptual Experience of Tone-mapped High Dynamic Range Videos through EEG. Proc 1st International Workshop on Perceptive Inspired Video Processing - PIVP '14. 2014;27–32.

[50] Kroupi E, Hanhart P, Lee J-S, Rerabek M, and Ebrahimi T. EEG correlates during video quality perception. In: Signal Processing Conference (EUSIPCO), 2014 Proceedings of the 22nd European. IEEE; 2014. pp. 2135–9.

[51] Korshunov P, and Ebrahimi T. Influence of Context and Content on Tone-mapping Operators. First Int Conf SME Work HDR imaging [Internet]. 2013;(2).

[52] Moon S-E, and Lee J-S. Implicit analysis of perceptual multimedia experience based on physiological response: a review. IEEE Trans Multimed. 2017;19(2):340–53.

[53] Kroupi E, Hanhart P, Lee J-S, Rerabek M, and Ebrahimi T. EEG correlates during video quality perception. Signal Process Conf (EUSIPCO), 2014 Proc 22nd Eur [Internet]. 2014;1–4.

Chapter 12
IoMT and healthcare delivery in chronic diseases

Yogesh Shelke[1]

Digital health broadly incorporates categories such as mobile health (mHealth), information technology comprising electronic health records, reimbursements (IT), wearable devices, telehealth and telemedicine. Recent advancements on this front includes Internet of Things (IoT) ecosystem, which provides a connected ecosystem for flawless information flow within various technologies involved at hardware, software and networking layer. These enabling technologies include devices embedded with sensor, actuator and communication protocol, which transmits and receives the data in real time. Along with other end applications such as smart energy transmission, smart homes, intelligent logistics and smart towns, healthcare provides an attractive opportunity area for successful implementation. Current estimates predict that nearly 60% of organizations a have implemented IoT in healthcare industry in partial or complete form, to deliver value to patients and transition from disjoint and reactive model towards interoperable and proactive service delivery model. Internet of medical things (IoMT)-enabled machine-to-machine interaction between devices in patient's body environment with enabling architecture, is predicted to provide higher impact in chronic disease care. Further, current topic would broadly review clinician side transformations of technology, explaining how IoT applications would create value for patients in different scenario and its relevance in clinical settings.

12.1 IoMT and healthcare delivery

Digital health broadly incorporates categories such as mobile health (mHealth), information technology comprising electronic health records, reimbursements (IT), wearable devices, telehealth and telemedicine [1]. Recent advancements on this front includes IoT ecosystem, which provides a connected ecosystem for flawless information flow within various technologies involve at hardware, software and networking layer [2]. These enabling technologies include devices embedded with sensor, actuator, and communication protocol which transmits and receives the data in real time [3]. Along with other end applications such as smart energy

[1]Aranca, Technology Research and Advisory Department, Mumbai, India

transmission, smart homes, intelligent logistics and smart towns, healthcare provides an attractive opportunity area for successful implementation [4].

Current estimates predict that nearly 60% of organizations have implemented IoT in healthcare industry in partial or complete form, to deliver value to patients and transition from disjoint and reactive model towards interoperable and proactive service delivery model [5]. IoMT-enabled machine-to-machine interaction between devices in patient's body environment with enabling architecture.

The value of this technology in chronic disease care can be judged by technology competency in addressing the clinical need to capture patient data, clinical effectiveness to modify the care in comparison to base care, cost-efficiency to be economically viable and practicality in implementation. This chapter discusses about evaluating the value of technology in healthcare delivery and clinical considerations as they pose critical milestones for further research investment decisions. The chapter covers the overall clinical workflow transformations due technology enablers and its impact on functional areas while diagnosing, imaging, treating and follow-up stages of care delivery. With the increasing emphasis on care delivery-based models, it is essential to evaluate the value created and unlocked due to implementation of IoT architecture in healthcare.

The second section of chapter covers the IoT effectiveness in high burden and potentially appealing disease condition such as diabetes, affecting developed and developing economies. Chapter reviews diabetes-specific research and clinical impact created in the changing era of fee-for-service (per visit) to value-based systems where payment is based on clinical quality of care and costs.

12.2 Impact of the IoMT in chronic disease treatment protocols/functional areas

With the patient centric architecture of the IoMT, conventional devices are enabled with sensing, monitoring and intervention functionalities, to provide timely required intervention in most of instances during routine clinical flow. The publications related to early implementation includes usage in medical nursing systems [6], rehabilitation system [7], disease detection [8], physiological condition monitoring [9], chronic diseased tracking [10], remote ECG monitoring and intervention [11], and home-based medical health monitoring system [12]. Significant transition due to IoMT implementation can be broadly considered for broader areas such as:

1. Remote clinical diagnosis and communication [13]
2. Product shopping/E-commerce [5]
3. Imaging and post-processing [14]
4. Drug/treatment planning [15]
5. Surgical procedure guidelines, follow-up and evaluation [16]
6. Practice administration/electronic health records [17,18]
7. Preventive health, wellness and patient education [19]

In each end application, IoMT would improve the quality of healthcare delivery, affordability and reliability in near future. Additionally, shared accountability in decision making in service delivery model would improve patient engagement and satisfaction. As a result of these value drivers, researchers predict faster technology adoption rates and growing market size to surpass $156 billion by 2020 [2].

12.2.1 Remote clinical diagnosis and communication

IoMT would impact clinical diagnostic workflow mainly at in-patient, outpatient and emergency room setups as outlined in Figure 12.1. Conventional in-patient diagnostic workflow would be potentially transformed in below functional areas:

- With the help of IoMT, in-patient follow-ups, response to treatment regime and diagnostic monitoring would be automated. The digital workflow in patient communication on medicine reminders and scheduling allows physician to improve adherence as well as capture patient data [15].
- Medical record management for patient medical files and patients drove communication facilitating patient participation in illness management, decision making and knowledge creation [20].
- Confirmatory diagnosis and peer-to-peer review to derive treatment guideline with experts with common expertise connect "virtually" to share patient records, ask treatment protocols-related queries or provide independent opinions [21].
- Virtual clinical checkup which facilitates the online transmission and video-based interactions with remote physicians and patient records simultaneously to establish a primary diagnosis using vital parameters tracked and correlating them with physical findings [22].
- In home care or outpatient, diagnosis could be transformed to enable self-assessment of individual at home, especially to keep track of between the two hospital visits [22].
- Triaging emergency: Access to the nearest emergency facility can be provided with patient mobile devices and interfacing with wearable technologies such as a wristband, spectacles, and rings. In such situations, real-time vital parameters monitoring is desired using wireless communication [22].
- Peer-to-peer data sharing: Professional networking to share second and third opinions which can remotely monitor and predict treatment course. Adherence and course correction based on inputs from other experts can be suggested [22].
- Workflow error reduction: Diagnosis process and inter-examiner treatment bias can be reduced in real time and a consensus from physician community can be obtained for developing treatment standards [22].
- Patient history retrieval before diagnosis: Blockchain-enabled communication about patient data and reimbursement codes, amounts would enable transparency and transmission security [20,22].

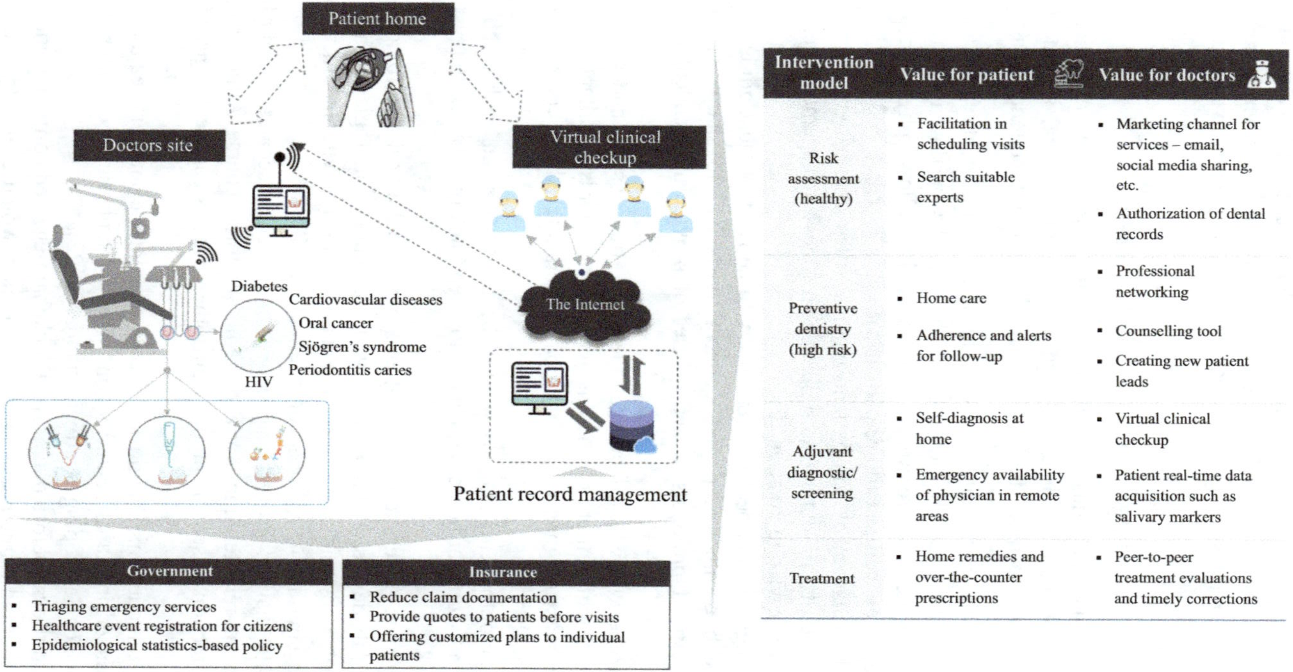

Figure 12.1 IoT impact on clinical diagnostic and communication workflow

- Reducing post-surgery follow-ups: Resource utilization and surgeons follow-up visits can be optimized based on the communicated data from patient devices such as implants, braces, etc. [15,22].
- Policy impact evaluation – Government reforms can be evaluated with data transmitted to public health providers to check preventive dental check-up impacts such as fluoride varnish application and social risk assessment [15].

12.2.2 Product procurement

IoT-based technologies are being implemented for asset management in hospitals and optimize the supply of resources. Also, the effective asset tracking data can be used for analyzing usage patterns and forecasting future demand of medical supplies throughout the hospital as outlines in Figure 12.2. Care providers could bring more transparency and informed decisions during buying cycle [23].

- Inventory management – Apart from device tracking, usage for inventory management and IoT-enabled tracking is used by hospitals in leveraging data to make decisions about resource capacity. Hospitals can order and store the required device volume based on historical usage and allocate budget for future procurement [23].
- Customer driven product development – Gathering unmet needs from the patient's device usage pattern, which can be input to prioritize R&D effort. It could enable products with multiple offerings, for example salivary biomarker devices for caries and cardiac risk.
- Related products marketing – Based on the patient consumption pattern, doctor prescription preferences, and device utility, a device manufacturer can formulate market penetration strategies/cross sell for related consumables.
- Antitheft solutions – Work piece thefts can be prevented using surveillance, object tracking (sensors) on devices embedded.
- On-demand 3-D printing – Customized, cheaper and on-demand device components can be manufactured using remotely enabled printers; this reduces device downtime and supply delay. The automated medical supply chain can bring in value for consignment, accurate clinical documentation, and product and workflow standardization across institutions [24].

12.2.3 Imaging and post-processing

Medical imaging has been used in diagnostics and treatment evaluations. With the advancements in IoT, research in high resolution transmission, and processing components such as computer assisted image analysis, enhancements, and segmentations has increased to provide accurate registration, visualizations and quantification of patient-specific anatomy as outlined in Figure 12.3. IoT has enabled remote cloud-based image analytics, connectivity of imaging devices and provide patient-specific intervention during imaging procedures [14].

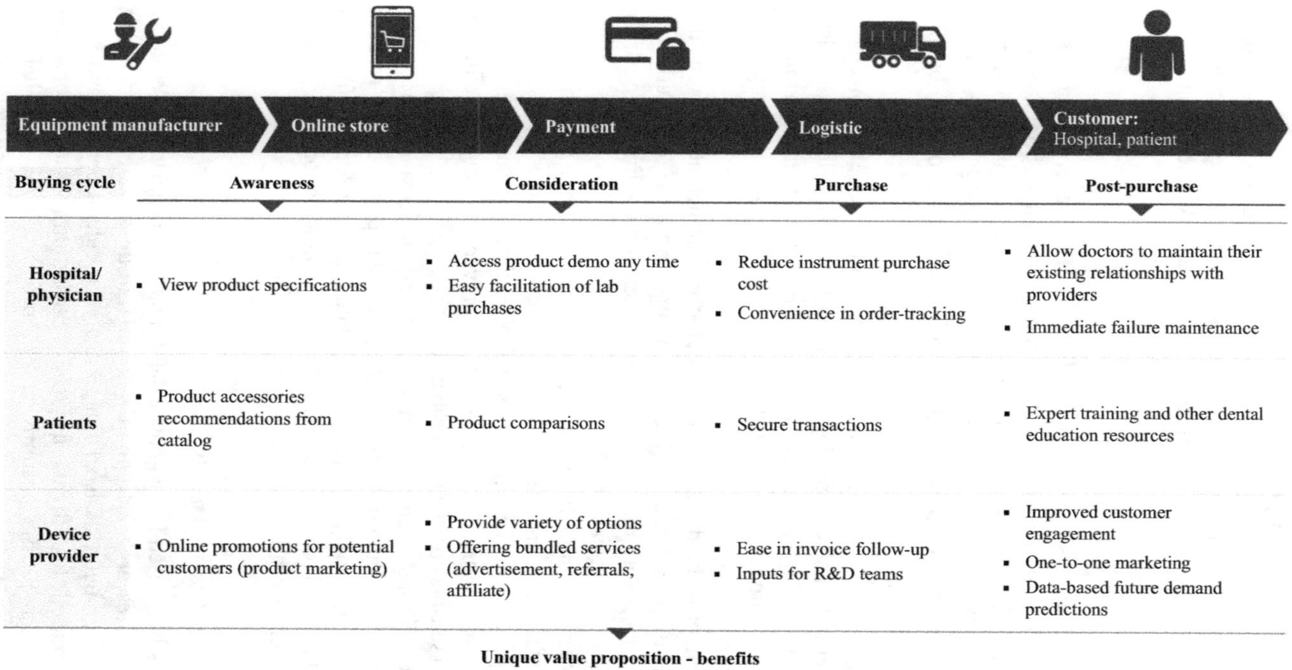

Figure 12.2 IoT impact on product procurement

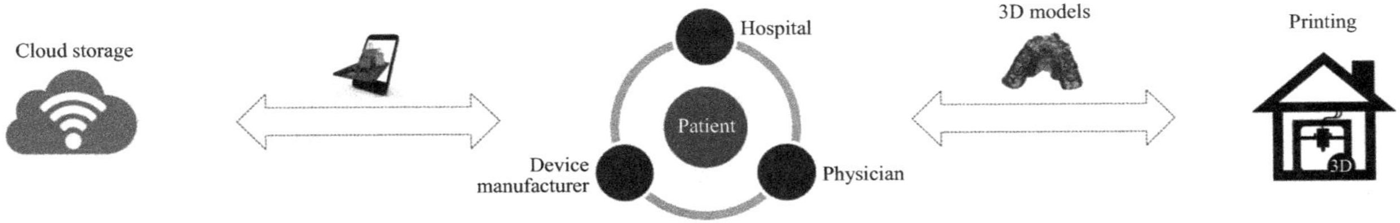

Practice scenario	Healthy	High risk/diagnosis	Treatment	Maintenance
Hospital/ physician	▪ Enhanced anatomical visualization of inaccessible areas ▪ Patient electronic health record	▪ Image-based disease and tissue damage estimation	▪ Quantification-based prognosis ▪ Simulations for patient before and after restoration	▪ High-resolution 3D virtual models at chairside design
Patients	▪ Educational tools	▪ Intraoral tissue mapping	▪ Removes discomfort for the patient during dental impressions	▪ Post implant checkups
Device provider	▪ Analyze demographic teeth details	▪ Insurance proof submission	▪ Eliminates drawback for plastic models – demand of physical storage space, fragility, degradation	▪ Accurate input for implant manufacturing ▪ Reduce supply downtime

Unique value proposition – benefits

Figure 12.3 IoT impact on product procurement

- Systemic disease diagnosis – Radiotracer-based imaging can be used to monitor tissue metabolism, mineral density and bacterial load, useful in osteoporosis/hypercalcemia diagnosis in home setups.
- Peer reviewed image interpretation – Data driven (patient history, lab findings) image analysis for differential diagnosis suggestion and expert verification on differential diagnosis and treatment modalities is being implemented with the connectivity of machine and standardization of procedures.
- Airway flow dynamics – CBCT imaging data can yield dynamic computational models of the airflow in the upper airway with the potential of employing this to patient-specific therapies.
- Future cost estimation – Implant stress analysis images would provide details on stress areas, fatigue level, fracture possibility which can be used to forecast future implant procurement estimations. Further, it provides R&D input for manufacturing with foreseen device failures images that can be shared with device manufacturers for product refinements.
- On-demand 3-D printing – Customized, cheaper and on-demand device components can be manufactured using remotely enabled printers; this reduces device downtime and supply delay.

12.2.4 Drug/treatment planning

IoMT-enabled devices offer promising alternatives to improve drug adherence by assisting patients in getting information on medications, alerting medication schedules, filling-up and dispensing drug, and reading labels on expiry and safety. Currently, IoT-enabled devices enables to monitor the vital parameters along with drug dynamics during the treatment period. Such devices are also used to monitor parameters such as blood pressure, random blood sugar levels, and weight and electrolyte concentrations inside the body after drug administration. The real-time vital data sourced by these devices is processed at a higher level and used for future treatment dose moderation and dose estimations, and to predict the prognosis with drug regimen [25].

- eHealth monitoring in homecare setups: RFID-enabled drug dispensing devices are prescribed at a health facility by physician to access patient drug prescriptions which would be read by hardware paired to it such as mobile devices, wearables, etc. Hence, it ensures the accurate dosages and timings of administrations [25].
- Drug supply chain management. Centralized data collection on prescribed medicine allows registration and retrieval of information related to drug availability problems and supply cost for a particular area with quality. Other solutions include incorporating this technology to medication; WuXiPharmaTech and TruTag Technologies have developed edible IoT “smart” pills, which help monitor drug doses and the patient’s pharmacodynamics. Such solutions may help drug companies mitigate risks and losses during supply chain and administration [26].

12.2.5 Preventive health, wellness and patient education

IoMT-enabled devices enable care providers with health supervision and monitoring systems as outlined in Figure 12.4 for diet, physical activity and quality of life in healthy and high-risk population [2].

- Advanced sensors, convertors and firmware in smart wearables and implants allow users to capture and correlate various daily events with health conditions at the local level. The same data is transmitted to remote physician or community information officers for analyzing the disease incidence risk and preclinical stage. In diseased individuals, data from network devices is registered at a central location at the physician's office. Compiling and processing patient-specific data enables healthcare automation, which analyzes fresh data against past records and decides the preventive approaches to avoid complications. This machine-enabled intelligence helps service providers transfer the tasks of routing, monitoring, and field administration to IoMT machines, thus saving the cost incurred from implementing follow-up resources and infrastructure utilization [2].
- Patient education: Awareness of disease condition, continuous monitoring and improving safety has been important for preventing treatment side effects after the patient is discharged from hospital, IoT-enabled devices are adopting inclusive approach with the involvement of patients in their health management. Such scenarios include drug adverse reaction monitoring, hospital acquired infections, hygiene-related patient counseling, and assisting vulnerable patients in home setups and predicting the risk of complication.

12.3 Chronic disease-specific implementation

12.3.1 Chronic disease monitoring as the lucrative application of IoMT

Considering the value consideration detailed above, the maximum potential to use IoT-based devices is in the field of chronic disease management. Key favorable drivers related to epidemiology, technical advancements, an economical and regulatory scenario which makes this a lucrative opportunity due to scarcity of healthcare resources and rising healthcare cost. Therefore, a trend to offer treatment at home has been explored and showing encouraging experimental results. Home-based solutions are initially introduced for chronic condition monitoring using vital parameters monitoring such as blood pressure, pulse rate and ECG in home setup. Additionally, it has been able to extend the offerings to tele-presence, remote visits and consult with professional experts over the connected environment. Technology further evolved to miniaturization and wearables to capture patient data along with web-based solutions to evaluate information and provide decisions to user, hence playing assistive roles in overall disease management.

Chronic disease monitoring appears to be high impact areas for early adoption of IoT due to additional reasons that, demographic shift towards ageing population

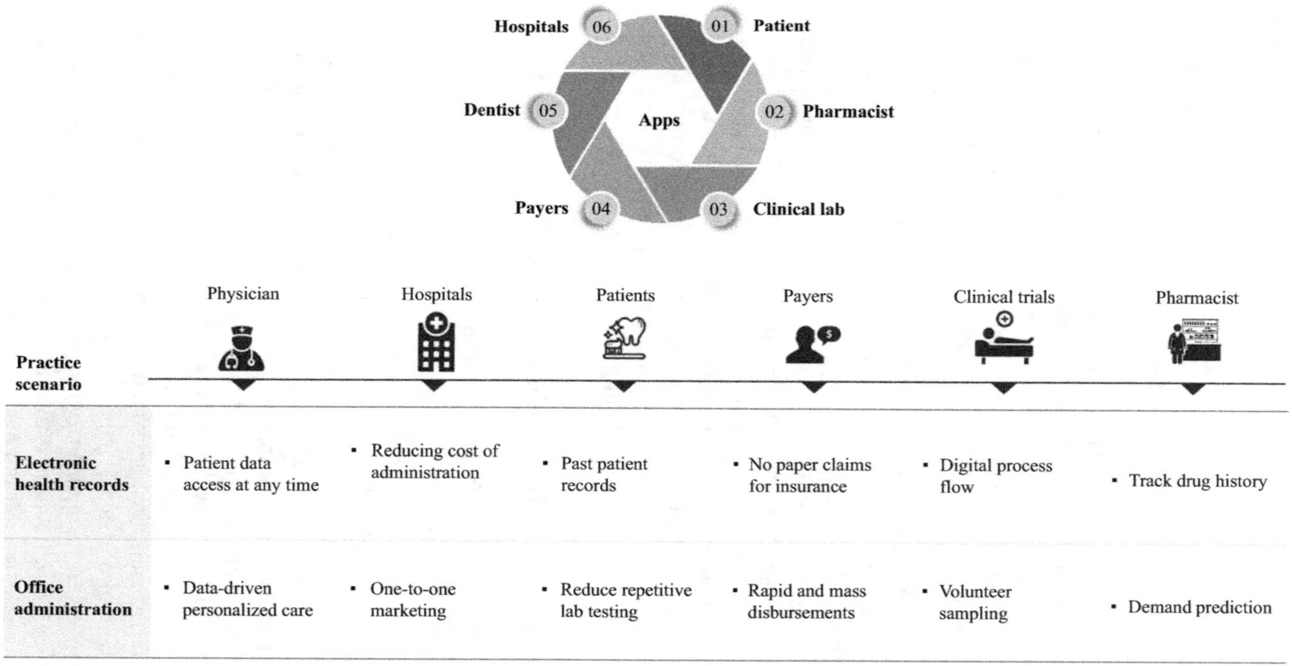

Figure 12.4 IoT impact on product procurement

in world. UN report in 2013 estimates that 21.1% of the world population would be above 60 years of age by 2050, exposing them to risk of age-related chronic conditions. Further this older population would be growing faster in developing economies that developed ones to reach as much as 8 out of 10 geriatric individuals would be from developing countries. This would be further supplemented by share of older persons above 80 years or over which would increase to 19 per cent by 2050 [27].

The third factor which necessitates the successful use case is prevalence of complications in chronic diseases and requirement of preventive monitoring. As per WHO consensus, diet- and nutrition-related chronic disease burden would increase to 57% by 2020 and half of the disease deaths would be attributed to complications of cardiovascular diseases, obesity, and diabetes in non-communicable disease type categories [44]. Another category, communicable chronic conditions such as human immunodeficiency virus/acquired immunodeficiency syndrome (HIV/AIDS), malaria and tuberculosis, along with other infectious diseases would predominate in sub-Saharan Africa but would be under control in rest of world due to advancements in treatments [28]. Mortality in non-communicable chronic conditions is estimated to almost three-quarters of all deaths worldwide, out-of-which, 71% of deaths attributed to ischemic heart disease (IHD), 75% to stroke, and 70% to diabetes. IoT presumably adds value in non-communicable chronic disease conditions by continuously monitoring vital parameters, increasing therapy adherence, avoid emergency hospitalization with regular virtual visits and post treatment follow-ups in the treatment regime.

Along with therapeutic benefits in disease population, IoT set to enable prevent the occurrence of disease in high risk population by timely wellness promotion and lifestyle changes. The economic impact is set to reduce about $190 billion to $1.2 trillion per year in next decade as per analyst estimates with these intervention and prevention approaches [29].

The system design ranges from in-home setups to wearables, ingestible, implantable or injectable to adopt to user requirements. Product variants including glucometer, point-of-care (PoC) devices, portable blood pressure monitoring system, activity tracking wearable, implantable heart rate monitoring devices, home care video systems, and diet and nutrition apps are particularly useful. In all chronic disease monitoring applications, all IoT architecture components including hardware and software such as sensors, gateways and microcontrollers are designed in a similar manner to capture vitals data accurately with case-specific customization of sensors.

One of the values of IoT at sensor level is enabling decision making through accurate classification of data. Real-time data acquired from sensors would be processed to analyze the health condition, one such approach by applying different classification algorithms such as Naive Bayes, J48, and SVM algorithms and their accuracy in detection of vital parameters in terms of precision, recall and *F*-measure reported by Raji *et al.* [30]. J48 and SVM have been found to achieve a precision of 1 in detecting diastolic blood pressure and systolic blood pressure, however, heart rate and temperature detection could achieve precision of 0.96.

Table 12.1 Accuracy measure of classification algorithm

Vital signs	Classification algorithms	Precision	Recall	*F*-measure
Temperature	Naïve Bayesian	0.824	0.750	0.747
	J48	0.922	0.958	0.939
	SVM	0.922	0.958	0.939
Heart rate	Naïve Bayesian	0.807	0.667	0.628
	J48	0.962	0.958	0.958
	SVM	0.971	0.975	0.964
	Linear regression	0.978	0.983	0.721
	Neural network	0.734	0.524	0.590
Systolic blood pressure	SVM	0.962	0.958	0.958
	Naïve Bayesian	1.000	0.857	0.921
	J48	1.000	0.952	0.975
	Neural network	0.882	0.859	0.869
	Multiple linear regression	0.723	0.862	0.981
Diastolic blood pressure	Naïve Bayesian	0.964	0.958	0.958
	J48	1.000	1.000	1.000
	SVM	1.000	1.000	1.000
	Neural network	0.901	0.871	0.832
	Multiple linear regression	0.923	0.795	0.834

Table 12.1 summarizes the physiological parameters monitored in chronic disease setups and their accuracy.

12.3.2 Implementation in diabetes

International diabetes federation estimates that in 2017, 425 million people that are currently leaving with diabetes conditions in with or without diagnosis established and set to increase to reach 629 million people by 2045 [31]. A major epidemiological factor to increasing disease burden is a sedentary lifestyle, genetic predisposition, increased lifestyle and poor care delivery infrastructure. IoT implementation in developed and emerging economies would impact to identify high risk population, provide healthcare definitive diagnosis and treatment, monitor vitals at regular intervals and predict complications [45]. The transformations would be primarily enabled through real-time sensor data and advancements in data processing techniques to turn data into meaningful insights [32]. Table 12.2 summarizes the key products implemented in diabetes and their clinical offering.

12.3.2.1 Therapy monitoring and risk prediction

Treatment protocol by professional bodies like the American Diabetes Association recommends measurement of blood glucose levels at least three times in a day to maintain in the euglycemic range 70–180 mg/dL. Current systems report the measurement error in the range of 4–6.5% [33], however, IoT-enabled systems theoretically allow the readings in real time from sensor and allows users to store vital signs on cloud systems.

Table 12.2 Current implemented products and unique clinical offering in diabetes monitoring

Product	Unique clinical offering
WellDoc	Digital platform for patients offering administrative functions such as educational coaching, based on real-time blood glucose values
Sugar IQ	Real-time personalized assistant based on user behavior with glucose patterns, food and patient awareness to predict values
iLet4	Closed-cycle system of glucagon and insulin delivery in response to CGM data. The system showed efficiency of bihormonal treatment group versus traditional pump therapy including average CGM glucose of 140 mg/dL vs. 162 mg/dL and only 0.6% vs. 1.9% of time spent with glucose less than 60 mg/dL, respectively
TypeZero	Analytical tool for monitoring blood glucose along with advisory applications for smart insulin pens and smartphone-based artificial pancreas systems that automatically regulate insulin delivery
MedicSen	Glucose prediction and personalized advice system which reported increase insulin permeability by up to 50 times inn studies; offers connectivity to a proprietary needle-free drug dispenser
MySugr	Digital platform with other device integration
BigFoot loop	Automatic titration; preparing for trial in 2019
CGS6 EasySense	Insulin patch pump with disposable CGM system
Next-Gen G6 Sensor	Long durability implantable sensing providing non-interference with Tylenol; FDA approved for users in more than two years old to facilitate glucose monitoring and remote data sharing
Basal-Bolus patch pump	Tubeless, Basal-Bolus insulin patch
Glooko	Synchronization of sensors and pumps
Cellnovo insulin pumps	insulin pump available only in Europe; Bluetooth enabled an adhesive device which also offers activity tracker and food library
t: slim X2	Low-glucose suspend (plgs) system
Contour. Next ONE	Virtual reality application for glycemic control
Eversense®	Durable implantable sensor (90 days) using an LED light source exciting the fluorescent polymer coating; mean absolute relative difference (MARD) is reported 8.8% in PRECISE II study
PEPPER	Patient empowerment through predictive personalized decision support
Hedia	Personal diabetes assistant based on AI
xbird	Biomarker tracking
GlucoWatchBiografer	Glucose monitoring system
Glucowise	Glucose level monitoring
Kaleido insulin pumps	Two rechargeable pumps

(Continues)

Table 12.2 (*Continued*)

Product	Unique clinical offering
Roche Accu-Chek Insulin Pumps	Offers insulin pump and smart glucometer; it facilitates user to change pump settings and bolus calculator using input through the Bluetooth connected glucometer
OmniPod	Uses Dexcom G6 CGM input and Insulet personal MPC algorithm. Efficiency in terms of increased time in euglycemic range and decreased hypoglycemia in adults, adolescents, and children of 69.5–73% and 0.7–2% values respectively.
Dana Diabecare R and DanaDiabecare RS insulin pumps	Connected glucometer and lightweight design which can be remotely controlling pump settings via android application
Medtronic CGM systems	Hybrid closed loop technology comprising Guardian Sensor 3 system and Medtronic 670G insulin pump; (MARD) is reported 8.7%
Abbott Freestyle CGM Systems	FDA approved in users of greater than 18 years; accuracy in terms of mean absolute relative difference (MARD) reported 9.4%
Sano	Low-profile patch glucometer

Additionally, IoT-enabled devices in development are able to monitor and predict diurnal sugar levels and the effect of current medications [7,46]. Bluetooth low energy (BLE)-based sensors-based system has been implemented to capture the personal data along with heart rate, blood pressure, weight and blood glucose in order to track blood glucose variations and predict complications and physicians' visits in case of critical situation. In treatment regimen, current approach is recommended with control/self-manage, diet, and physical activities to targeted populations that are currently euglycemic or suffering from chronic hyperglycemia.

12.3.2.2 Medication and drug dosage administration

In the clinical workflow, physicians evaluate the dosage decisions and insulin infusion protocols based on glycemic levels at clinics and educate patients or caregivers about same in home care setup. However, lack of real-time sugar levels, calculation errors, and diurnal variations lead to administration of inaccurate dosages in some instances, leading to hypoglycemic or hyperglycemic states. IoT-enabled administration devices such as pumps, smart pens, and patches release the drug to maintain euglycemic state, tracks on-board drug amount, make dosing recommendations and send treatment data to treating physicians located at remote location. Devices provide clinical value with improved adherence, adequate insulin initiation, and intensification leading to fewer complications and unscheduled visits to health care providers [43]. One such intervention includes AP@home project, an initiative funded by the European Union, reported a patient perception of 80% usefulness of system in their responses [34].

12.3.2.3 Educational and patient communication tool

United States National Standards for Diabetes Self-Management Education and Support (DSMES) emphasizes patient awareness and skill development are important for Self-management of diabetes. Self-management can be enabled with patient generated health data including glucose data, lifestyle data and feedback loop from treating physicians. Technology-enabled diabetes self-management education and support interventions have shown promising results in reduction in serum markers such as HbA1c [35].

Communication aspects in patient treatment regime consist of engagement between patient and physician in one- or two-way communication. Studies have suggested that one-way communication has not affected the outcome of disease prognosis [36], however results are encouraging in two-way communication-based systems, especially which are addressing patient tele-advising and shared decision-making cohorts [37]. Tele-monitoring programs delivered by physicians are found to be more effective than non-monitored ones [38,39]. The involvement of the parents and peer group is also important in establishing trust and suitability about patient education platforms [40].

12.3.2.4 Complication reduction

Continuous vital monitoring aids in identifying the daily variations in blood glucose levels and estimate the disease prognosis, especially the occurrence of diabetic complications in patients. Although glycolated Hb is currently considered as gold standard in evaluating glycemic control, it does not reflect measure of magnitude or frequency of daily fluctuations in blood glucose. Both hyperglycemia and hypoglycemia are risk factors for cardiovascular disease (coronary heart disease or stroke) along with other complications. Data captured from sensors are utilized to detect early warning signals to diagnose such cardiovascular, renal, retinal and other metabolic complications in patients.

Long term clinical studies report a reduction of cardiac mortality in insulin pump treated populations [41]. An observational study showed a reduction of 45% for fatal coronary heart disease, 42% for fatal cardiovascular disease, and 27% for all-cause mortality in diabetes type I patients treated with insulin pumps. The effectiveness is attributed to better control of HbA1c and LDL cholesterol due to periodic monitoring offered by IoT.

Other common complications in the diabetic population such as retinopathy, peripheral nerve abnormality, Microalbuminuria which are associated with higher HbA1c. Patients with continuous monitoring have significantly lower risk of retinopathy progression compared with control group in type I diabetes population [42].

Metabolic complications such as hypoglycemia, diabetic ketoacidosis, and coma risk appear to be lowered in long term observational studies using insulin pumps in the type I diabetic population. Events of hypoglycemia are reported with 10.30 vs. 15.53 per 100 patient-years and hypoglycemic coma at 2.26 vs. 3.43 per 100 patient-years, lower that conventional injection therapy. Diabetic ketoacidosis was also reported at incidence of 3.64 vs. 4.26 per 100 patient-years which further observed severe form of clinical representation at 2.29 vs 2.80 per 100 patient-years.

12.3.3 Implementation challenges

Although early feasibility results of IoT implementation in chronic monitoring seems encouraging, it has to evolve over the coming years in order to provide value in different clinical scenarios and various socio-economic conditions, technological, security and infrastructural requirements.

Along with common challenges IoT implementation challenges such as infrastructure, communication protocols, IoMT applications would face additional domain-specific challenges such as interoperability, integration and data security and privacy.

- Device interoperability: Due to lack of data standards for connected health devices data generated by monitoring devices from different manufacturers cannot be harnessed to its full potential due to various schemas for data storage and retrieval, which further makes it difficult to aggregate in universally recognizable format.
- Integration: Device data requires to be integrated with third party systems especially hospital or governmental electronic health records to facilitate the propagation and exploration of data. Open EHR, HL7 or their simplified versions FHIR are few current standards that are facilitating this bottleneck. EHR adoption has been rising for nearly a decade and reached around 96% for registered hospital setups.
- Security: An IoMT application requires to guarantee the security of their solutions and privacy during data acquisition, transmission and further processing. HIPAA or FDA's recommendations are providing guidelines on these requirements to design secure future devices.

12.3.4 Future for IoMT in chronic disease monitoring

The IoT-based technology is currently in a nascent stage of implementation to revolutionize clinical workflow. The implementation of this technology is likely to have a number of advantages in various heath conditions, especially in chronic diseases. Most importantly, it is expected to increase the use of network devices, enable real-time responses from remote locations, and enhance operational efficiency to track vitals in real-time in-home care setup. Similar to other industries, IoT-based connected devices are anticipated to bring significant change in chronic disease healthcare delivery on operational aspects by enabling transparent data flow from the lower physical device layer to the upper layers of cloud and data analytics. Such data-driven decision making is likely to empower caregivers to accurately monitor patients' health statuses, predict unforeseeable events, and immediately respond to emergency situations. The interconnected systems are forecast to reduce cost for patients, increase patient compliance, and offer the advantage of locally smart devices that can control heath automatically.

Although automation in healthcare monitoring would increase operational efficiency, it may pose serious risks during implementation, such as data theft, insecure data transfers and irregular network connections. These challenges, combined with regulatory hurdles, are projected to drive growth in IoT-based solutions.

Government initiatives such as the Patient Protection and Affordable Care Act, which focuses on authenticated electronic health records (EHRs), might improve the quality and efficiency of care and promote consistency in caregiving. There is still scope to improve device and international data standards across the industry, which would enable data handling on a consistent basis.

12.4 Conclusion

Considering the above benefits and challenges, IoMT seems a promising solution to improve healthcare monitoring and treatment outcomes in chronic diseases like diabetes. By providing individual data-driven treatment regimens and optimized devices as per physiological requirements, this technology is set to promote personalized care and improve living standards. Moreover, recent research in the sensor, network, cloud, mobility, and big data domains is expected to give rise to the creation of affordable medical devices and a connected health ecosystem.

References

[1] U.S. Food and Drug Administration. Digital Health (2019).

[2] Yogesh, S., Internet of Medical Things IoMT Aranca-Special-Report, Aranca library Available, 2016.

[3] Pallavi, S. and Smruti R. Sarangi, Internet of Things: Architectures, Protocols, and Applications, Journal of Electrical and Computer Engineering, (2017).

[4] Muruganandam, M., Balamurugan, D. and Khara, D., Design of Wireless Sensor Networks for IOT Application: A Challenges and Survey. International Journal of Engineering and Computer Science (2018), 7(03), pp. 23790–5.

[5] Low, I., Healthcare of the Future: Rapid Adoption of IoT Reshaping Healthcare Industry (2018).

[6] Huang, C.-H *et al.*, Bulletin of Networking, Computing, Systems, and Software (2014) – ISSN 2186–5140, 3(1), pp. 20–4.

[7] Fan, Y.J., Yin, Y.H., Xu, L., Zeng, Y. and Wu, F., IoT Based SR, IoT-Based Smart Rehabilitation System. IEEE Transactions on Industrial Informatics (2014), 10, pp. 1568–77.

[8] Divya Krishna, K., Akkala, V., Bharath, R., Rajalakshmi, P., Mohammed, A., Merchant, S. and Desai, U., Computer Aided Abnormality Detection for Kidney on FPGA Based IoT Enabled Portable Ultrasound Imaging System. IRBM (2016), 37(4), pp. 189–97.

[9] Sundhara, K. and Bairavi, K., IoT Based Health Monitoring System for Autistic Patients. Proceedings of the 3rd International Symposium on Big Data and Cloud Computing Challenges (ISBCC – '16) (2016), pp. 371–6.

[10] Ghose, A., Sinha, P., Bhaumik, C., Sinha, A., Agrawal, A. and Dutta Choudhury, A., UbiHeld. Proceedings of the 2013 ACM conference on Pervasive and Ubiquitous Computing Adjunct Publication – UbiComp '13 Adjunct (2013).

[11] Pallavi, C., Prerna, M., Neha, T., Shraddha, Y. and Pallavi, D., ECG – Remote Patient Monitoring using Cloud Computing. Imperial Journal of Interdisciplinary Research (IJIR) (2016), 2(2) , ISSN: 2454-1362.

[12] Iuliana, C., Oan A Geman, An Approach of a Decision Support and Home Monitoring System for Patients with Neurological Disorders using Internet of Things Concepts, Wseas Transactions on Systems (2014), 13, E-ISSN: 2224-2678.

[13] Catherwood, P., Steele, D., Little, M., Mccomb, S. and Mclaughlin, J., A Community-Based IoT Personalized Wireless Healthcare Solution Trial. IEEE Journal of Translational Engineering in Health and Medicine (2018), 6, pp. 1–13.

[14] Chae, S., Moon, D., Lee, D. and Pan, S., Medical Image Segmentation for Mobile Electronic Patient Charts using Numerical Modeling of IoT. Journal of Applied Mathematics (2014), pp. 1–8.

[15] Zanjal, S. and Talmale, G., Medicine Reminder and Monitoring System for Secure Health Using IOT. Procedia Computer Science (2016), 78, pp. 471–6.

[16] Davis, C. and Rosenfield, L., Looking at Plastic Surgery through Google Glass. Plastic and Reconstructive Surgery (2015), 135(3), pp. 918–28.

[17] Hillestad, R., Bigelow, J., Bower, A. *et al.*, Can Electronic Medical Record Systems Transform Health Care? Potential Health Benefits, Savings, and Costs. Health Affairs (2005), 24(5), pp. 1103–17.

[18] Chinmay, C., Gupta, B. and Ghosh, S.K., A Review on Telemedicine-Based WBAN Framework for Patient Monitoring. International Journal of Telemedicine and e-Health, Mary Ann Libert Inc (2013), 19(8), 619–26.

[19] Handel, M., mHealth (Mobile Health)—Using Apps for Health and Wellness. EXPLORE, (2011), 7(4), pp. 256–61.

[20] Winkelman, W., Patient-Perceived Usefulness of Online Electronic Medical Records: Employing Grounded Theory in the Development of Information and Communication Technologies for Use by Patients Living with Chronic Illness. Journal of the American Medical Informatics Association (2005), 12(3), pp. 306–14.

[21] Eysenbach, G., Powell, J., Englesakis, M., Rizo, C. and Stern, A., Health Related Virtual Communities and Electronic Support Groups: Systematic Review of the Effects of Online Peer to Peer Interactions. British Medical Journal (2004), 328(7449), p. 1166.

[22] Tachakra, S., Wang, X., Istepanian, R. and Song, Y., Mobile e-Health: The Unwired Evolution of Telemedicine. Telemedicine Journal and e-Health (2003), 9(3), pp. 247–57.

[23] Man, L., Na, C. and Kit, N., IoT-Based Asset Management System for Healthcare-Related Industries. International Journal of Engineering Business Management (2015), 7, pp. 19.

[24] Health, C., 3 tips to utilize the Internet of Things (IoT) in the healthcare supply chain: With the novelty of the Internet now considered the norm, we must place a greater focus on how to thrive in the age of the Internet of Things (IoT) (2018).

[25] Laranjo, I., Macedo, J. and Santos, A., Internet of Things for Medication Control: Service Implementation and Testing. Procedia Technology (2012), 5, pp. 777–86.

[26] Harpham, B., How the Internet of Things is changing healthcare and transportation (2015).

[27] United Nations report, World Population Ageing, Department of Economic and Social Affairs Population Division (2013).

[28] WHO, Report on global burden of chronic, accessed in 2019.

[29] McKinsey & Company, Unlocking the potential of the Internet of Things (2015).

[30] Raji, A., Jeyasheeli, P. and Jenitha, T., IoT based classification of vital signs data for chronic disease monitoring. 10th International Conference on Intelligent Systems and Control (ISCO) (2016).

[31] International diabetes federation report, International Diabetes Federation – Facts & figures (2017).

[32] Alfian, G., Syafrudin, M., Ijaz, M., Syaekhoni, M., Fitriyani, N. and Rhee, J., A Personalized Healthcare Monitoring System for Diabetic Patients by Utilizing BLE-Based Sensors and Real-Time Data Processing. Sensors (2018).

[33] Cohen, M., Boyle, E., Delaney, C. and Shaw, J., A Comparison of Blood Glucose Meters in Australia. Diabetes Research and Clinical Practice (2006), 71(2), pp. 113–18.

[34] Lanzola, G., Losiouk, E., Del Favero, S. *et al.*, Remote Blood Glucose Monitoring in mHealth Scenarios: A Review. Sensors (2016), 16(12), p. 1983.

[35] Greenwood, D., Gee, P., Fatkin, K. and Peeples, M. A Systematic Review of Reviews Evaluating Technology-Enabled Diabetes Self-Management Education and Support. Journal of Diabetes Science and Technology (2017), 11(5), pp. 1015–27.

[36] Jimison, H., Gorman, P., Woods, S. *et al.*, Evid Rep Technol Assess (Full Rep) (2008), Nov (175), pp. 1–1422.

[37] Greenwood, D., Young, H. and Quinn, C., Telehealth Remote Monitoring Systematic Review. Journal of Diabetes Science and Technology (2014), 8(2), pp. 378–89.

[38] Chinmay, C., Mobile Health (m-Health) for Tele-wound Monitoring, *IGI: Mobile Health Applications for Quality Healthcare Delivery* (2019), Ch. 5, pp. 98–116, ISBN: 9781522580218, DOI: 10.4018/978-1-5225-8021-8.

[39] Peyrot, M., Rubin, R., Funnell, M. and Siminerio, L., Access to Diabetes Self-management Education. The Diabetes Educator (2009), 35(2), pp. 246–63.

[40] Nordfeldt, S., Ängarne-Lindberg, T., Nordwall, M. and Krevers, B., Parents of Adolescents with Type 1 Diabetes – Their Views on Information and Communication Needs and Internet Use. A Qualitative Study. PLoS ONE (2013), 8(4), p. e62096.

[41] Steineck, I., Cederholm, J., Eliasson, B. *et al.*, Insulin Pump Therapy, Multiple Daily Injections, and Cardiovascular Mortality in 18 168 People

with Type 1 Diabetes: Observational Study. British Medical Journal (2015), 350(1), pp. h3234–h3234.

[42] Zabeen, B., Craig, M., Virk, S. *et al.*, Insulin Pump Therapy Is Associated with Lower Rates of Retinopathy and Peripheral Nerve Abnormality. PLoS ONE (2016), 11(4), p. e0153033.

[43] Vinaytosh, M. and Naik, M.K.P., Use of wireless devices and IoT in management of diabetes, National Conference on Emerging Trends in Science, Technology and Management (2017), ISBN: 978-93-5281-325-4.

[44] WHO, Report on cardiovascular diseases, accessed in 2019.

[45] Plamenka, B., DesislavaIvanova, Ivo Draganov, Serdica Journal of Computing, Bulgarian Academy of Sciences Institute of Mathematics and Informatics (2018).

[46] Al-Taee, M., Al-Nuaimy, W., Al-Ataby, A., Muhsin, Z. and Abood, S., Mobile health platform for diabetes management based on the Internet-of-Things. IEEE Jordan Conference on Applied Electrical Engineering and Computing Technologies (AEECT) (2015).

Chapter 13

Transform domain robust watermarking method using Riesz wavelet transform for medical data security and privacy

Gajanan K. Birajdar[1], *Vishwesh A. Vyawahare*[1], *Smitha Raveendran*[1] *and Pooja Patil*[1]

Rapid progress of digital multimedia content has tremendously improved different forms of information and its processing. New digital technologies help to store, transmit and process the information in a quick and accurate way. However, digital data in the form of videos and images can be effortlessly manipulated and redistributed using the computers. Violation of ownership rights and verifying the integrity of the digital content can be significantly improved by the watermarking approaches. Watermarking algorithms embed additional information for verifying the authenticity and trustworthiness. Security and privacy of medical data in the form of image or other *1-D* signals are of prime importance and has become an emerging area in the field of biomedical information technology. Biomedical image watermarking algorithms enable transmission of medical records and patient history in a secure way. The aim of this book chapter is to propose a new watermarking approach using a transform domain for medical image security. Riesz wavelet transform (RWT) and singular value decomposition (SVD) is employed for embedding the watermarking in the cover medical image at the transmitter side. At the receiver, the embedded information is recovered successfully using the watermarking extraction algorithm. The RWT-SVD algorithm is tested on different types of medical images like X-ray, CT scan, MRI and retinal images. The watermark is extracted at the receiver without the original image. Imperceptibility evaluation using several metrics (SNR, PSNR, WPSNR, SSIM, MSSIM, SC) shows the improved performance of the proposed approach. In addition to this, robustness analysis is also carried in terms of correlation coefficient.

13.1 Introduction

Rapid progress in the field of digital technology has boosted access to digital data in a simple and easy way. Digital multimedia of very good quality can be stored

[1]Department of Electronics Engineering, Ramrao Adik Institute of Technology, Navi Mumbai, India

efficiently and can be processed easily by using computers. Moreover, digital information can be transmitted and disseminated in a rapid and cost-effective way through the Internet without losing their quality. However, this may lead to unlawful duplication and production of digital data. Redistribution and modification of such digital data have become extremely simple in today's scenario. The detection of such activities has also become difficult. Therefore, it creates issues like copyright violation of multimedia data and proving ownership [1,2].

In the present era, the digitization of information has been promoted in many fields like telemedicine, banking, shopping, office work, broadcasting, etc. which leads to the accessibility of person's data in the public. The transmission of medical information has increased manifold with the use of telemedicine. Important consultations by remote specialists are possible due to telemedicine. This has greatly impacted the health care system by allowing instant availability of patient information along with loss-free and improved communication [3]. The threat on privacy of patient information is manifold due to ease of data distribution and access.

The World Health Organization (WHO) defines telemedicine as "healing from a distance". Telemedicine makes use of telecommunications and information technologies to provide inaccessible medical services to the patient [4]. Telemedicine is used by doctors for the transmission of digital images, consultations through video conferencing, and providing medical diagnosis remotely [5]. Nowadays people have access to basic telemedicine devices like mobile phones and computers. Monitoring of vitals to glucose levels can be easily done by caregivers with the help of home-use medical devices. The physician can collect crucial medical information and make efficient diagnosis without patients having to schedule visits to doctors to receive treatment [6]. Moreover, elderly people who struggle to get healthcare options can avail of telemedicine solutions.

Privacy of an image is always an important issue in the management of patient's medical records. Efforts are constantly being made to provide security solutions to ascertain that (a) unauthorized agents cannot access transmission of medical images ensuring confidentiality, (b) images are not altered during transmission of medical images ensuring confidentiality, (c) images are not during transmission which ensures integrity, and (d) pictures have originated from the right sources, decoded by the claimed receivers which ensure authentication [1]. To preserve privacy, patient data can be embedded into the medical images. The patient information can be used as a watermark.

There are numerous methods for concealing information in digital media. They are used for several purposes as well as copyright protection. Cryptography and steganography are the basic methods used for information hiding. The name steganography is defined as "cover writing" and cryptography refers to "secret writing". Steganography is the process in which digital media is used to embed the message. Embedding is carried out in such a way that the hidden message can be interpreted only by the sender and the intended receiver.

The cover which is a digital media can be detected by anyone, but the message which is hidden in the cover can solely be discovered by the individual having the particular key. Thus steganography actually refers to covering point-to-point communication between two parties. Text, audio, or video file is used for concealing the information. These files are given as input to a steganography system which creates a new file. The created stego object is not distinguishable from the old one and it is not possible for a third person to detect concealed information. In the process of using the watermarking system, the embedded information can only be identified or detected but it is not possible to remove the information or to replace it [7].

In digital watermarking, an image (logo) is embedded into the host image in advance at the transmitter end [8]. At the receiver end, the process of extraction of the embedded watermark is carried out. In order to maintain copyright protection, the conditions of invisibility and robustness must be met by the watermark. When the watermarked image is extracted very well from the distorted image due to attacks like statistical attacks, cropping, JPEG compression attack, noise addition and geometrical attack, the watermark is said to be robust. Robust watermarking has been a major research problem for many years [9].

Typical watermarking framework is depicted in Figure 13.1. The host signal can be a video, image or audio whereas the watermark can be a logo, image or other information which is to be inserted in the host signal. Usually, these inputs are converted into a binary sequence prior to the process of embedding. Based on the steps of embedding, the watermark is embedded in the original data in the embedding stage generating a watermarked signal. Different attacks that modify the watermarked data are tested to verify the robustness of the system. Finally, the extraction step recovers the original watermark using the extraction algorithm. Extraction algorithms can be: blind, non-blind or semi-blind. Security is enhanced by adding a secret key mechanism. Additionally, the visual quality and accuracy of the recovered watermark will be assessed by comparing original and extracted watermark using various evaluation parameters.

The broad classification of digital watermarking schemes can be done as: spatial and transform domain [10]. In the spatial domain, the pixel values are manipulated and then hidden in the host image. This process has less computational cost, and the implementation process is simpler. Spatial domain watermarking is found to be less secure and its ability to resist image processing attacks is limited.

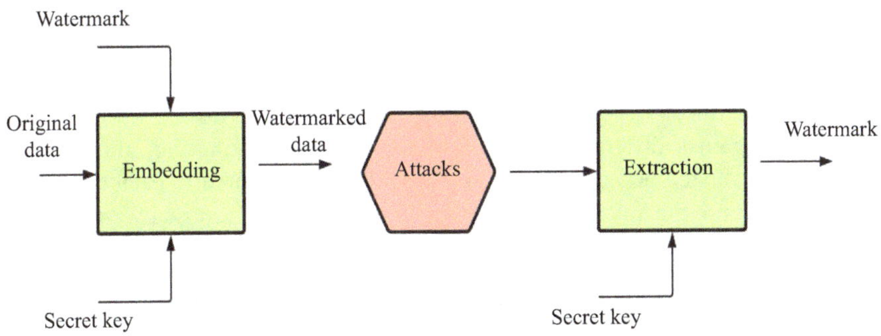

Figure 13.1 Typical watermarking scheme

Another important feature of this technique is that a small watermark can be embedded several times, hence the possibility of eliminating all watermarks by any kind of attack is very low. The watermarking methods based on transform domain are computationally complex, but these methods are found to be more robust against different attacks.

Another watermarking algorithm classification is based on the information required at the receiver for watermark extraction and there are three types: (1) blind, (2) non-blind and (3) semi-blind [4]. Blind watermarking techniques do not require watermark or original image at the decoder to pull out the watermark whereas, in non-blind watermarking, watermark extraction step requires both the original image and the original watermark. In semi-blind watermarking approach, the watermark is extracted using either whole watermark-embedded watermark or partial of it.

In transform domain watermarking, the transform coefficients of the host image are modulated to embed the watermark. In transform domain techniques, before embedding the watermark, a transformation like DCT, DFT, contour let, DWT, DT-DWT is applied to the host image to create the coefficients [10]. However, DWT-SVD combination is a popular choice for watermarking algorithms in variety of applications [3,4,11–13]. The transform domain is found to be more robust and provides better visual quality in comparison to spatial domain.

The transform domain medical image watermarking algorithm is proposed using the RWT in this chapter. The RWT is a higher extension of the Hilbert transform. The Riesz transform is scale and translation-invariant. Remarkably, the RWT is also found to be rotation-invariant. Another useful and important property for the image analysis of isotropic features is the reconstruction property of Riesz transform. Implementation of this transform can be easily be done in the Fourier domain [14].

Biomedical image watermarking algorithms enable transmission of medical records and patient history in a secure way. The aim of this book chapter is to propose a new watermarking approach using transform domain for medical image security. RWT and SVD are employed for embedding the watermark in the medical image at the transmitter side. At the receiver, the embedded information is recovered successfully using the watermarking extraction algorithm. Singular values (SVs) of higher and lower frequency bands of RWT are utilized to optimize the perceptual quality and robustness against various types of attacks. Moreover, a secret key authentication mechanism (signature) is added in order to strengthen security. Perceptual quality assessment is performed using various evaluation parameters like Peak-signal-to-noise ratio (PSNR), signal-to-noise ratio (SNR), root-mean-squared error (RMSE) and structural similarity index (SSIM) [15]. Robustness against different types of attacks including filtering, rotation and scaling are evaluated and correlation coefficients are computed in each case.

Following are the advantages and disadvantages of the proposed watermarking technique:

- The presented biomedical image watermarking algorithm has optimized perceptual image quality (PSNR, SNR, RMSE and SSIM) and robustness against different attacks because of the combination of SVs and RWT sub-bands.

- The method achieves high PSNR and SSIM demonstrating superior performance that is useful for biomedical image watermarking applications.
- Watermark is inserted by modifying the RWT sub-bands that retain the structural information such as texture or gradient contour and it guarantees perfect reconstruction and closeness thereby enhancing the perceptual image quality.
- The method requires RWT sub-band decomposition and subsequent SV replacement step resulting in slightly higher computational complexity.

The rest of this book chapter is organized as follows: background work and different medical image watermarking approaches are explained in Section 13.2. Then, Section 13.3 describes the proposed watermarking framework using the RWT and SVD. First, data embedding procedure is elaborated followed by data extraction procedure. Section 13.4 introduces RWT and its usage in the proposed watermarking scheme in addition to the SVD and its applications in security. Experimental results in Section 13.5 demonstrate the robustness and efficiency of the proposed watermarking algorithm using several performance evaluation parameters and Section 13.6 concludes the chapter.

13.2 Background work

As the chapter presents RWT- and SVD-based watermarking scheme, this section reviews the literature related to transforming domain and SVD approaches proposed for medical image watermarking. Research in digital watermarking can be categorized in two classes: spatial and frequency domain. In the first method, pixel values of original image are manipulated to embed the watermark inside host image. In the second domain the watermark is embedded by altering the coefficient values. Different frequency domain techniques are primarily focused on DFT, DCT and DWT [1].

Medical images that can be viewed, transmitted and extracted can be manipulated both within as well as outside of a secure medical environment. Organizations across the world have invested profoundly in Picture Archiving and Communication Systems (PACS), which facilitates data security [16]. Images and records are extracted from PACS for a broad range of acceptable practices, like patient data requests, transmission to medical experts, external second opinion, etc. Therefore, it is very essential to confirm trustworthiness within various medical imaging workflows.

Medical image integrity can be attained by digital watermarking. The identification of information origin and ensuring that the data relates to the correct patient is referred to as authenticity. The ability to ascertain that the information has not been distorted without authorization is called integrity [1]. The ever-growing need to share medical digital images among hospitals and specialists for enabling accurate and precise diagnosis has also increased the need to protect the patient's privacy. This leads to the urgent need for medical image watermarking (MIW) [10].

In [17], a new watermarking method which is also reversible is proposed to address the security issues of medical images. In this research work, a recursive dither modulation (RDM) algorithm based on signature information and text insertion was employed into the original medical images. This process was initiated after wavelet transform (WT) and SVD. The use of a differential evolution algorithm was suggested to develop the quantization steps and optimal control of watermark strength. In [4], DWT-SVD combination-based blind image watermarking method is proposed. The extraction of watermark contents is done successfully using blind watermarking method. The contents of watermark are successfully extracted under various attacks.

The DWT, DCT, bacterial foraging optimization (BFO) and particle swarm optimization (PSO) are used for watermarking of medical images, and the performance of all these transforms is analyzed in [18]. An improved version of wavelet-based watermarking approach is illustrated in [12]. This technique decomposes the cover medical image into region-of-interest (ROI) and non-region of interest (NROI) regions and three watermarks are embedded into the (NROI) band of the cover image.

In [19], DWT and a chaotic-based medical image watermarking approach are proposed. In this research work, medical image is used as a binary watermark image and the details corresponding to the patient's illness is embedded in the medical image. DWT is applied to the medical image, which in turn decomposes the image into four different sub-bands of low and high frequencies. The chaotic watermark is obtained from watermark image and a logistic map is used to obtain the chaotic watermark. An IWT-based watermarking technique is proposed in [20] and it achieves the accurate identification of the tampered blocks.

Text and image watermarks are embedded into the same multimedia object in [21] using DWT and SVD. Error correction codes like Hamming code, Reed-Solomon code and BCH are applied to the ASCII representations of text. The algorithm is found to be very robust against various types of attacks and correctly extracts the watermarks. The watermarked image is found to be of excellent quality without any kind of degradation. In [22], two watermarks are embedded in the HL and LH bands using DWT and SVD. Evaluation of simulation results demonstrates that the proposed technique is able to endure various attacks. Cryptography, steganography and digital watermarking, when combined together, can hide the image with watermark logo inside the cover image which is proposed in [23]. This is achieved by using DCT, DWT, RSA and SVD approach. DCT is used to encrypt the watermark logo which is hidden inside a secure image, this results in the formation of a stego image. DWT-SVD is used to hide the stego image inside the cover image.

Singh *et al.* [24] have developed a hybrid watermarking method based on DWT-DCT-SVD combination. In this research work, SVs of the cover image DWT sub bands are used for the purpose of embedding. Experimental results demonstrate that this technique can withstand various signal processing attacks. LWT-DCT-based method of watermarking is used for maintaining confidentiality and for authentication, which is presented in [25] using MD5 and BCH codes.

Thakur *et al.* [26] transformed the host image using fusion of three challenging transformation techniques, and SV replacement method is used to generate the watermarked image. The chaotic encryption algorithm is used to encrypt the watermarked image by using the secret key. This leads to the generation of an encrypted watermarked image. Douglas *et al.* [27] proposed a hybrid data hiding algorithm combining DWT HH sub-band and SVD.

13.3 Proposed medical image watermarking algorithm using RWT

This work presents a medical image watermarking algorithm using RWT and SVD. Figure 13.2 illustrates different stages during the embedding procedure. The image watermarking algorithm involves two major steps: (a) watermark embedding stage and (b) watermark extraction stage. Riesz wavelet decomposition decomposes the image into various frequency bands and scales. The watermark is replaced with first sub-band and third sub-band of first level is used for secret key embedding. Experiments are also performed while embedding watermark in last sub-band.

13.3.1 Watermark embedding steps

1. Get the host medical image $h(i, j)$ and decompose into different scales using RWT. Extract first sub-band SB_1
2. Compute SVD of extracted SB_1

$$S_1 = U_H * S_H * V_H^T \tag{13.1}$$

3. Get watermark image $w(i, j)$ and apply SVD.

$$W_1 = U_W * S_W * V_W^T \tag{13.2}$$

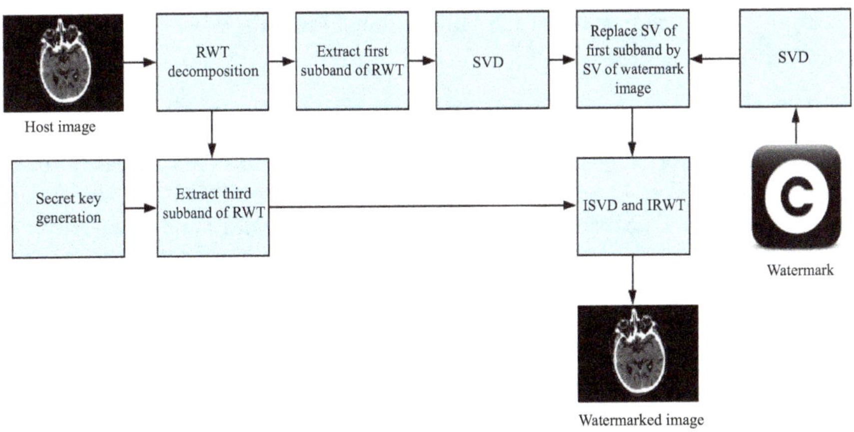

Figure 13.2 RWT-SVD-based watermarking scheme

4. SVs of the SB_1 sub-band are replaced with the SVs of the watermark image.
5. Modified SB_1 sub-band is obtained by applying inverse SVD.

$$S_1 = U_H * S_W * V_H^T \tag{13.3}$$

6. Select a secret key and generate the signature of length *K* bits and insert these *K* coefficients in the third sub-band SB_3.
7. Compute the inverse RWT using modified SB_1 and SB_3 sub-band to generate the watermarked image *w*(*i*, *j*).

13.3.2 Watermark extraction steps

1. Get the watermarked image *w*(*i*, *j*) and decompose using RWT. Extract first sub-band SB_1.
2. Compute SVD of extracted SB_1.

$$S_1 = U_H * S_H * V_H^T \tag{13.4}$$

3. Obtain SVs of SB_1 sub-band.
4. Extract the original watermark using SVs of SB_1 sub-band and U_W and V_W of the original watermark.

$$W_1 = U_W * S_H * V_W^T \tag{13.5}$$

5. Select *K* coefficients from SB_3 using shared secret key and extract the signature. Compare this signature with signature generated using U_W and V_W.
6. Obtain *U* and *V* from the original logo, for signature generation at the receiver end, and compare it with extracted signature for authentication.

13.4 RWT and SVD

This section briefly describes the RWT and SVD used in this study. The Riesz transform is a generalization of the Hilbert transform with $d > 1$ and is a type of singular integral operator [28,29].

13.4.1 Generalized Riesz wavelet transform (GRWT)

The structural information of texture and gradient contour could be easily maintained in the higher order Riesz transform proposed in [29]. The steerability property of GRWT enables random-order steerable wavelet family generation in the case of $d \geq 2$ [30]. The preservation of the frame bounds while trying to map one wavelet frame into another is an important property of Riesz transform and its higher order generalization [31].

For *N*th-order RWT with $d = 2$, there are $N + 1$ individual components [31]. The Riesz wavelet coefficients are expressed as,

$$C_i^{(n_1,\ldots,n_d)}[k] = (S, R^{(n_1,\ldots,n_d)}\varnothing_{i,k}) \tag{13.6}$$

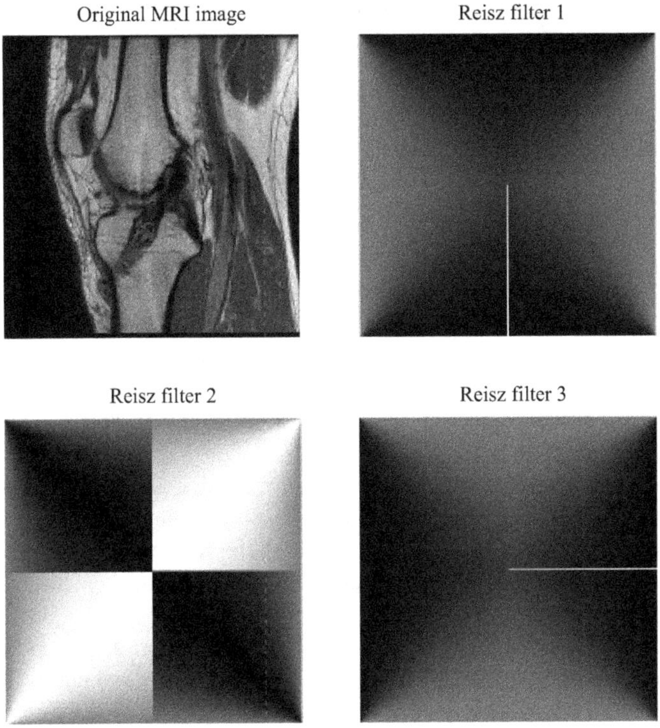

Figure 13.3 Original MRI image and different Riesz filters

where k stands for the location of multi-resolution transformation and i stands for current decomposition level. Because of the properties of RWT (as described above), the use of RWT is suggested for the medical image watermarking in this chapter. RWT retains the structural information such as texture or gradient contour and it guarantees perfect reconstruction and closeness. Figure 13.3 shows sample MRI images and corresponding Riesz filter configurations.

13.4.2 Singular value decomposition

SVD is commonly used in image compression, image hiding, restoration and image reconstruction. SVD is one of the most powerful and well recognized mathematical transform which allows the representation of data into a lower dimension. The image information can be effectively represented using a few SVs [32].

SVD results in a real or complex rectangular matrix decomposition A, with useful properties employed in image processing applications [33]. Each matrix A can be decomposed into a product of three matrices as $A = USV_A^{\mathrm{T}}$ where U and V are orthogonal matrices. In this matrix, SVs S are the diagonal component of matrix A, $S = \mathrm{diag}(\sigma_1, \sigma_2, \ldots, \sigma_r, 0, \ldots, 0)$ [34,35].

SVD decomposition is expressed using the following equation as,

$$A = U_A S_A V_A{}^T \tag{13.7}$$

where U_A and V_A are the Ath column of U and V, respectively [32]. SVs provide us the information related to the energy in the image. It also gives us the detailed knowledge of how the energy is distributed in the image. SVD is used in watermarking as it helps to achieve better transparency and hence is said to be very robust.

13.5 Simulation results and discussions

The proposed RWT-SVD-based watermarking technique is tested using five types of medical images: (1) retina images [36], (2) brain tumor images [37], (3) CT scan images, (4) X-ray images and (5) computed tomography (CT) images. Each type consists of a total of five images with dimension of 512 × 512. The watermark image which is embedded in the cover medical image is shown in Figure 13.4. Number of scales and number of levels of RWT decomposition are set to 2. As described above, embedding is performed using the first band.

The original (host) and watermarked images along with their histogram representation are depicted in Figures 13.5–13.9. Figure 13.5 shows retinal images, Figure 13.6 depicts five images of X-ray, MRI test images are shown in Figure 13.7, brain tumor images in Figure 13.8 and finally five CT images in Figure 13.9. In each of the figure, first row corresponds to the original host images, second row illustrates its histogram, watermarked images are depicted in row three and row four shows its corresponding histogram. It is evident from these figures that, perceptual quality is not degraded by the proposed algorithm, even after embedding the watermark in the host image. All the watermarked image histograms closely match with the original image histograms revealing better performance of the proposed approach.

PSNR, RMSE, SNR, weighted PSNR (WPSNR), structure similarity measure index (SSIM), multiscale SSIM (MSSSIM), structural contents (SC), normalized absolute error (NAE) and average difference (AD) are used to measure the

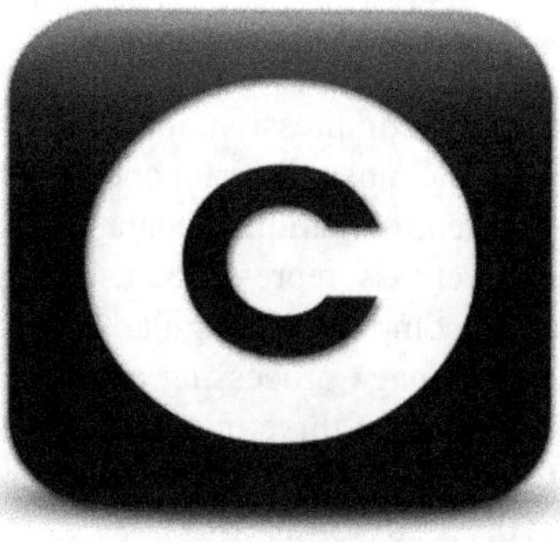

Figure 13.4 Watermark image

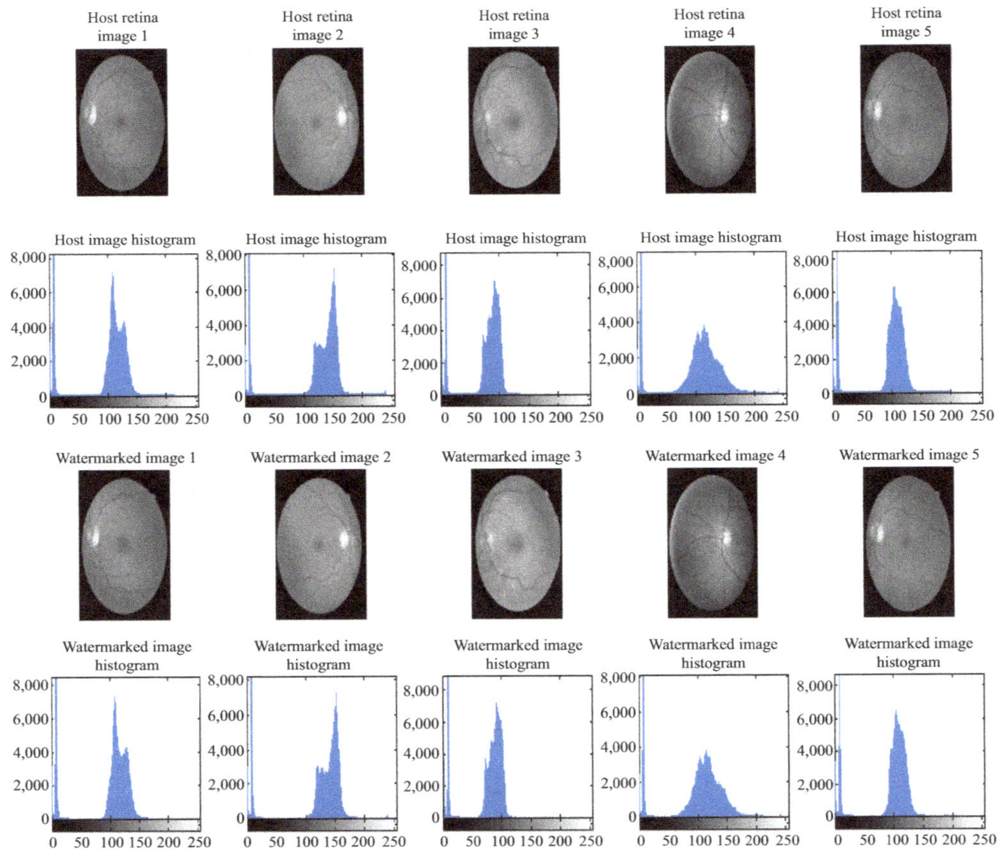

Figure 13.5 Original and watermarked images with corresponding histogram representation using retinal images

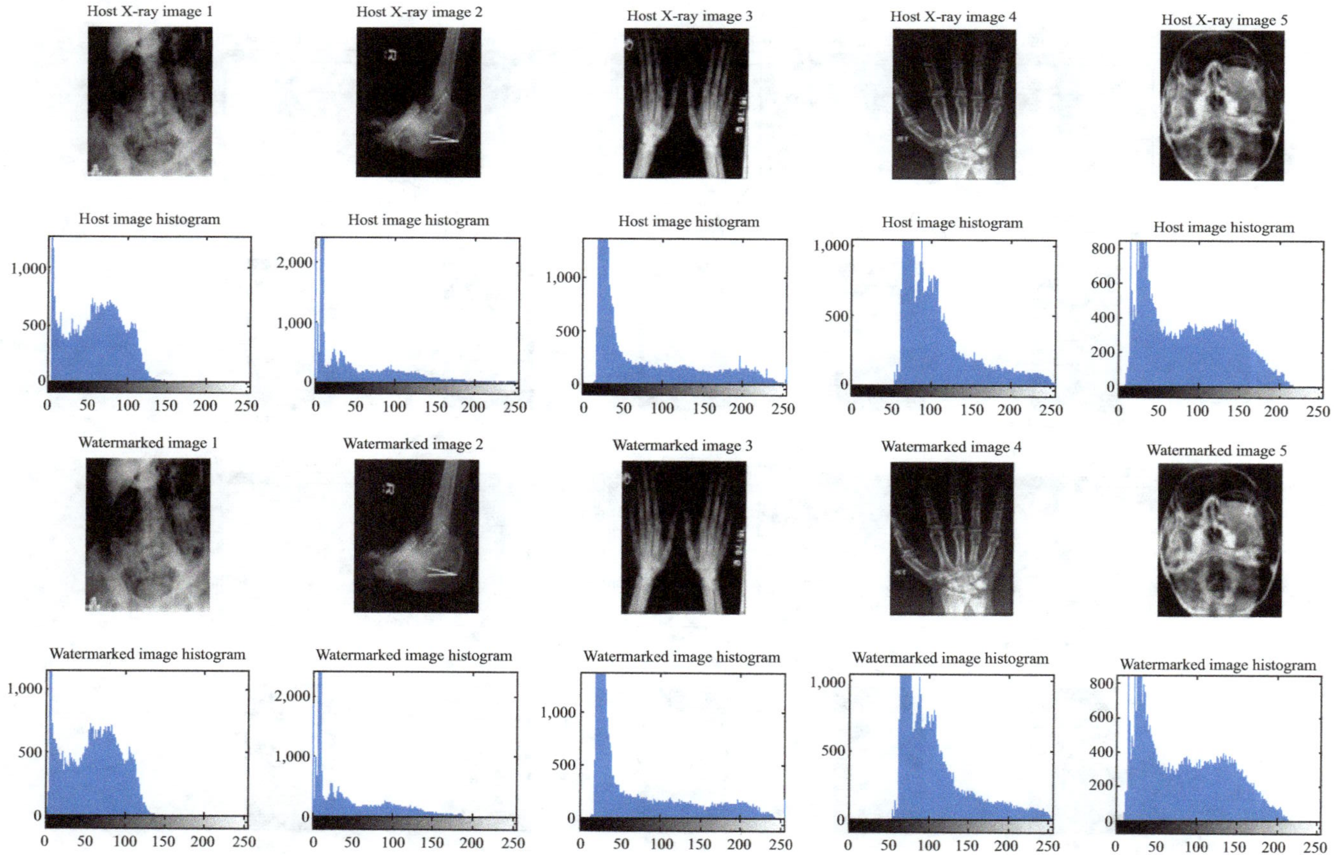

Figure 13.6 Original and watermarked images with corresponding histogram representation using X-ray images

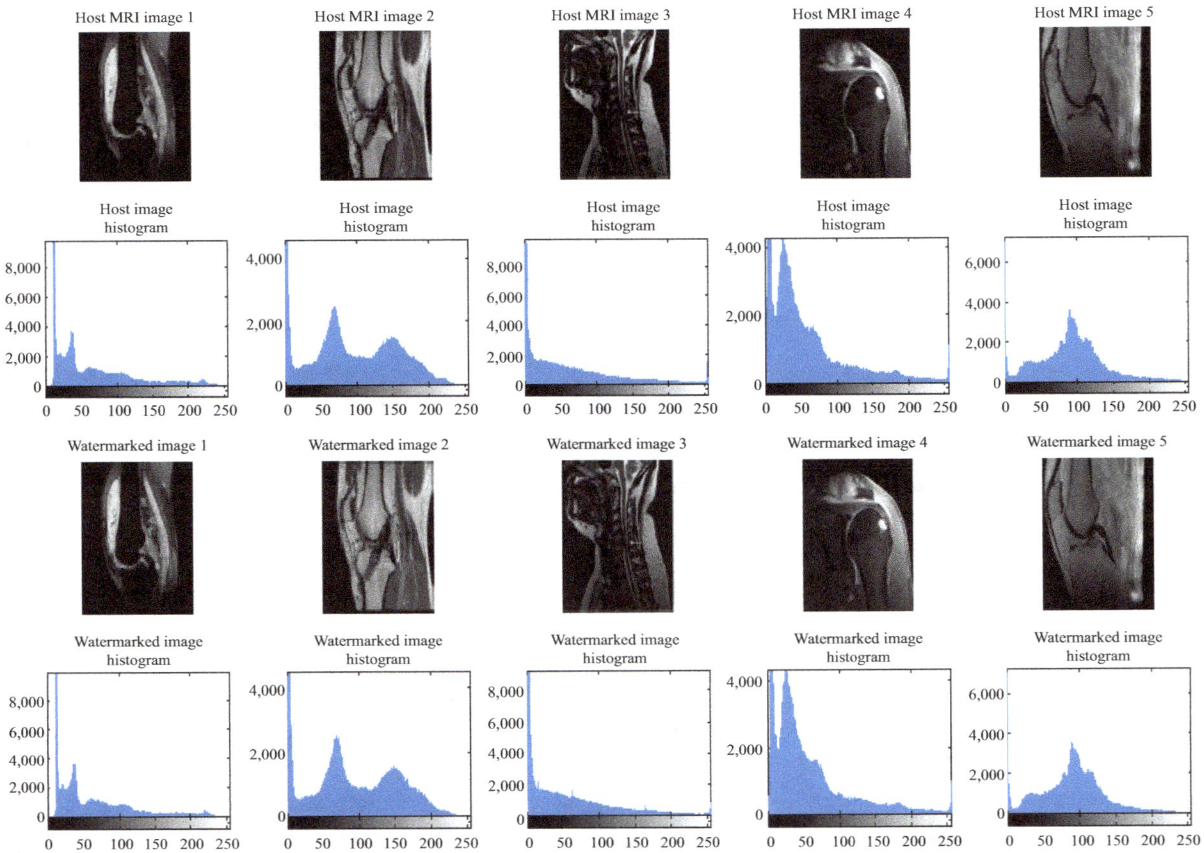

Figure 13.7 Original and watermarked images with corresponding histogram representation using MRI images

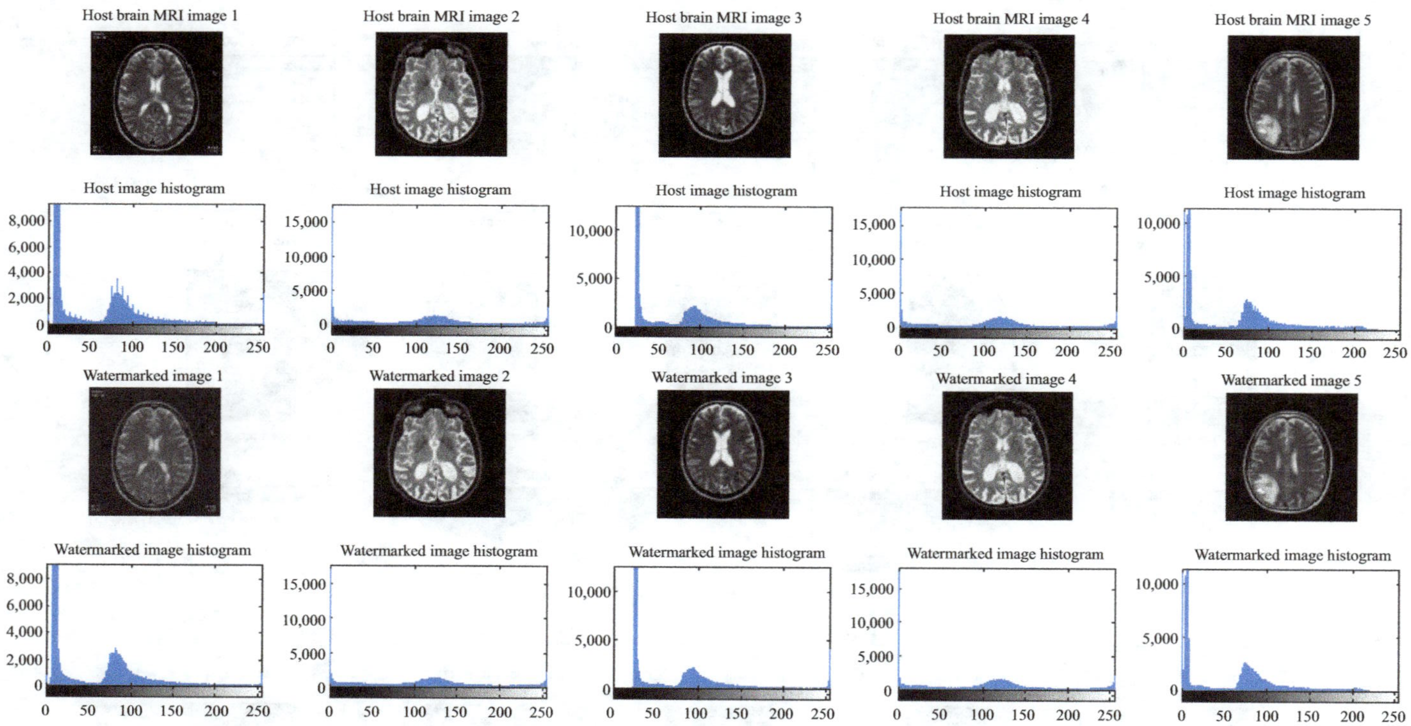

Figure 13.8 Original and watermarked images with corresponding histogram representation using brain tumor MRI images

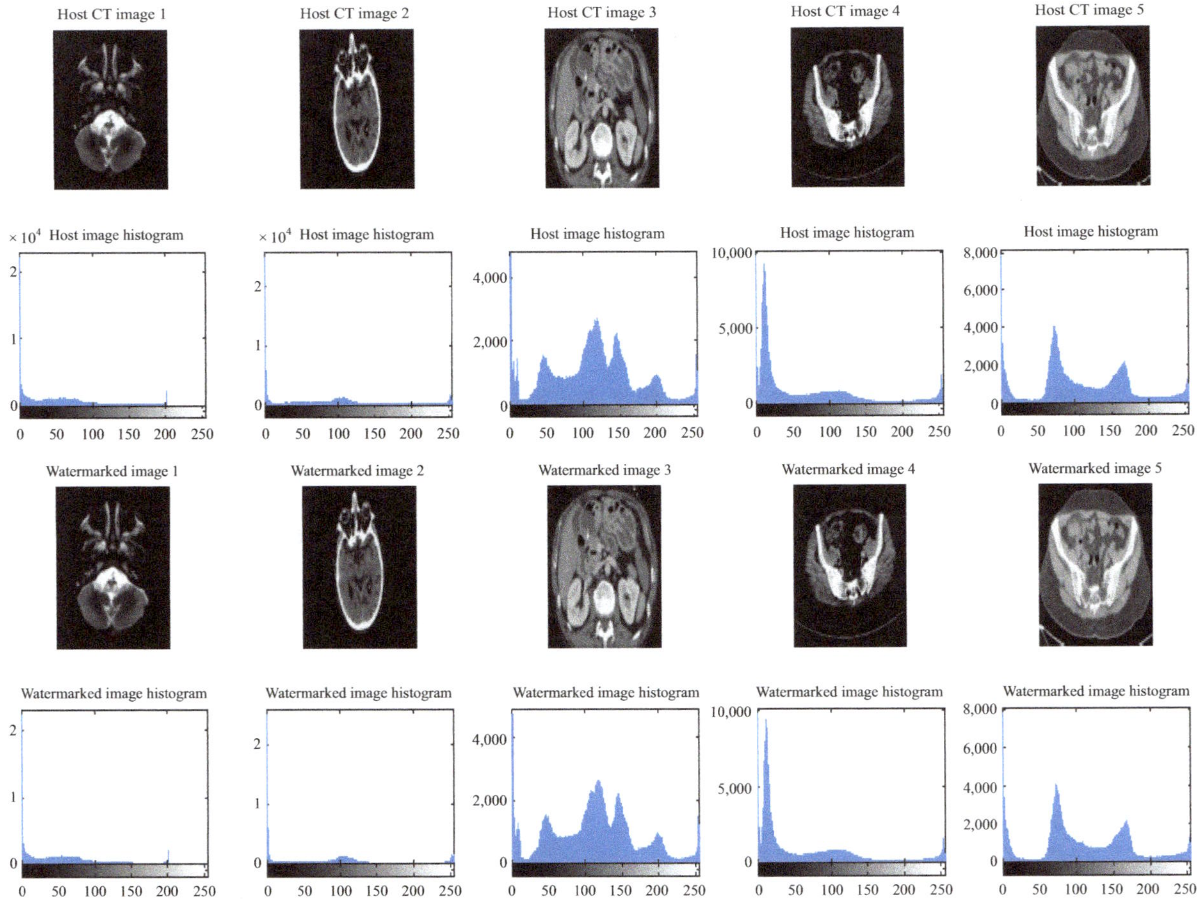

Figure 13.9 Original and watermarked images with corresponding histogram representation using CT images

performance and imperceptibility of the proposed approach. These parameters are computed as:

- RMSE: Computes the error between host and watermarked images. Lower values of RMSE is expected for better visual quality watermarked images (producing low visual distortion).

$$\text{RMSE} = \sqrt{\frac{1}{M \times N}\sum_{i=0}^{N-1}\sum_{j=0}^{M-1}[(h(i,j) - w(i,j)]^2} \tag{13.8}$$

  where $h(i, j)$ and $w(i, j)$ are the hosts and watermarked images, respectively, and the image size is N_M.
- PSNR: Higher PSNR values result in higher imperceptibility.

$$\text{PSNR} = 10\log_{10}\left(\frac{255^2}{\text{MSE}}\right) \tag{13.9}$$

  where maximum pixel value is 255 and MSE is mean squared error.
- Weighted PSNR (WPSNR) involves noise visibility function (NVF) based on the Gaussian model and is obtained as [4],

$$\text{WPSNR} = \frac{255^2}{\text{NVF} \times \text{MSE}} \tag{13.10}$$

- Signal-to-noise ratio (SNR) in dB is expressed as,

$$\text{SNR} = 10\log_{10}\frac{\sum_{i=0}^{N-1}\sum_{j=0}^{M-1}[h(i,j)]^2]}{\sum_{i=0}^{N-1}\sum_{j=0}^{M-1}[h(i,j) - w(i,j)]^2} \tag{13.11}$$

- Structure similarity measure index (SSIM) evaluates imperceptibility in the range $[-1, +1]$ and is obtained as [38],

$$SSIM(h, w) = \frac{(2\mu_w\mu_h) + (C_1) + (C_2 + 2\sigma_{hw})}{(\mu_h^2 + \mu_w^2 + C_1)(\sigma_h^2 + \sigma_w^2 + C_2)} \tag{13.12}$$

  where μ_h is the average of h, μ_w is the average of w, σ_h^2 the variance of h, σ_y^2 is the variance of w, σ_{hw} is the covariance of h and w, $c_1 = (k_1L)^2$ and $c_2 = (k_2L)^2$ are the two variables, dynamic range is L, $k_1 = 0.01$ and $k_2 = 0.03$.
- The multiscale similarity measure index (MSSIM) is evaluated using multiple scales and is also computed in this chapter [39].
- Structural content (SC) is obtained as,

$$\text{SC} = \frac{\sum_{i=0}^{N-1}\sum_{j=0}^{M-1}(h(i,j)^2)}{\sum_{i=0}^{N-1}\sum_{j=0}^{M-1}(w(i,j)^2)} \tag{13.13}$$

- NAE is computed as,

$$\mathrm{NAE} = \frac{\sum_{i=0}^{N-1}\sum_{j=0}^{M-1}|h(i,j) - w(i,j)|}{\sum_{i=0}^{N-1}\sum_{j=0}^{M-1}|h(i,j)|} \tag{13.14}$$

- Average difference (AS) is expressed as,

$$\mathrm{AD} = \frac{\sum_{i=0}^{N-1}\sum_{j=0}^{M-1}(h(i,j) - w(i,j))}{M \times N} \tag{13.15}$$

- The correlation coefficient (CC) analyses the similarity between original and extracted watermark in the range [0, 1] and is calculated by,

$$\mathrm{NC} = \frac{\sum_{i=0}^{N-1}\sum_{j=0}^{M-1}w(i,j)w(i,j)}{\sqrt{\sum_{i=0}^{N-1}\sum_{j=0}^{M-1}w(i,j)^2\sum_{i=0}^{N-1}\sum_{j=0}^{M-1}w(i,j)^2}} \tag{13.16}$$

The performance of the proposed watermarking algorithm is assessed using different performance metric including PSNR, SNR, SSIM, RMSE, WPSNR, NAE, MSSIM, SC and AD. These performance parameters are computed using five different types of image modalities, and types and are tabulated in Tables 13.1–13.5. In Table 13.1, the performance verification of the proposed medical image watermarking scheme using a retinal image database is computed between original and watermarked image. As it can be seen from the table that for all the images, PSNR values are greater than 46 dB (in the range of 46–49 dB) whereas, weighted PSNR values are also in a similar range. SSIM and multiscale SSIM are close to 1 for each of the images. Also, SC value is not more than 1.01 indicating better perceptual quality.

The different performance metric is obtained using X-ray and MRI images in the next experiment. Tables 13.2 and 13.3 depict the evaluation parameters using

Table 13.1 Performance verification of the RWT watermarking scheme using retinal image database

Metric Image	Retina image 1	Retina image 2	Retina image 3	Retina image 4	Retina image 5
RMSE	1.0518	1.141	0.8743	0.9172	1.0659
PSNR	47.692	46.985	49.298	48.882	47.577
WPSNR	47.033	50.51	38.817	50.862	48.494
SNR	39.384	40.299	38.176	39.464	40.339
SSIM	0.99453	0.9467	0.99515	0.99552	0.99569
MSSIM	0.9905	0.99909	0.99912	0.99926	0.99925
SC	1.0003	1.0003	1.0004	1.0003	1.0003
NAE	0.0060537	0.0049334	0.0070535	0.0055939	0.0055063
AD	9.85E−15	1.58E−14	9.41E−16	1.64E−15	4.3157e−15

Table 13.2 Performance verification of the RWT watermarking scheme using X-ray image database

Metric/ Image	X-ray image 1	X-ray image 2	X-ray image 3	X-ray image 4	X-ray image 5
RMSE	0.43805	1.4582	2.0448	0.47152	0.5983
PSNR	55.3	44.854	41.918	54.661	52.592
WPSNR	38.746	32.049	42.748	56.059	60.421
SNR	43.784	32.391	33.29	47.956	44.483
SSIM	0.99953	0.99492	0.99612	0.99915	0.999
MSSIM	0.99992	0.99917	0.9995	0.99989	0.999
SC	1.0001	1.0014	1.0008	1	1.0001
NAE	0.002781	0.012155	0.0089978	0.002018	0.0033
AD	1.42E−14	6.17E−17	6.15E−15	2.79E−14	1.84E−16

Table 13.3 Performance verification of the RWT watermarking scheme using MRI image database

Metric/ Image	MRI image 1	MRI image 2	MRI image 3	MRI image 4	MRI image 5
RMSE	0.71587	3.1565	6.4514	2.3685	0.91426
PSNR	51.034	38.147	31.938	40.641	48.909
WPSNR	59.594	30.906	31.31	33.691	42.517
SNR	40.318	30.493	21.221	30.216	40.109
SSIM	0.99725	0.97678	0.97447	0.98071	0.99673
MSSIM	0.99951	0.99611	0.9967	0.99655	0.9995
SC	1.0005	1.0022	1.0153	1.0021	1.0002
NAE	0.0078752	0.022946	0.50676	0.023277	0.0060199
AD	1.10E−16	5.20E−17	1.98E−14	1.49E−14	1.33E−15

Table 13.4 Performance verification of the RWT watermarking scheme using brain MRI image database

Metric/ Image	Brain MRI image 1	Brain MRI image 2	Brain MRI image 3	Brain MRI image 4	Brain MRI image 5
RMSE	5.5138	1.0876	1.4985	1.0548	2.3643
PSNR	33.302	47.401	44.617	47.668	40.657
WPSNR	24.477	40.632	40.432	38.795	35.414
SNR	22.568	39.56	34.892	39.714	29.883
SSIM	0.98482	0.99729	0.99578	0.99743	0.99022
MSSIM	0.9975	0.99951	0.99935	0.99953	0.99834
SC	1.0117	1.0006	1.0011	1.0006	1.0027
NAE	0.032255	0.0089769	0.010128	0.0087268	0.022083
AD	8.27E−17	5.26E−16	1.58E−16	5.30E−16	3.52E−16

Table 13.5 Performance verification of the RWT watermarking scheme using CT image database

Metric/Image	CT image 1	CT image 2	CT image 3	CT image 4	CT image 5
RMSE	0.4848	1.9835	1.1223	1.1934	0.9286
PSNR	54.42	42.182	47.128	46.595	48.774
WPSNR	50.056	35.783	46.54	37.9	36.557
SNR	40.336	31.229	40.648	36.439	41.878
SSIM	0.99906	0.99477	0.99495	0.99613	0.99615
MSSIM	0.99988	0.99928	0.99934	0.999943	0.99942
SC	1.0002	1.0017	1.0002	1.0006	1.0002
NAE	0.0079271	0.018938	0.0064809	0.012869	0.0055211
AD	5.40E−15	1.68E−16	2.40E−14	5.79E−15	4.11E−15

Table 13.6 Different medical image watermarking algorithm comparison

Algorithm	Transform	PSNR	SSIM
[3]	DWT-SVD	49.93	0.962
[8]	Integer WT	51.9	0.9998
[9]	Shear let transform	45.27	0.997
[4]	DWT-SVD	44.62	–
[40]	DCT-DWT	51.24	0.997
[18]	DWT	55.23	–
[41]	DWT	49.58	0.995
[42]	Integer WT	52.13	0.9824
[24]	DWT-SVD	3.62E+01	0.9993
[43]	DWT	42.453	0.9891
Proposed	RWT-SVD	55.3	9.95E−01

proposed medical image watermarking scheme for X-ray and MRI images, respectively. Medical image perceptual quality is a prime factor in watermarking algorithm. From Tables 13.2 and 13.3, the best PSNR and MSSIM value are 54.661 dB (51.034 dB) and 0.99953 (0.99955) for X-ray (MRI) images, respectively. Higher the PSNR values and MSSIM close to 1, better is the perceptual quality of the watermarked image. Additionally, NAE and AD values are very small in both images' types, clearly indicating better fidelity.

Last experiment computes various metric using brain MRI and CT images and values are shown in Tables 13.4 and 13.5, respectively. It is important to mention that the performance of the watermarking approach is superior in this case also.

The average values of PSNR, WPSNR, SNR, SSIM, NAE are 44.56, 34.73, 33.67, 0.9993 and 0.00056 dB, and 48.84, 42.47, 38.93, 0.9994 and 0.00034 dB, respectively, for brain MRI and CT images.

To validate the RWT-SVD approach with the existing state-of-the-art, the method is compared with various proposed techniques. Table 13.6 shows different medical image watermarking algorithm comparison. As seen from the table, most of the techniques employed discrete wavelet transform watermarking. The maximum PSNR value is obtained by using RWT-SVD combination. Also, SSIM is better compared to most of the DWT-based approaches. Comparative result analysis shows that the RWT-SVD method outperforms other state-of-art watermarking algorithms.

Robustness of the RWT watermarking algorithm is also evaluated to measure the watermark logo reliability in terms of correlation coefficient (CC). Four different attacks are tested against the watermarked image: (1) filtering, (2) cropping, (3) noise and (4) rotation. The first signal processing attack is average filtering using the mask size of 3_3. Second, a cropping attack with 25% of the total image dimension is applied to the watermarked medical image. In noise attack, Gaussian noise with mean zero and variance of 0.005 is applied. Finally, the watermarked image is rotated by 15° under the image rotation attack. For each case, correlation coefficient between original and extracted logo after attack is computed.

Figures 13.10 and 13.11 show extracted log using the proposed approach under different attacks. Filtering and cropping attack, image after attack and extracted logo image are shown in Figure 13.10. Correlation coefficient values are 0.745 and 0.793 in filtering and cropped attack, respectively. Figure 13.11 depicts Gaussian noise and rotation attacked images and extracted watermark images with CC of 0.897 and 0.762.

The biomedical image watermarking algorithm is presented in this book chapter which involves three major steps: (1) RWT image decomposition, (2) watermark embedding and (3) watermark extraction. The simulations are performed using Core-i5(8 Generation) processor working at 2.4 GHz with 4 GB DDR4 RAM. The RWT image decomposition step took 0.245 s, whereas watermark embedding and extraction steps required 0.627 s and 0.411 s, respectively. In this work, a single watermark is embedded in RWT sub-band by modifying its SVs at the transmitter. The method can further extend for embedding multiple watermarks into different RWT sub-bands. Additionally, optimization techniques can be explored for selecting the region of interest in order to improve the robustness against the attacks and also for improving the perceptual image quality.

High-end technology-based sensors, health monitors, touch-screen technology and websites are used daily to record patient vitals, heart patterns, blood pressure and glucose levels. These types of monitoring help a lot in chronic health management. Readings taken from the monitoring systems are logged into personal health records, and alerts are sent wirelessly to health-care providers when readings fall beyond their normal range. Telemedicine allows us to check in with your patient's medications more readily and allows us to ensure that they are complying with proper medication regimens. The communicative nature of the technology that is used in telemedicine is what makes it the most effective in treatments.

Doctors rely extensively on images in the form of CT scans, MRI, ultrasound and X-rays for diagnostic purposes. Due to the expansion of Tele diagnosis, every hospital has their own database systems in which they store medical images. Exchange of medical images with other hospitals and doctors may help in concluding good treatment methods. However, while exchanging images extreme care has to be taken in terms of security, copyright and secrecy. In order to avoid misuse or infringement it is

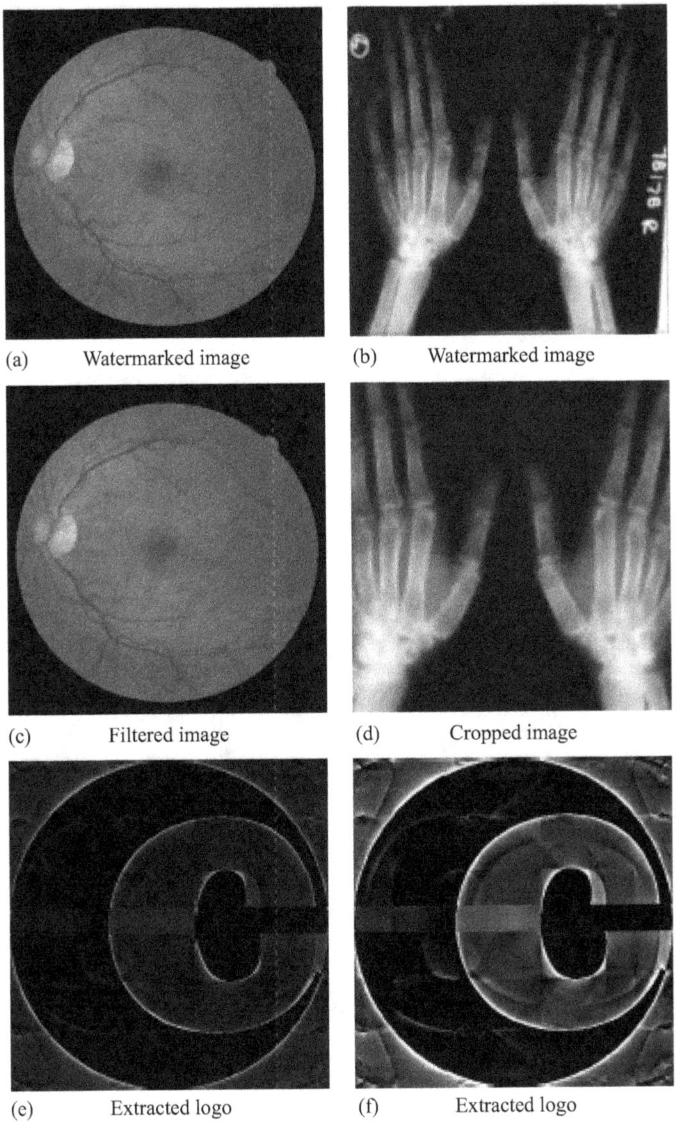
(a) Watermarked image (b) Watermarked image

(c) Filtered image (d) Cropped image

(e) Extracted logo (f) Extracted logo

Figure 13.10 Filtering and cropping attack and watermark extraction

very important that efficient security solutions are provided. Solutions can be provided in the form of watermarking. In this book chapter, a new watermarking scheme is presented for medical image security. Typical architecture of watermarking for data security in telemedicine applications is shown in Figure 13.12. RWT and SVD are used to embed the watermark in the image. The embedded information is recovered successfully by using the extraction algorithm.

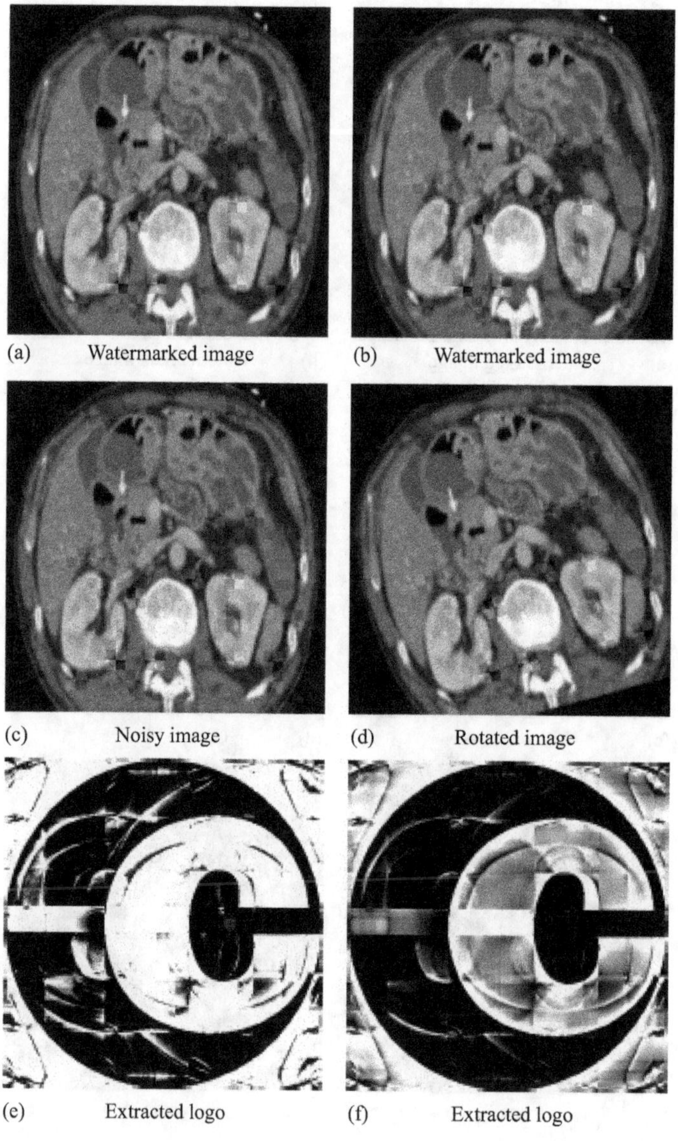

Figure 13.11 Gaussian noise and rotation attack and watermark extraction

13.6 Conclusion

RWT-based medical image watermarking technique is presented in this book chapter. The use of RWT for embedding the watermark resulted in better perceptual quality images with higher values of PSNR and SSIM. The experimental results indicate the effectiveness of the proposed algorithm measured in terms of

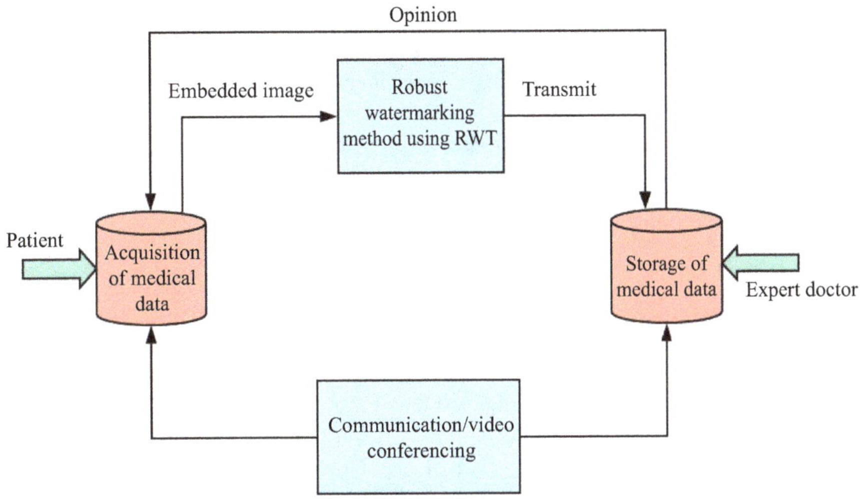

Figure 13.12 Typical architecture of watermarking for data security in telemedicine applications

different performance metrics and robustness analysis. The higher value of PSNR represents that the image quality is not degraded and provides excellent visualization. The proposed algorithm provides imperceptibility and security in medical image with minimum distortion.

References

[1] Qasim AF, Meziane F, and Aspin R. Digital watermarking: applicability for developing trust in medical imaging workflows state of the art review. Computer Science Review. 2018;27:45–60.

[2] Gangadhar Y, Akula VSG, and Reddy PC. Adaptive digital medical image watermarking approach in 2D-wavelet domain using speed-up robust feature method. International Journal of Biomedical Engineering and Technology. 2019;29(3):273–92.

[3] Singh HV, and Rai A. Medical Image Watermarking in Transform Domain. In: Tiwari S, Trivedi MC, Mishra KK *et al.* editors. Smart Innovations in Communication and Computational Sciences. Singapore: Springer Singapore; 2019. pp. 485–93.

[4] Thakkar FN, and Srivastava VK. A blind medical image watermarking: DWTSVD based robust and secure approach for telemedicine applications. Multimedia Tools and Applications. 2017;76(3):3669–97.

[5] Chakraborty C, Gupta B, and Ghosh SK. A Review on telemedicine-based WBAN framework for patient monitoring. International Journal of Telemedicine and e-Health, Mary Ann Libert, Inc. 2013;19(8):619–26.

[6] Mishra KN, Chakraborty C, Farsi M *et al.* editors. In: A Novel Approach Toward Enhancing the Quality of Life in Smart Cities Using Clouds and IoT-Based Technologies. Cham: Springer International Publishing; 2020. pp. 19–35.

[7] Balu S, Babu CNK, and Amudha K. Secure and efficient data transmission by video steganography in medical imaging system. Cluster Computing. 2018 Mar.

[8] Tamal TA, Saha C, Hossain MF *et al.* Integer Wavelet Transform Based Medical Image Watermarking for Tamper Detection. In: 2019 International Conference on Electrical, Computer and Communication Engineering (ECCE); 2019. pp. 1–6.

[9] Al-Azzawi, and Ahmed N. Security in Telehealth Applications: Issues in Medical Image Watermarking Scheme Through the Shearlet Transform. In: Proceedings of the International Conference on Information and Communication Technology. ICICT '19. New York, NY, USA: ACM; 2019. pp. 160–4.

[10] Mousavi SM, Naghsh A, and Abu-Bakar SAR. Watermarking techniques used in medical images: a survey. Journal of Digital Imaging. 2014;27(6):714–29.

[11] Gupta A, and Raval M. A robust and secure watermarking scheme based on singular values replacement. Sadhana. 2012;37(4):425–40.

[12] Chauhan DS, Singh AK, Kumar B *et al.* Quantization based multiple medical information watermarking for secure e-health. Multimedia Tools and Applications. 2019;78(4):3911–23.

[13] Nair UR, and Birajdar GK. Audio watermarking in wavelet domain using Fibonacci numbers. In: 2016 International Conference on Signal and Information Processing (IConSIP); 2016. pp. 1–5.

[14] Unser M, and Van De Ville D. Wavelet steerability and the higher-order Riesz transform. IEEE Transactions on Image Processing. 2010;19(3):636–52.

[15] Chakraborty C, and Gupta B. Adaptive filtering technique for chronic wound image analysis under tele-wound network. International Journal of Communication, Navigation, Sensing and Services. 2016;1(1):57–76.

[16] Choplin RH, Boehme JM, and Maynard CD. Picture archiving and communication systems: an overview. Radio Graphics. 1992;12(1):127–9.

[17] Lei B, Tan EL, Chen S *et al.* Reversible watermarking scheme for medical image based on differential evolution. Expert Systems with Applications. 2014;41(7):3178–88.

[18] Bharati S, Rahman MA, Mandal S *et al.* Analysis of DWT, DCT, BFO & PBFO Algorithm for the Purpose of Medical Image Watermarking. In: 2018 International Conference on Innovation in Engineering and Technology (ICIET). IEEE; 2018. pp. 1–6.

[19] Moniruzzaman M, Hawlader MAK, and Hossain MF. Wavelet based watermarking approach of hiding patient information in medical image for medical image authentication. In: 2014 17th International Conference on Computer and Information Technology (ICCIT). IEEE; 2014. pp. 374–8.

[20] Eswaraiah R, and Reddy ES. Robust medical image watermarking technique for accurate detection of tampers inside region of interest and recovering original region of interest. IET Image Processing. 2015;9(8):615–25.

[21] Singh AK, Dave M, and Mohan A. Hybrid technique for robust and imperceptible dual watermarking using error correcting codes for application in telemedicine. International Journal of Electronic Security and Digital Forensics. 2014;6(4):285–305.

[22] Joseph A, and Anusudha K. Robust watermarking based on DWT-SVD. International Journal on Signal & Image Security. 2013;1(1).

[23] Patel P, and Patel Y. Secure and authentic DCT image steganography through DWT-SVD Based Digital Watermarking with RSA Encryption. In: 2015 Fifth International Conference on Communication Systems and Network Technologies. IEEE; 2015. pp. 736–9.

[24] Singh AK, Dave M, and Mohan A. Hybrid technique for robust and imperceptible multiple watermarking using medical images. Multimedia Tools and Applications. 2016;75(14):8381–401.

[25] Singh A. Robust and distortion control dual watermarking in LWT domain using DCT and error correction code for color medical image. Multimedia Tools and Applications. 2019;78(11):30523–33.

[26] Thakur S, Singh AK, Ghrera SP *et al.* Multi-layer security of medical data through watermarking and chaotic encryption for tele-health applications. Multimedia Tools and Applications. 2019;78(3):3457–70.

[27] Douglas M, Bailey K, Leeney M *et al.* Using SVD and DWT based steganography to enhance the security of watermarked fingerprint images. Telkomnika. 2017;15(3).

[28] Zhang X, Li X, and Feng Y. A new image fusion performance measure using Riesz transforms. Optik-International Journal for Light and Electron Optics. 2014;125(3):1427–33.

[29] Unser M, and Van De Ville D. Wavelet steerability and the higher-order Riesz transform. IEEE Transactions on Image Processing. 2010;19(3):636–52.

[30] Zhang L, and Li H. Encoding local image patterns using Riesz transforms: with applications to palmprint and finger-knuckle-print recognition. Image and Vision Computing. 2012;30(12):1043–51.

[31] Dogra A, Goyal B, and Agrawal S. Bone vessel image fusion via generalized Reisz wavelet transform using averaging fusion rule. Journal of Computational Science. 2017;21:371–8.

[32] Ansari IA, Pant M, and Ahn CW. SVD based fragile watermarking scheme for tamper localization and self-recovery. International Journal of Machine Learning and Cybernetics. 2016;7(6):1225–39.

[33] Bhandari A, Soni V, Kumar A *et al.* Cuckoo search algorithm based satellite image contrast and brightness enhancement using DWT-SVD. ISA Transactions. 2014;53(4):1286–96.

[34] Nouri R, and Mansouri A. Digital image steganalysis based on the reciprocal singular value curve. Multimedia Tools and Applications. 2017;76(6):8745–56.

[35] Birajdar GK, and Mankar VH. Blind image forensics using reciprocal singular value curve based local statistical features. Multimedia Tools and Applications. 2018;77(11):14153–75.

[36] Staal J, Abramoff MD, Niemeijer M *et al.* Ridge-based vessel segmentation in color images of the retina. IEEE Transactions on Medical Imaging. 2004;23(4):501–9.

[37] Prastawa M, Bullitt E, and Gerig G. Simulation of brain tumors in MR images for evaluation of segmentation efficacy. Medical Image Analysis 2009;13(2):297–311.

[38] Wang Z, Bovik AC, Sheikh HR *et al.* Image quality assessment: from error visibility to structural similarity. IEEE Transactions on Image Processing. 2004;13(4):600–12.

[39] Wang Z, Simoncelli EP, and Bovik AC. Multiscale structural similarity for image quality assessment. In: The Thirty-Seventh Asilomar Conference on Signals, Systems Computers, 2003. vol. 2; 2003. pp. 1398–402.

[40] Mehto A, and Mehra N. Adaptive lossless medical image watermarking algorithm based on DCT & DWT. Procedia Computer Science. 2016;78(C):88–94.

[41] Moniruzzaman M, Hawlader MAK, and Hossain MF. Wavelet based watermarking approach of hiding patient information in medical image for medical image authentication. In: 2014 17th International Conference on Computer and Information Technology (ICCIT); 2014. pp. 374–8.

[42] Eswaraiah R, and Sreenivasa Reddy E. Robust medical image watermarking technique for accurate detection of tampers inside region of interest and recovering original region of interest. IET Image Processing. 2015;9(8):615–25.

[43] Sharifara A, and Ghaderi A. Medical Image Watermarking using 2D-DWT with Enhanced security and capacity. CoRR. 2017;abs/1703.05778.

Chapter 14

Conclusion

This book presents new telemedicine approaches for healthcare data analysis and diagnosis of medical conditions. Telemedicine technologies play an important role in the fields of biomedical sensors, wireless body sensor networking, computer-aided diagnosis methods, signal and image processing, and analysis, automation and control, virtual and augmented reality, multivariate analysis and data acquisition devices. The book provides practical examples for stakeholders in telemedicine while highlighting the factors that are essential in the development, implementation and data evaluation of telemedicine applications. Technologists, engineers, scientists and clinicians can advance future development in the field by expanding their understanding of low-cost, high-performance, highly efficient, deployable telemedicine systems.

Recent advancements in signal/image processing techniques along with the system and network design for healthcare applications are discussed. Real-life case studies in the areas of neuroscience and cardiovascular systems have been presented. Another example in the area of health monitoring is heartbeat detection being sent to a remote platform using wireless technology and enhanced by telemedicine applications to improve accuracy. Data mining is another very efficient method in knowledge discovery, and the trustworthiness of decisions is bringing further success to telemedicine. Data is collected and stored in the cloud, then structured and organised into forms that can be fed into a data mining engine. The data mining engine is enabled with data analytics techniques to process structured data and discover knowledge. As the development of information and communication technologies advance, data mining will move closer to achieving its full potential in the discovery of knowledge hidden within medical data. Thus, the integration of data mining techniques into the telemedicine systems will bring two-way advantages for both healthcare professionals and patients.

Through innovative telemedicine platforms and using communication and information exchange across local, national and global networks, cost-effective solutions can be tailored for complex health services. As an example, telemedicine is providing innovative and cost-effective solutions for health services to be provided to 'hidden' patients in under-serviced rural and remote areas. Tele-social work now provides the scope for social workers to deliver services in rural areas where governments are unlikely to provide or deliver on-the-ground services. Tele-social work has the potential to transform the profession of social work and increase the accessibility and flexibility of services. However, tele-social work must complement rather than replace the provision of face-to-face service. The book demonstrates examples of how seriously ill patients with conditions such as epileptic episodes, heart attack, stroke and diabetic attack can be remotely monitored outside of an intensive care unit by telemedicine technologies. The use of smartphones with remote patient monitoring system is also enhancing the healthcare patients can receive.

To highlight the development in the area of health monitoring a novel content-based high dynamic range image quality prediction model using EEG features has been introduced. Riesz-wavelet transform-based medical image watermarking technique is also demonstrated. The experimental results indicate the effectiveness of the proposed algorithm measured in terms of different performance metrics and robustness analysis. The proposed algorithm provides imperceptibility and security in the medical image with minimum distortion. Tone-mapping-operators provide a useful means for converting high dynamic range images to low dynamic range images for maintaining standard displays, but this may impact the visual quality-of-experience for end-user.

Finally, telemedicine applications can effectively monitor the health of remote patients and this advancement has been made possible by the use of the Internet of Things (IoT). Telemedicine systems using IoT-cloud are also being used to great effect in the healthcare sector, especially for older people with limited mobility, and for those requiring home-based health solutions. The Internet of medical things is another fast-developing solution to improve healthcare monitoring and treatment outcomes for chronic diseases, such as diabetes. While telemedicine applications reflect advancements in providing improved health services, it should be remembered that well-organised structures and standards still need to be followed. The fail-safe use of telemedicine technologies and assured services is not guaranteed, and it very much depends on the health service provider and health experts.

Index

www.ingramcontent.com/pod-product-compliance
Lightning Source LLC
LaVergne TN
LVHW011847200926
848484LV00002B/415